MANUAL
OF
NATURAL
THERAPY

A Practical Guide
to Alternative Medicine

Moshe Olshevsky, C.A., Ph.D.
Shlomo Noy, M.D.
Moses Zwang, O.M.D., Ph.D.
with Robert Burger

Foreword by Dr. Ted Kaptchuk

A CITADEL PRESS BOOK
Published by Carol Publishing Group

To our parents and students

*Grateful acknowledgment is made
to Abraham and Judy Aven-Hen
for their help in
preparing the nutrition sections.*

First Carol Publishing Group Edition 1990

By arrangement with Facts on File

A Citadel Press Book
Published by Carol Publishing Group
Citadel Press is a registered trademark of Carol Communications, Inc.

Editorial Offices: 600 Madison Avenue, New York, NY 10022
Sales & Distribution Offices: 120 Enterprise Avenue, Secaucus, NJ 07094
In Canada: Canadian Manda Group, P.O. Box 920, Station U, Toronto,
Ontario, M8Z 5P9, Canada

Queries regarding rights and permissions should be addressed to:
Carol Publishing Group, 600 Madison Avenue, New York, NY 10022

Manufactured in the United States of America
ISBN 0-8065-1202-4

Carol Publishing Group books are available at special discounts
for bulk purchases, for sales promotions, fund raising, or
educational purposes. Special editions can also be created to
specifications. For details contact: Special Sales Department,
Carol Publishing Group, 120 Enterprise Ave., Secaucus, NJ 07094

10 9 8 7 6 5 4 3 2

Library of Congress Cataloging-in-Publication Data

Manual of natural therapy.
    Bibliography: p.   Includes index.
      1. Therapeutics, Physiological. 2. Alternative medicine.
I. Olshevsky, Moshe.
RM700.M36   1989   615.5   88-24410

CONTENTS

FOREWORD

Describing the origin of medicine, Hippocrates in Ancient Medicine *wrote: "For the art of medicine would never have been discovered to begin with, nor would any medical research have been conducted—for there would have been no need for medicine—if sick men had profited by the same mode of living and regimen as the food, drink and mode of living of men in health, and if there had been no other things for the sick better than these."*

As long as there has been life on earth, disease has been a fellow-traveler. Fossil shells of 350 million years ago show signs of parasites and trauma. The 200-million-year-old bones of dinosaurs are marked with evidence of arthritis, tumors, and dental caries (Ackerknecht, 1982). Examinations of wild apes have found a wide assortment of diseases, including sinusitis, hernia, malaria, spina bifida, fractures, periodontal diseases, congenital birth defects, parasites, and arthritis (Bramblett).

Human life, also, has never escaped instances of dysfunction, disfigurement, and discomfort. Prehistoric remains of our species reveal various pathologies (Ackerknecht, 1982). Egyptian mummies safeguard evidence of osteomyeltis, arthritis, tuberculosis, tumors, kidney stones, anthracosis, pneumonia, pleurisy, and poliomyelitis (Sigerist). Pre-Columbian Indian bones are imprinted with distortions caused by disease (Goldstein). When scientists, in 1972, discovered a preserved human body from China's ancient times, their X-ray examination showed that this 2000-year-old noblewoman had tuberculosis scars, a poorly set fracture of her right forearm, and spinal problems that might have caused lumbago. Internal organs contained gallstones and parasites. The much-delayed autopsy determined that the cause of death was heart disease—a severely occluded left coronary artery (Hall).

Animals react to disease and depend on instinct. Humans respond to disease. Having less-reliable instincts and an increased awareness of the threat of annihilation, humans counter illness with consciousness, creativity, and accumulated experience. Concrete evidence for herbal medicine going back 60,000 years has been discovered by archaeologists in a Neanderthal burial mound in what is now northern Iraq (Solecki). Stone Age tools were made of sharpened flint, and skulls from that era have been discovered that show signs of having undergone the difficult operation of trepanning, the surgical opening of the skull usually performed to relieve pressure on the brain (Bishop). Egyptian medical papyrus contain over 500 different medical substances (Ackerknecht, 1973), and the first compilation of the Aztec Indian *materia medica* lists 1,200 substances (Thorwald). The Chinese noblewoman was buried with herbs that are still used to treat heart disease in hospitals in China today (Bensky). In fact, every culture has created an approach, if not several different avenues, to counter the inevitability of disease.

The history and accumulated experiences of the human engagement with illness is vast. Human beings have perceived many different sources of potential power and transformation in the world. Various techniques, methods, theories, and all-encompassing systems have been created or discovered. Some approaches emphasize the mind, belief, and will; some stress various types of remedies and medicaments; others concentrate on mechanical manipulation and restructuring. Alliances between these three styles can develop. The fact that so many approaches exist and continue to exist—in both cooperation and competition—seems to indicate that none has a completely satisfactory answer.

In modern times, easily the most successful and widespread medical system is that of scientific biomedicine. It is available throughout the globe and is an important option, in some form, for most of the world's peoples. Scientists and clinicians from every nation have contributed. Its achievements are awesome. Insulin can sustain most diabetics, antibiotics control most bacterial infections, anesthesia has removed the terror of surgery, lithium balances many manic-depressives, organ transplants replace impaired organs, and many cancers have lost their horror.

Yet despite biomedicine's obvious accomplishments, much disenchantment has developed. John Knowles characterized the situation in the title of a recent book: *Doing Better and Feeling Worse*. National surveys commissioned by the American Medical Association show a steady decline in public opinion concerning the biomedical profession. In 1984, 68% agreed that "people are beginning to lose faith in doctors," compared with 62% two years earlier (Hume). The sources of this paradox are many-faceted and include: 1) unrealistic expectations and overselling of scientific medicine's capabilities (Ingelfinger); 2) the fact that many diseases resist cure, or even palliative care (Inglis); 3) economic factors that, despite increased allocation of resources, have only been marginally affected (Powles); 4) the perceived side effects of highly technological (Schimmel) and drug-oriented (Lasagna) interventions; 5) the exclusion of many types of treatment that some people believe in from examination and possible usage within the dominant system for ideological and political reasons (Wolpe).

Recently there has been a veritable renaissance in what are called "alternative" therapies in the United States, "complimentary" therapies in Great Britain, and "parallel" therapies in France. Sometimes these therapies are called "natural" because they are relatively less dependent on modern science and technology; at other times the word "holistic" is applied as a catch-all. This rubric embraces a vast assortment of techniques, and even elaborate integrated systems. Its practitioners can encompass a wide variety of people, from yoga teachers and health-store advisers to chiropractors, homeopaths, and even practitioners qualified in biomedicine. Though unified in not being an integrated part of the conventional scientific system, these various approaches are disparate and can be uncommunicative or even competitive with one another.

The authors of this book have undertaken an ambitious task. They have tried to bring together some of the most important available alternative techniques in one volume. Ecumenical in spirit, pluralistic in ideology, and noncompetitive in practice, this book provides a useful service. Too often health-care systems are contending factions rather than cooperative alliances. By compiling in one place what is usually scattered in many places, practitioners and patients have an opportunity to see a wide gamut of possible therapeutic paths. It provides a rare overview of options. By keeping the illness categories in modern medical terminology, the authors have left open the possibility of dialogue and cooperation with the biomedical world. At the same time, it is important to remember that although this volume is comprehensive in scope, it is not a complete answer. Eclecticism is never a substitute for expert medical advice and rigorous clinical training.

—Ted Kaptchuk

REFERENCES

Ackerknecht, Erwin, *A Short History of Medicine*. Baltimore: Johns Hopkins University, 1982.

————, *Therapeutics: From the Primitives to the Twentieth Century*. New York: Hafner, 1973.

Bensky, D., A. Gamble and T. Kaptchuk, *Chinese Herbal Medicine*. Seattle: Eastland Press, 1986.

Bishop, W. J., *The Early History of Surgery*. London: Robert Hale, 1960.

Bramblett, Claud, "Pathology in the Darajani Baboon," *American Journal of Physical Anthropology*, 26(1967), 331–340.

Goldstein, Marcus, "Skeletal Pathology of Early Indians in Texas," *American Journal of Physical Anthropology*, 15(1957), 299–311.

Hall, Alice J., "Lady for China's Past," *National Geographic* (May 1974).

Hume, Ellen, "The AMA is Laboring to Regain Dominance over Nation's Doctors," *The Wall Street Journal*, June 13, 1986.

Ingelfinger, Franz J., "Medicine: Meritorious or Meretricious," *Science*, 200(1978).

Inglis, Brian, *The Diseases of Civilization*. London: Granada, 1981.

Lasagna, Louis, "The Diseases Drugs Cause," *Perspectives in Biology and Medicine*, 7(1964), 457–470.

Powles, John, "On the Limitations of Modern Medicine," *Science, Medicine and Ethics*, 1(1973), 1–30.

Schimmel, Elihu, "The Hazards of Hospitalization," *Annals of Internal Medicine*, 60(1964), 100–110.

Sigerist, Henry E., *A History of Medicine*. New York: Oxford University Press, 1951.

Solecki, Ralph S., "Shanidar IV, a Neanderthal Flower Burial in Northern Iraq," *Science*, 190(1975).

Thorwald, Jurgen, *Science and Secrets of Early Medicine*. New York: Harcourt, Brace and World, 1962.

Wolpe, Paul Root, "The Maintenance of Professional Authority: Acupuncture and the American Physician," *Social Problems*, 32(1985), 409–424.

INTRODUCTION
THE ALTERNATIVE
MEDICAL ARTS—
THEIR PLACE IN
MODERN TREATMENT

The trend toward self-care and informed patients has been clearly established in the last two decades. The modern layman wants to know more—not just about alternative medicine, but about the chemicals in foods, the drugs his physician prescribes, and the latest in the *New England Journal of Medicine*. "Second opinion" is the order of the day.

At the same time that this quest for medical information has reached a fever pitch, the alternative therapies such as acupuncture, applied nutrition, and homeopathy seem to have lost their punch. The half dozen or so of these "renegade" treatments caused some excitement in recent years, stirred some thinking, then were relegated once more into the category of splinter movements. Each new book proclaimed a certain approach as the key to every ailment of mankind: the thyroid, or sugar, or exercise, or vitamin C, or stress reduction through meditation. Splintered, these alternatives have become will-o'-the-wisps—unless, as some have tried to do, one lumps them all together under the name "holistic." In order to understand or evaluate any of them, a patient in need of treatment would have to devote a college education to its literature and critics.

This book begins with the simplifying premise that there is *some* truth, and a lot of help, in *all* of the major alternative therapies. We have not attempted to proselytize for any of them; we do not wish to raise the issue of better or worse. But we do know, from our own experience in treatment and from our study of the literature, that for the vast majority of common medical problems each of these therapies is helpful—and quite cost-effective. None of them has to be king.

Our second premise is that these therapies work well together. There is no reason why one should not use them all for any given ailment. In some cases, in fact, there is a combined effect that is greater than the sum of the parts. Some therapies promote the effectiveness of others in a synergistic way.

It should be clear from a brief thumbing of the following pages that our purpose is treatment, not theory. We have limited our description of each therapy to the following summary; the bibliography contains ample references to the history or theoretical underpinnings of each type of treatment.

All of these therapies, with the clear exception of acupuncture, can be easily administered by oneself. This fact is the key to their usefulness and inexpensiveness. No physician or nurse could afford the time to carry out the multiple applications most of them require over the course of a day. On the other hand, it is not always easy to obtain the materials necessary for various therapies, such as color therapy or Bach flowers. Most major cities have sources for Chinese and Western herbs. We suggest that the reader use the bibliography to locate sources for the rest. This is not a catalog, but it does provide the first level of help in locating remedies.

Finally, we must address the question of the place of alternative therapies, as a whole, in modern medical practice. Clearly, most of these treatments are outside the sphere of the M.D. (Acupuncture received some notice in medical groups after James Reston's publicity for his appendectomy in China some fifteen years ago, but few hospitals have access to this technique today.) The M.D. is trained in acute medicine: drugs, surgery, and sometimes radiation. Often, acute medicine is what is needed—and fast. Quite often, too, acute medicine is administered when the patient would be better off with a more cautious and *patient* approach. Alternative medicine provides that important *alternative*. Sometimes, as in the case of the common cold, the sore throat, or indigestion, alternative medicine is the *only* sensible approach. In our frantic search for pill-popping answers to everything, we have neglected, if not forgotten, the wisdom of the past. Each alternative medicine has a legitimate place in the maintenance of health—primarily in self-care, and especially when the drug alternative is not that urgent, has side effects, or is just too expensive.

A WORD ABOUT THE THERAPIES

The following therapies are considered for the various medical conditions covered in this book. In most cases, all of them have some degree of application for each condition. For a comprehensive history of these therapies and the rationale for their use, refer to the bibliography at the end of the book.

Acupuncture, Acupressure (Reflexology)

Although these two time-honored Eastern therapies are based on a theory of the inner connections of all parts of the body, they differ radically in what those connections are and how they should be put to use. Acupuncture employs needles to penetrate well beneath the skin—to reach nerve endings or other sites that control pain. This is *not* a self-administered therapy; even a skillful acupuncturist would not treat himself or herself as a matter of choice. Acupressure, on the other hand, is a massagelike therapy based on precise pressure points on the feet, hands, and ears. These extremities are the sites of treatment because they are the "end points" of the "ten meridians" that run from the head through the body to the hands and feet. Known in Japan as shiatsu, and in Western countries as reflexology, usually referring to corresponding body organs in the feet, this therapy is designed to "unblock" various pathways that are claimed to be the source of relief from virtually every type of illness or discomfort. Unlike acupuncture, acupressure is primarily a self-care treatment, requiring patient massaging of the suspected pressure point several times during the day. In reflexology, "x" indicates how many times to press.

Applied Nutrition

Often called simply "nutrition" or "diet," this approach is the primary self-care therapy. Nutrition has generally been denied any place in therapy, being considered for the most part "preventive" only. It is called "applied nutrition" here to emphasize its new therapeutic role. (See also "Diet" below.) A list of the diets recommended in the text of this book is found in the Appendix.

Aromatherapy

The use of the scents of various plants and flowers to alter mood is a minor but often helpful treatment. The importance of aroma in healing is usually emphasized by the *negative* in Western culture: the smell of gases and antiseptics in hospitals, for example. That the sense of smell can have positive applications in health care is recognized in many cultures.

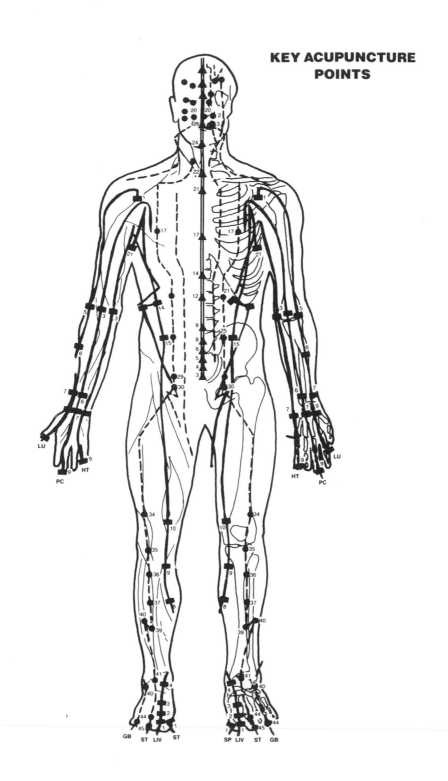

KEY ACUPUNCTURE POINTS

KEY ACUPUNCTURE POINTS

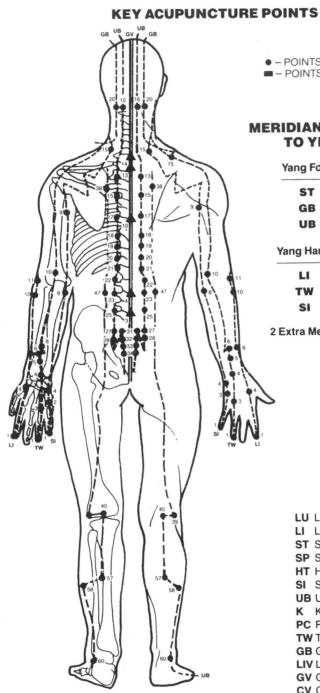

● – POINTS ON YANG MERIDIAN
■ – POINTS ON YIN MERIDIAN

MERIDIANS ACCORDING TO YIN-YANG

Yang Foot	Yin Foot
ST	SP
GB	LIV
UB	K

Yang Hand	Yin Hand
LI	LU
TW	PC
SI	HT

2 Extra Meridians: GV
CV

INDEX

LU LUNG
LI LARGE INTESTINE
ST STOMACH
SP SPLEEN
HT HEART
SI SMALL INTESTINE
UB URINARY BLADDER
K KIDNEY
PC PERICARD
TW TRIPLE WARMER
GB GALL BLADDER
LIV LIVER
GV GOVERNING VESSEL
CV CONCEPTION VESSEL

KEY ACUPUNCTURE POINTS

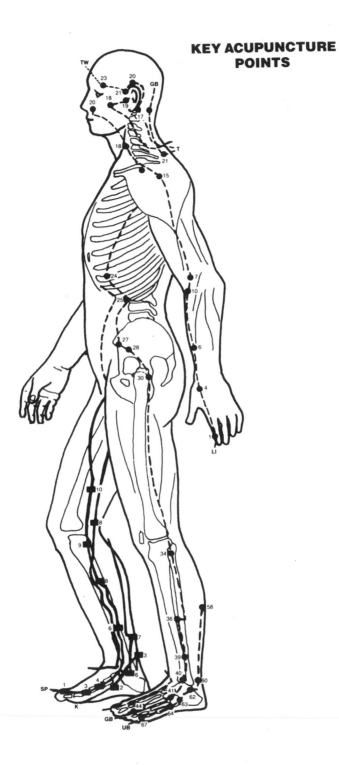

ATLAS OF REFLEXOLOGY

THE TEN MERIDIANS

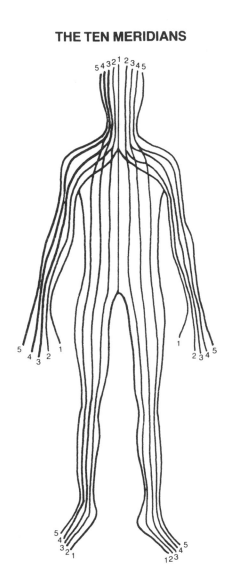

1 Sinus	44 Uterine Tube;
2 Pituitary	Spermatic Duct
3 Cerebrum	45 Groin
4 Cerebellum	46 Ovary; Testicle
5 Nose	47 Uterus; Prostate
6 Eye	48 Vagina; Penis
7 Temple	49 Sex-Hormones
8 Neck	50 Tonsils
9 Ear	51 Thymus
10 Throat	52 Autonomic Nervous
11 Parathyroid	System
12 Spine	53 Waist
13 Thyroid	54 Cranial Nerves
14 Shoulder	55 General Pain;
15 Trapezius	Toothache
16 Lung; Chest; Breast	56 Energy
17 Solar plexus	57 Buttocks
18 Heart	58 Fingers
19 Spleen	59 Stomach Disorders
20 Adrenal Gland	60 Urethra
21 Kidney	61 Mouth
22 Pancreas	62 External Nose
23 Duodenum	63 Internal Nose
24 Liver	64 Forehead
25 Gall Bladder	65 Tongue
26 Stomach	66 Skin
27 Transverse Colon	67 Hypertension
28 Ascending Colon	68 Appetite
29 Descending Colon	69 Elbow
30 Sigmoid Colon	70 Vertex
31 Small Intestine	71 Fever
32 Urinary Tract	72 Medulla Oblongata
33 Bladder	73 Alcoholism
34 Leg; Knee; Hip;	74 Stop Smoking
Lower Back	75 Neurasthenia
35 Sciatic	76 Cheek
36 Hemorrhoids	77 Ribs
37 Rectum	78 Vocal Chords
38 Ileo Cecal Valve	79 Thirst Control
39 Appendix	80 Wrist
40 Jaws	81 Hormonogenic
41 Diaphragm	82 Breathing
42 Upper Lymph	Difficulties
Glands	83 Jaundice
43 Lower Lymph	84 Hair Problems
Glands	

ATLAS OF REFLEXOLOGY

RIGHT AND LEFT EAR

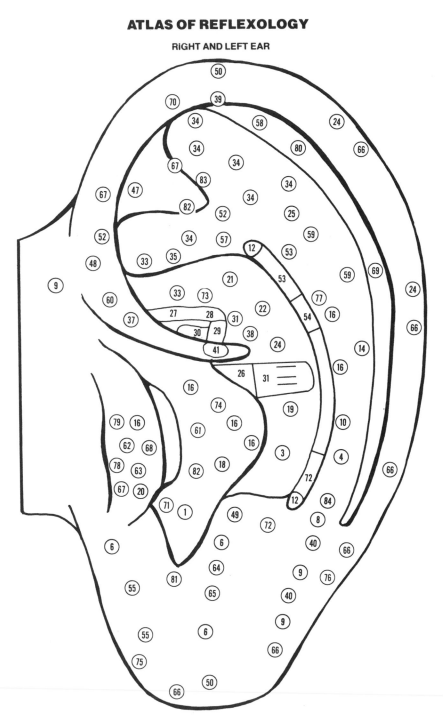

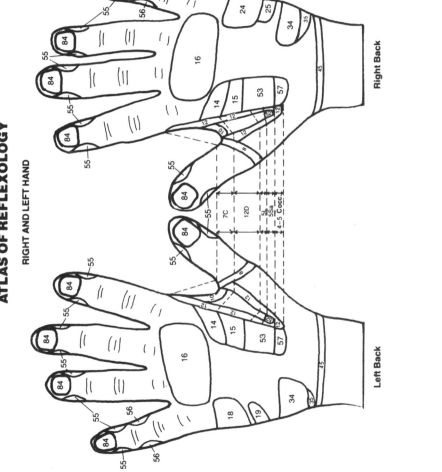

ATLAS OF REFLEXOLOGY

RIGHT AND LEFT HAND

Left Back

Right Back

ATLAS OF REFLEXOLOGY

RIGHT AND LEFT HAND

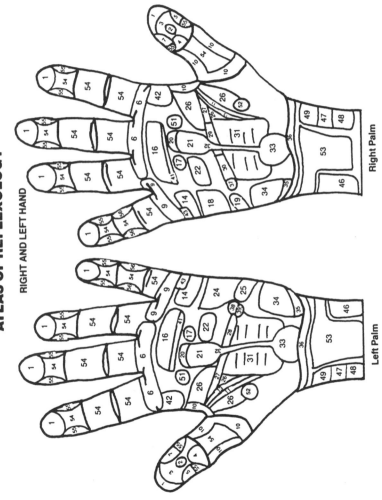

Left Palm

Right Palm

ATLAS OF REFLEXOLOGY

RIGHT AND LEFT FOOT (1–2–3)

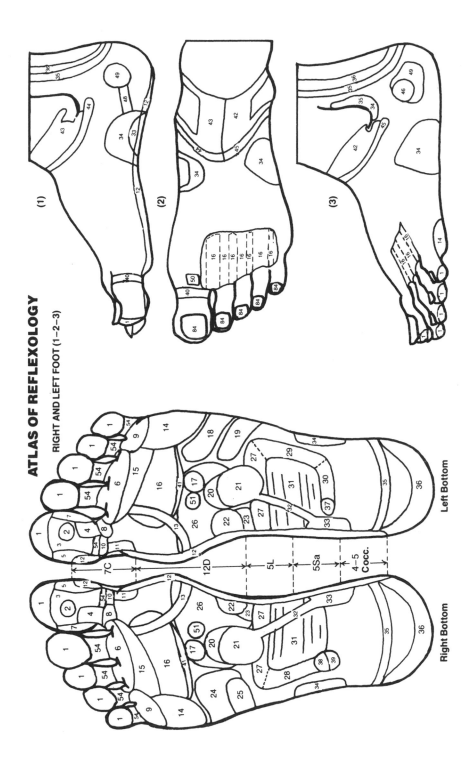

Right Bottom

Left Bottom

(1)

(2)

(3)

Bach Flowers

In the 1930s a doctor extracted oils from thirty-eight flowers of various plants and tested them for their effect on mood. Now known by his name, these flowers are not harmful or habit-forming (as are the essences of such plants as marijuana). Yet they have been effective in altering such moods as fear, worry, anger, or depression—all of which can cause illness or retard normal healing.

In general, Bach flowers are used in doses of four drops, three times a day—morning, noon and evening—and are taken on an empty stomach. Treatment should be continued up to six or seven weeks or until improvement is shown.

Breathing Therapy

The importance of adequate air is now recognized in medicine as an active factor in healing. Once considered only an autonomic response, good breathing techniques can be consciously acquired. Normal exercise that raises the heartbeat to moderate levels for about thirty minutes is popularly known as "aerobics." Deep breathing can also be practiced by itself and can have many therapeutic consequences.

Along with nutrition, exercise and breathing are the basic forms of self-care that can be undertaken by virtually anyone at no cost. (See Appendix under "Yoga and Other Breathing Therapies".)

Color Therapy

It has been known in every culture that certain colors are calming and others agitating. Yet only recently has there been a direct effort to use colors in healing. As described in the bibliography, specialized equipment is needed to display the proper colors effectively.

Diet: Macrobiotics and Fasting

These are two of the more extreme forms of dietary therapy. Both have their supporters and detractors. It is important to understand the reason for choosing these treatments and to make sure of an adequate intake of nutrients before attempting either program. (See also the appendix for a list of additives that are considered safe in foods and for guidelines for a gluten-free diet.) The denial of various types of foods, or the occasional two- to four-day fast from solids, can be an important therapeutic tool against allergies.

Herbs—Chinese and Western

The use of extracts from plants (and occasionally animals) for direct medicinal purposes is the oldest form of therapy. It is also the basis of modern pharmacology, although the synthetic creation of drugs is now virtually the sole occupation of pharmaceutical companies. (It should be remembered that when penicillin was commercially developed in the United States during World War II, the best source for the proper mold turned out to be a batch of rotten peaches.) Chinese herbs have been developed and codified over many centuries; Western herbs are still undergoing experimentation. The important difference between herbology and the "magic bullet" drugs of modern medicine is that the former are relatively weak against virulent disease or illness, yet they have the advantage of virtual absence of disastrous side effects. Herbs are taken in a wide variety of forms, including tinctures, teas, pills, tablets, and pressed juices for internal use and ointments and shampoos for external use.

Tinctures

These are comparatively low concentrations of the primary ingredients of an herb, in an alcohol solution. Take ten to twenty drops with a few tablespoons of water, three times a day, one half hour before meals.

Combined Teas

Herbal teas, combined in specific proportions, are often a pleasant form of medication for certain ailments. As with any medical prescription, it is important that the chemical and botanical compatiblity of the herbs be taken into account. Pour *boiling* water over one to two teaspoons of dry herbs and let stand for ten to fifteen minutes.

Ointments

The ointment form of herbs is very effective in treating the skin and speeding the healing process, such as with hemorrhoids. Apply externally only.

Pressed Juices

Juices made from fresh plants are useful primarily for their rich content of vitamins and minerals. They can be taken like tinctures—diluted with a few tablespoons of water, three times a day about a half hour before meals.

A complete catalog of Chinese herbal prescriptions, referred to in the text of this book, is found in the Appendix.

Note that the German health ministry does not recommend the use of *tussilage farfara* (coltsfoot), *eupatorium* (agrimony), or *symphytum* (comfrey) as they may be cancer-causing agents.

Homeopathy

By its name, this treatment is designed to pit "like" against "like" rather than "unlike" (drugs) against illness, or "allopathy." Developed in the early nineteenth century, homeopathy focuses on an exhaustive casebook of each type of illness to determine its essential features, then to recreate the conditions causing it. The therapy has been criticized for its insistence on minimal doses—so small in many cases as to amount to a few molecules. Yet it has had success for almost two centuries. Remedies can be administered as 1) drops of tincture, 2) granules, 3) powder or 4) tablets. For use at home we recommend the low potencies. And because homeopathic medicines are *energetic* medicines, avoid "anti-dotes," such as coffee, camphor, toothpaste, cough drops and the like while using homeopathic remedies. Also *never* touch the actual remedy with your hands, and keep the remedy out of sunlight or intense lighting.

In case of acute symptoms, use the remedy more often, and use the remedy for 2–3 days to get results. If symptoms return, change remedy. We recommend the decimal potencies marked with the letter "X." "X" potency equals "d" potency in Europe. There is also a centesimal system marked as "c," which is common in Europe. Where potencies are *not* mentioned please use 6X = 12X potency.

Hydrotherapy

Mineral baths for general therapy—although no longer as popular as in the great days of the European spas—have great benefit. But "water therapy" also consists of extended baths or showers in the home. Relief of muscular soreness in saunas or hot tubs is also a part of hydrotherapy and relaxation.

Psychotherapy

Numerous theories of the mind and consciousness have led to equally numerous forms of therapy. Freudian insights are still dominant in the field, although "organic" therapies, such as orthomolecular psychiatry, have achieved scientific acceptance.

Autosuggestion (Self-Hypnosis)

The power of suggestion, of imaging, and of "psyching up" has been popularized by several recent books dealing with life-threatening illness. This process involves the repetition of reassuring phrases and the calling up of positive images to counteract fears in the face of disease.

Schuessler Tissue Salts

Minerals have only recently come into prominence, along with vitamins, as essential elements for most bodily functions. The Schuessler salts were developed to provide those minerals in controlled amounts for specific deficiencies.

HOW TO USE THIS BOOK FOR BEST RESULTS

At the start we must emphasize that the purpose of this book is to augment, not replace, the services of a qualified physician. By all means see your doctor for any condition that requires immediate medical attention. The authors make no claims, direct or implied, for any treatment in this book. But we do invite you to participate in any of these forms of self-care, based on our practical experience with them as well as on our medical studies.

It should be noted that any therapy, conventional or not, may be dangerous if used improperly, or useless if practiced incorrectly. We therefore suggest that you pay close attention to the following rules before using this book.

1. For best results, use as *many* of the therapies suggested for each ailment as you find convenient. These "modalities," as they are called, work best in concert. Try not to be a devotee of a particular treatment.
2. Try to employ *first* the therapy that is recommended as most efficacious for the particular ailment. Because of variations between individuals, there is no absolute "first." *As a guide to priority of treatment, we have used stars, from one to four,* to indicate the relative value of a treatment in each case. As in film and restaurant reviews, four stars is top priority. Evaluations are not made for Bach flowers, which are used for mood effect rather than direct organic reaction.
3. Some of the therapies discussed here require supplies, which, though inexpensive, may take time to obtain (note the sources at end of book). So you should start at once with those therapies that require no special supplies: nutrition, exercise, breathing, reflexol-

ogy, and acupressure. These activities also lay the groundwork for a more receptive attitude toward other therapies.

4. The only therapy recommended here that should not be self-applied is acupuncture. Both acupressure and reflexology are similar in theory to acupuncture and can be applied by oneself.

5. Three major therapies that require supplies are herbal remedies, homeopathic remedies, and Bach flowers. We will also refer occasionally to other modalities requiring special equipment. Be sure to follow the instructions accompanying these supplies. A full description of these therapies appears below, along with appropriate charts for acupressure and reflexology.

6. Finally, note that this book is not intended as a polemic for or against any form of treatment, but as *a manual for use*. The rationale for each modality can be gathered from the sources cited in the bibliography.

NOTE TO THE READER

At the beginning of each section there is a general discussion of the causes and related symptoms of each illness treated in that section. For the benefit of practical application of various remedies, specific *symptoms* are described immediately before the presentation of those remedies. Where symptoms are obvious (e.g., nosebleed) symptoms are not described.

· 1 ·
THE DIGESTIVE SYSTEM

Medical practice is most often concerned with gastrointestinal problems, for our digestive system is the source of our ability to sustain life. Small disorders in the complex process of turning food into living cells can disrupt our lives and, worse, can mean the difference between merely surviving and living in the full glow of health.

Five organs of the body make up the gastrointestinal tract, and each has a special role in preparing food molecules to be distributed throughout the cells of the body:

1. The *mouth*. Here the first of the digestive juices, saliva, softens food as it is chewed, changing some of the starches into sugars by means of enzymes (pytalin and amylase).
2. The *esophagus* carries the softened food to the stomach in a regulated way.
3. The *stomach*. Here gastric juices containing various enzymes (such as the enzyme pepsin) act on fats, starches, or protein. An important gastric juice is hydrochloric acid, which activates pepsin, softens connective tissue in meat, and kills harmful bacteria.
4. The *small intestine*. As food is liquefied it enters the small intestine, where nutrients are "snagged" by minute projections of its walls and passed through tiny capillaries into the bloodstream. These projections, known as villi, also contain lymphatic capillaries (lacteals), which absorb most of the fats.
5. The *large intestine*. Food particles not ingested in the small intestine

pass to the large intestine, where they are moved slowly toward defecation. The intestines are some thirty feet in length, and most of the problems we refer to as being in our stomach are in fact below the stomach in the intestinal tract.

The gastrointestinal (G.I.) tract contains many necessary bacteria— the intestinal flora—that fight certain opportunistic infections, aid in water absorption to prevent diarrhea, reduce the accumulation of gas, and help in the digestion of such foods as milk and the absorption of such minerals as calcium. Beyond the G.I. tract are two critical organs, the liver and the pancreas, which continue the absorption process. The largest organ in the body, the liver has two well-known roles: to store glucose in the form of glycogen, and to detoxify such harmful substances as alcohol and other drugs. The pancreas is best known as the maker of insulin, which regulates blood sugar. Both organs have other important functions, both in digestion and in hormonal activity. Their importance is such that they cannot be considered in themselves, but only as part of many bodily functions.

The most common symptom of a gastrointestinal problem, indigestion, is the result of poor eating habits—too much, too fast; excessive fats; foods such as wheat and milk that may cause allergic reactions; or meals consumed under conditions of stress. Abdominal fullness, pressure, heartburn, belching, bad breath, and flatulence commonly accompany indigestion.

Gum and mouth diseases are less common symptoms, but quite a bit more serious. Gingivitis and pyorrhea are both diseases of the gums— the latter degenerative—that can be brought on by malnutrition or problems in the nervous system or the gastrointestinal tract. High fevers, menses, and pregnancy are also causes to be suspected. Other stresses, including the use of antibiotics for a prolonged period, can cause sores and ulcers in the mouth.

The annoying but otherwise minor problems of belching and hiccuping can result from irregularities in the esophagus or the stomach, but no specific etiology has as yet been identified.

The much-publicized syndrome of anorexia—the unwillingness to eat sufficiently to maintain weight—can be the result of a gastrointestinal disease or a psychological state (nervosa). The latter is often accompanied by voluntary vomiting, whereas nausea almost always precedes spontaneous vomiting.

The most common disturbance of the stomach is the painful, episodic illness *gastritis*. Chemical irritants are the usual cause: alcohol, salicylates, nicotine, or allergy-causing foods; but bacterial and viral infections can also be the villain, as in food poisoning or hepatitis.

Peptic ulcers create similar symptoms but are usually the result of heredity, stress, or problems with gastric juices.

In the stomach, the small intestine, and the large intestine, a weakness in the digestive wall (a pouch, or diverticulum) may cause inflammation or buildup of waste materials: diverticulosis, or, in the inflammed state, diverticulitis. Improper diet and heredity are presumed causes. An equally serious inflammation, primarily of the small intestine called regional enteritis occurs mainly in young adults and can do widespread damage to the intestines.

Irregularity in the large intestine—due to infection, food poisoning, irregular eating habits, or stress—is seen as diarrhea: frequent, liquid bowel movements. Signs of blood in the stool—tar-blackness—should be immediately brought to the attention of a physician. The opposite condition—infrequent stools, or constipation—can be uncomfortable but is usually unthreatening. Constipation may be simply the result of infrequent activity or change of diet, but it can also have deep-seated emotional or biological causes.

Both diarrhea and constipation may be accompanied by flatulence— the excess of gas expelled from the intestines. Often this is merely the result of the swallowing of air in eating and drinking, but excessive food gases are usually the result of the inappropriateness of certain foods for each individual, including the promotion of the wrong bacteria in the colon (intestines).

When the large intestine becomes inflamed, primarily in young people, bouts of alternating constipation and diarrhea may result—a condition known as colitis. Colitis may be ulcerative if blood appears in the diarrhea.

An essential part of the defecation process is the passage of fecal matter by veins located around the rectum. These veins are known as hemorrhoids, or piles, but we commonly use the same names to signify the excessive enlargement, hardening, and bleeding of these vital organs. Piles can therefore be quite painful as they lose their proper place and their function.

Beyond the gastrointestinal tract, the most common ailment associated with digestion is gallstones (Cholecystitis). These are indeed "stones"—pebbles, so to speak—that form probably from the precipitation of bile into small crystals. These stones are sometimes "passed," or excreted through the intestines. The pain of gallstones that are not excreted can be such as to require an emergency operation in many cases, but for the most part these pains are episodic. The excessive deposit of cholesterol in the gall bladder by the liver is the most recent explanation for the prevalence of this ailment in Westernized countries.

DYSPEPSIA (INDIGESTION)

SYMPTOMS

Improper digestion may result from many different causes, but it is identified by the same symptoms: a sudden appearance of bad breath and belching, often flatulence, and subjective feelings of pressure in the abdomen and heartburn in the chest and throat.

SUGGESTED TREATMENT

Acupuncture and Acupressure **

Li 4, ST 25, ST 36, ST 37
With flatulence, add:
BL 20, BL 60, SP 6

Applied Nutrition ****

Drink: distilled water with honey or pure fruit juices, four to six glasses daily.
Eat: well-cooked whole rice, low-fat milk, yogurt, low-fat cheese, boiled vegetables, fresh apples, fresh bananas. Normally the diet should be adjusted to the age and weight of the patient. An example of a diet for a person of average weight, thirty years old (overall intake should decrease with age and weight):

2000 calories	100 mg vitamin B_1 (thiamin)
42 g protein	100 mg vitamin B_2 (riboflavin)
90 g fat	100 mg niacin
255 g carbohydrate	1500 mg vitamin C (ascorbic
800 mg calcium	acid)
15 mg iron	10 mg zinc
20,000 IU vitamin A	

Aromatherapy *

For general symptoms of indigestion, inhale **basil** *(Ocymum basilicum)* singly or in combination with **black pepper** *(Piper nigrum),* **camomile** *(Matricaria camomila),* and **lavender** *(Lavendula officinalis).* Place two drops on the back of the wrist and inhale through the mouth or nose three times daily.

Autosuggestion

Indigestion is often the result of anxiety and feelings of general malaise. Repeat the following affirmation at least ten times daily:

> *I take in the new and easily assimilate it.*

Bach Flowers ***

Agrimony: When indigestion is accompanied by anxiety and nervous tension, take as a tincture, three to five drops daily.
Horn beam: For low vitality, add to agrimony treatment, also in tincture, four drops every half hour in acute cases, otherwise a few drops daily.

Color Therapy

Yellow is the color of choice to soothe the stomach. Meditate and visualize yellow color warming the abdomen, or use a yellow screen on the abdominal area fifteen minutes daily.

Herbs ***

Western

Meadowsweet *(Filipendula ulmaria):*   To reduce excess acidity and calm the stomach, use one teaspoon per one cup of boiled water. Leave the cup covered for ten minutes, filter, and drink the liquid only once or twice a day before meals. Honey may be added for taste.
Peppermint *(Mentha)* or **aniseed** *(Pimpinella):*   In cases where flatulence accompanies indigestion, add to meadowsweet infusion.
Lavender *(Lavendula)* or **camomile** *(Matricaria camomila):*   In cases where nervous tension accompanies indigestion, add to meadowsweet infusion.

Chinese

Hoelen and **alisma:**   Take as tea or in tablets. The tablets are manufactured and consist of the following recommended ratio of ingredients:

65 g hoelen	6 g alisma
4.5 g plyporus	3 g cinnamon
4.5 g atractylodes	

Homeopathy **

The recommended remedies can be taken as tinctures or globules. The lower simillimums are advised unless otherwise prescribed by a homeopathic physician.

Nux vomica: Use in cases of heartburn, heaviness after meals, flatulence, and lingering bitter taste in mouth, 6X potency.

Lycopodium: Use in cases where heartburn accompanies daily or chronic indigestion, as instructed by a homeopathic physician, at night and in the morning, 6X potency.

Pulsatilla: Use in cases of white-coated tongue, and for cravings for rich food, 6X potency.

Reflexology **

Massage in round movements, clockwise, the following points on each foot, five to ten minutes daily:
26, 27, 28, 29, 30, 31, 37, 38, 39.

Schuessler Tissue Salts **

Calcarea phosphorica: In chronic cases of indigestion, pain after eating and excessive gas in the stomach, take one tablet in 3X potency.

GUM AND MOUTH DISEASES (GINGIVITIS, PYORRHEA, AND SORES)

SYMPTOMS

Agrimony: In cases where mouth sores may be caused by anxiety, use in tincture, four drops daily.

SUGGESTED TREATMENT

Acupuncture and Acupressure *

The general recommendation for pressure is:
    ST 4, ST 25, ST 36, GV 4, CV 12, CV 23, BL 20, BL 23
For pyorrhea, add:
    Li 20, BL 10, Li 11
For mouth ulcers, add:
    CV 24

Applied Nutrition ***

Drink: Distilled water, three to five cups daily
Eat: Food rich in B-complex vitamins, such as whole grains, seeds, etc., and foods rich in proteins. An example of a diet for a person of average weight, thirty years old:

2200 calories	800 IU vitamin E
42 g protein	100 mg vitamin B_1
70 g fat	100 mg vitamin B_2
340 g carbohydrates	120 mg niacin
1400 mg calcium	50 mg vitamin B_{12}
12 mg iron	5000 mg vitamin C
30,000 IU vitamin A	400 mg vitamin D

Aromatherapy *

For general symptoms of gingivitis, inhale either singly or in combination **camomile** *(Matricaria camomilia)* and **myrrh** *(Commiphora molmol)*, two drops, three times daily between meals. For pyorrhea, inhale **cypress** *(Cupressus sempervirens)* as above, instead of camomile.

Bach Flowers ****

Agrimony: In cases where mouth sores may be caused by anxiety, use in tincture, four drops daily.
Hornbeam: Add to treatment to increase strength.
Impatiens: Add to treatment to soothe anxiety or restlessness.

Color Therapy

Blue light radiation is effective as a bacteriocidal and is useful in treating infections and ulcerations. Use for thirty minutes followed by ultraviolet light, two to three times daily.

Herbs ****

Western

Myrrh *(Commiphora molmol):* In gingivitis, wash the mouth with a tincture and massage the gums before bed with eucalyptus oil. In cases of pyorrhea, drink a tea combined with echimacea.
Red sage *(Salvia officinalis):* In cases of mouth ulcers or aphtae, use as a mouthwash, twice daily.

Chinese

Pinellia, ginseng and **ginger:** Use as tea or in tablets, twice daily.

Homeopathy **

Plantago major *(plantain):* Use in cases of pyorrhea in tincture in the lower potencies of 3X to 6X. (Plantago major is also effective in treating toothache).

Staphysagria *(stavesacre):* In cases of gingivitis, or other symptoms of spongy gums and lacerated tissues, use in tincture three times daily.

Borax *(borate of sodium):* In cases of aphtae with white funguslike growth or in cases of bleeding ulcers on the gums, use in tincture in potency of 1X to 3X.

Reflexology *

Massage the upper surface of the big toes of both feet, beginning just below the toenail, and continue all the way down to the base of the toe for fifteen to twenty minutes twice daily.

Schuessler Tissue Salts

Calcarea Phosphorica: For imflamed gums, pyorrhea, and mouth ulcers, use three times daily at 6X potency.

BELCHING AND HICCUPS

SUGGESTED TREATMENT

Acupuncture and Acupressure ****
The recommended points are:
   Li 17, ST 11
Also:
   CV 12, CV 14, CV 15

Aromatherapy *
Inhale or sniff six drops each of **basil** *(Ocymum basilicum)* or **sandalwood** *(Santalum album),* singly or in combination.

Herbal ***

Dill weed: Make a tea by boiling a teaspoonful of seed in one cup of water for fifteen minutes, strain, and drink.

Homeopathy **

Rathnia *(Krameria mapato):*   For violent hiccups, take in 3X to 6X potency.
Ginseng tincture: For all sorts of hiccups, take a general dosage.
Ignatia (St. Ignatius bean):   In cases of loud and noisy hiccups, take a general dosage.

Schuessler Tissue Salts ***

Magnesium phosphorica: In cases of acute attacks, use in 3X to 6X potency every fifteen minutes.

ANOREXIA, NAUSEA, VOMITING

SYMPTOMS

The unwillingness to eat or the fear of gaining weight is commonly accompanied by forced vomiting and other obvious signs of psychological obsession with weight loss.

SUGGESTED TREATMENT

Acupuncture and Acupressure ****

Anorexia: ST 36, LV 4, CV 12, BL 20, BL 21 (**)
Nausea and Vomiting: PC 6, ST 11, ST 36, CV 12

Applied Nutrition ***

Although rapid symptomatic alleviation of these symptoms is best effected with acupressure, homeopathy, and herbs, applied nutrition is an excellent preventative method. Vitamin B_6 or pyridoxine is a natural specific for nausea associated with pregnancy, but only in cases where the nausea extends past the first three months. For a person of average weight, thirty years old, follow the Rejuvenating Diet (see Appendix).

Bach Flowers ****

Red chestnut and **Rock rose:**   Use in cases of anorexia accompanied by anxiety and nightmares.

Willow and **Holly:**　Use in cases of appetite loss as a psychological product of poor self-esteem.

Color Therapy

Green or red colors are recommended as therapy for these symptoms. Use color filters for fifteen to thirty minutes once or twice daily for the duration of the problem.

Herbs **

Western

Mugwort *(Artimesia vulgaris):*　In cases of anorexia, use twice daily.
Calamus (acorns):　Take as tea twice daily half an hour before meals.
Centaury *(Centaurium erythraea)* and **burdock** *(Arctium lappa):*　In cases of anorexia, take as a combination tea.
Black horehound *(Ballota nigra):*　In cases of nausea and vomiting, take as a tea or infusion. This can be combined with **meadowsweet** and **camomile.**

Chinese

Pinellia and Ginseng Six Combination:　For cases of anorexia as well as for nausea and vomiting, use in following formula:

Pinellia 4g	Coptis 3g
Hoelen 4g	Scute 3g
Ostrea 4g	Citrus 2g
Atractylodes 4g	Licorice 1g
Ginseng 4g	

Homeopathy **

Nux vomica:　For nausea and vomiting, use twice daily in 6X potency.
Tabacum or **Cocculus indicus:**　In cases of nausea and vomiting due to motion sickness, use before or during travel three times daily at 6X potency.
Ipecac root *(Ipecacuanha):*　In cases of persistent nausea and vomiting, use in 6X to 12X potency.
China *(Cinchona officinalis):*　In cases of anorexia, and for cases of flatulence, use in 6X potency.

Reflexology ***

Massage the stomach, large intestine, and pituitary area for thirty minutes twice daily.

PEPTIC ULCER AND GASTRITIS

SYMPTOMS

Sensations of burning, often sharp pains in the stomach and intestines may indicate either gastritis or peptic ulcers. It is difficult to distinguish between gastritis caused by food poisoning and that caused by improper diet. In both conditions there may also be diarrhea or constipation, but the site of the pain can be approximated by touching the affected area.

SUGGESTED TREATMENT

Acupuncture and Acupressure ***

BL 17, BL 19, BL 20, BL 21, CV 12, CV 14

Applied Nutrition ****

Avoid known irritants that stimulate hydrochloric acid secretions—e.g., coffee, tea, alcohol, cigarettes, spicy or fried foods. Eat bland food of an alkaline nature. Use the following formula three times daily:

aloe vera gel 1/2 oz.
predigested protein 4g
raw egg

vitamin C 500 mg
cream 1 oz.
water 3 oz.

Blend together at high speed and avoid foaming. Take two tablespoons of liquid acidophilus between meals.
When burning and discomfort abate, yogurt, avocados, natural processed cheese, and whole-grain foods may be added to the diet.

Aromatherapy

Geranium *(Pelargonium odorantissimum)* or **camomile:**   Inhale two drops three times daily.

Bach Flowers **

Agrimony: Use five drops three times daily.
White chestnut and **gentian:**   Add in cases where depression or anxiety are present.

Color Therapy
Use blue and yellow filters combined or alternating twice daily for fifteen minutes.

Herbs **

Western

Comfrey root *(Symphytum officinale)*, **marshmallow root** *(Althaea officinalis)*, **meadowsweet** *(Filipendula ulmaria)*, and **golden seal** *(Hydrastis canadensis):* In cases of gastritis and peptic ulcers, use in one to one ratio of all herbs either in tea or in capsules.
Valerian *(Valeriana officinalis)* or **Hops** *(Humulus lupulus):* In cases of severe nervous tension, add to above herbs.

DIVERTICULITIS AND DIVERTICULOSIS

SYMPTOMS

It is difficult to distinguish the causes of pain in the abdomen. The inflammation of the small and large intestines, if prolonged and unrelated to a specific food intake, may also be regional enteritis as well as diverticulosis.

SUGGESTED TREATMENT

Acupuncture and Acupressure ***

CV 4, CV 6, GV 1, GV 4, GV 20
SP 6, BL 31–BL 34, ST 25, ST 36
In diverticulitis, best results will be obtained by a combination of acupuncture, nutrition, and herbs.

Applied Nuttrition ****

Eat: Bland and low-fiber demulcent-rich foods (which supply mucilage and can soothe and protect irritated or inflamed internal tissue)—e.g., *slippery elm*. The dietary approach seems paradoxical. In spite of the fact that diverticulosis is caused from a lack of roughage in the diet over a period of time, when the inflammation is in an acute stage roughage might aggravate the condition and should be avoided.
    The following foods should constitute the mainstay of the diet:

low-fat milk	cooked vegetables
yogurt	cooked fruits and apples
low-fat cheese	little quantity of seeds

An example of a diet for an adult of average weight:

1700 calories	800 IU vitamin D
38 g protein (less than the rec-	500 mg vitamin B_1
ommended quantity in the begin-	500 mg vitamin B_2
ning)	500 mg vitamin B_3 (niacin)
60 g fat	300 mg pantothenic acid
252 g carbohydrates	300 mg paba (para-aminobenzoic
1000 mg calcium	acid)
10 mg iron	800 IU vitamin E
50,000 IU vitamin A	3000 mg vitamin C

Aromatherapy

Inhale two drops of **hyssop,** an abdominal relaxant, three times daily.

Bach Flowers

Use of **crabapple** for cleansing and general promotion of health is recommended. When the person is self-concerned, **heather** is suggested.

Color Therapy

Yellow and blue filters alternating are recommended for fifteen minutes twice a day.

Herbs **

Western

An effecient herb mixture can be made from:

Wild yam *(Dioscorea villosa)*—3 g	Marshmallow *(Althaea officin-*
German camomile *(Matricaria ca-*	*alis)*—1 g
momila)—2 g	Calamus *(Acornus calamus)*—1 g

Drink the mixture as tea twice daily. If diverticulitis is accompanied by flatulence, add **ginger** *(Zingiber officinale)*. If diverticulitis is accompanied by constipation, add **senna pods** *(Cassia senna)*.

Reflexology *

Massage the painful, sensitive, and crystallized areas along the alimentary canal.

Schuessler Tissue Salts *

Natrum sulphorica: 3X twice daily is recommended.

REGIONAL ENTERITIS

SYMPTOMS

The most disabling and discouraging affliction of the small intestine known to the practitioner is regional enteritis, which is a chronic inflammatory disease that may involve the entire alimentary tract, especially the small intestine (ileum). It generally occurs in young adults and runs an intermittent clinical course with mild to severe disability and frequent complications. The disease is characterized by granulomatous response of the submucosa to unknown agents by lymphoid tissue thickening, encroachment upon the lumen, scarring of the muscle, mucosal ulceration, and fistula formation between bowel loops themselves and the skin. The causes are unknown, though genetic and familial factors play a role.

SUGGESTED TREATMENT

Acupuncture and Acupressure *

   CV 4, CV 6, CV 13, Li 11, SP 6, ST 25, ST 36.
If patient has fever, add GV 14.

Applied Nutrition ****

Eat: A diet consisting of high roughage, cereals, well-cooked legumes, and seeds. Green cooked vegetables are excellent, but avoid strong-tasting vegetables such as onions, garlic, pepper, radish. An example of a diet for an adult of average weight:

2400 calories	300 mg vitamin B_1
48 g protein	350 mg vitamin B_2
60 g fat	325 mg vitamin B_3 (niacin)
41 + g carbohydrate	600 IU vitamin E
800 mg calcium	300 mg pantothenic acid
15 mg iron	400 mg paba
30,000 IU vitamin A	4,000 mg vitamin C
1,000 IU vitamin D	

Aromatherapy

Inhale two drops, three times daily, **rosemary** *(Rosmarinus officinalis),* an antispasmodic, astringent oil to aid digestion.

Bach Flowers ***

Crabapple: For general strength and promotion of vitality.
Cerato: Recommended for the person who doubts his or her own ability and distrusts himself or herself.

Color Therapy

Use blue filter directed toward the abdomen for fifteen minutes twice daily.

Herbs ***

Western

Comfrey root *(Symphytum officinale)*—2 g

Marshmallow root *(Althaea officinalis)*—2 g

American cranesbill *(Geranium maculatum)*—1 g

Echimacea *(Echimacea augustifolia)*—1 g

Golden seal *(Hydrastis canadensis)*—1 g

Wild yam *(Dioscorea villosa)*—1 g

Drink this mixture twice daily. To prepare the tea, boil the water and leave the herbs inside a covered cup for ten to fifteen minutes. Filter and drink.

Chinese

Use the pinellia combination, which consists of:

Pinellia 6.0 g

Scute 3.0 g

Coptis 2.0 g

Ginseng 3.0 g

Jujube 3.0 g

Ginger 3.0 g

Licorice 3.0 g

Homeopathy **

Croton oil seed *(Croton tiglium):*   Best in acute enteritis where diarrhea with copious, watery stools, gurgling in the intestine, and skin problems are present, 30 potency.
May apple *(Podophy ilum):*   Best in acute cases where colicky pains, bilious vomiting, and watery, jellylike mucous stools are present.

Arsenic trioxide *(Arrenicum album):*   In chronic cases where stool is greenish with offensive and putrid odors, 6X potency.
Sublimated sulphur: Use when the abdomen is very sensitive to pressure and the mouth and lips are very dry. This is a very good remedy for chronic cases and in finishing acute ones, 12X potency.

Schuessler Tissue Salts

Ferrum phosphorica: Use 3X potency twice daily until the condition improves.

DIARRHEA

SYMPTOMS

Diarrhea might be acute or chronic and may be considered as the frequent passage of unformed stools. The acute, sudden onset of loose stools in a previously healthy person commonly is due to an active infection and less often to the ingestion of toxins, poisonous chemicals, drugs, or psychological stress.

SUGGESTED TREATMENT

Acupuncture and Acupressure **

BL 23, BL 25, CV 12, ST 25, ST 34, ST 36, Li 4, Li 11
Use a moxa stick over these points for ten minutes.
Also apply to CV 8 once.

Applied Nutrition ****

Drink: Increased amounts of water, preferably mineral water, to replace lost fluids. In the beginning avoid fruit juices.
Eat: Whole-wheat toast and take 1200 mg of potassium daily. Avoid fats and oily food. If you are in a generally healthy state, a twenty-four-hour fast with unlimited water intake may do wonders.
The main foods should be cooked cereals, such as brown rice, whole wheat, corn, cornflakes, oats, and barley, and food containing cellulose, such as vegetables lightly cooked. Avoid fresh fruits in the first two days, and avoid refined foods such as white sugar, white wheat

products, chocolate, and milk products such as milk yogurt, cottage cheese, yellow cheese, etc. An example of a diet for an adult of average weight:

1600 calories	15 mg iron
35 g protein	50,000 IU vitamin A
40 g fat	1,000 IU vitamin D
275 g carbohydrate	4 tablets per day B_{50} complex
1200 mg potassium	400 IU vitamin E
1100 mg calcium	

Aromatherapy

At separate times inhale two drops, three times a day, of **rosemary** *(Rosmarinus officinalis)* and **black pepper** *(Piper nigrum).*

Bach Flowers

When diarrhea is accompanied by uncertainty, indecisiveness, and hesitancy, **scleranthus** should be tried. For stress, tension, and strain, **vervain** is recommended.

Color Therapy

Alternating red and yellow filters are best due to their astringent action. Use these filters three times daily, accompanied by the above therapies.

Herbs *

Western

Meadowsweet *(Filipendula ulmaria):* The best digestive astringent, which can safely be used in all cases of diarrhea.

For an acute attack, an effective mixture can be made of the following herbs in equal parts:

Meadowsweet *(Filipendula ulmaria)*	Bayberry *(Myrica cerifera)*
American cranesbill *(Geranium maculatum)*	Oak bark *(Quercus robur)*

This tea should be drunk every hour until the symptoms subside and then before every meal until digestion is normal.

Single Herb

Black currant juice: Take a glass, unsweetened, three times daily.

Chinese

A general Chinese herbal formula to ease diarrhea is the "digestive tea" (Pingweisan), which is composed of:

Magnoliae cortex—3.0 g
Atracotylodis rhizoma—4.0 g
Citri reticulatae pericarpium—3.0 g

Zingiberis rhizoma—1.0 g
Geycyrrhizae radix—1.0 g
Zizyphi sativae fructus—2.0 g

Homeopathy *

In cases of severe chronic diarrhea the remedy of choice is **podophyllum** taken at 3X to 6X potency a few times daily, until the condition improves. For pale, mucotic diarrhea, often worse at night and after eating fruits, the remedy of choice is **china**: 3X to 6X potency a few times daily. For early morning ("5 A.M.") diarrhea, use **sulphur** in 3X to 6X potency. In very chronic diarrhea **goat bush** *(Chapparo amargoso)* in 32X potency might be useful.

Reflexology

Diarrhea can be relieved by foot massage. The massage may increase circulation, relax the muscle tone, and regulate the bowels. Massage the reflex areas of the intestines ten minutes a few times daily until the sensitivity in the reflex areas diminishes. Emphasize the small intestine, pylorus, and ilio-cecal valve. Add general massage to stomach, large intestine, liver, gall bladder, and pancreas areas.

Schuessler Tissue Salts *

An effective mixture in equal parts is *natrum sulphorica, kali phosphorica,* and *ferrum phosphorica* in 3X potency a few times daily until the diarrhea improves.

CONSTIPATION

SUGGESTED TREATMENT

Acupressure and Acupuncture *

This treatment is designed to stimulate bowel movements and regulate the peristalsis. The points to use are:
    BL 22, 25, 27, CV 12, ST 25, ST 36.

Applied Nutrition

Drink: Pure water—6–8 glasses with lemon. Avoid alcohol.
Eat: A high-roughage diet—e.g., bran, whole wheat, whole grains,

seeds, etc. (Refer to our recommended general R.N.H. Diet.) This will increase peristaltic movement and regulate the well-being of the intestinal tract and thus prevent recurrences of constipation. Eliminate low-fiber products like refined sugar, canned foods, and processed edibles. The main foods to consume while suffering from constipation are: brown rice, (five parts water to one part brown rice); whole wheat; seeds such as sesame; oils such as olive oil, soybean oil, peanut oil; fresh fruits; fresh vegetables; dairy products; eggs. Avoid refined foods, processed foods, etc. An example of a diet for a person of average weight:

2200 calories
42 g protein
70 g fat
351 g carbohydrate
800 mg calcium
300 mg potassium
18 mg iron
30,000 IU vitamin A

400 IU vitamin D
800 IU vitamin E
500 mg vitamin B_1
500 mg vitamin B_2
2 tablets per day vitamin B complex
6,000 mg vitamin C

The supplements suggested are ten to fifteen dietary supplement tablets a day. If the liver is involved, add bowel salt formula—two per each meal. In case of suspected low gastric secretions add two multiple enzyme tablets per meal.

Aromatherapy

Inhale five drops, three times daily of **marjoram** *(Origanum marjorana)*. Also helpful is a **rose bath** *(Rosa gallica),* the least toxic of essences: use ten to fifteen drops in a full tub, three or four times a week.

Bach Flowers

Willow: in cases where resentfulness and bitterness accompany constipation.
Star of Bethlehem: when constipation is an aftereffect of mental or physical shock.
Pine: in cases where guilt feelings, self-reproachfulness, and despondency accompany constipation.

Color Therapy

Blue is the color of choice, to be focused at the abdomen fifteen minutes, a few times daily.

Exercise

Habitual constipation is mitigated by round muscle and anal sphincter exercises. Lying on your back, elevate your knees to your chest and breathe out with a beelike sound, through clenched teeth, for as long as possible.

Herbs ***

Western

From a naturopathic and herbal point of view, the muscles of the intestine have to be retrained to move the fecal matter.

Cascara sagrada *(Rhammus purshiane):*   To restimulate the peristaltic movement.

Rhubarb root *(Rheum palmatum):*   The best purgative in large doses. In small doses promotes appetite and can disperse any gas that develops.

The following mixture combines a number of favorable actions:

Barberry *(Berberis vulgaris)*—2 g   Licorice *(Glycyrrbiza glabra)*—1 g
Boldo *(Pemus boldo)*—2 g   Rhubarb *(Rheum palmatum)*—1 g
Cascara sagrada *(Rhammus pur-*   Ginger *(Zingiber officinale)*—1 g
shiane)—1 g

Chinese

The most effective herbs, according to Chinese herbology, are:

Persica semen   Trichosanthia semen
Rhubarb

The compound formula recommended is:

Cannabis indica seeds 28.5%   Aralia cordata 14.3%
Fructose persica 28.5%   Rheum officinale 14.3%
Peucedanum decursivum 14.3%

Homeopathy

The most commonly recommended homeopathic remedies for constipation are:

Plumbaum, bryonia, and nux vomica: To be taken separately in 3X to 6X potency, three times daily between meals until constipation improves.

Alumina (oxide of aluminum):   Useful in cases of dryness of stool with complete and total lack of intestinal activity.

Reflexology

Foot massage tends to increase the circulation, relax the muscles, and regulate the bowels. Symptomatic zones are the large intestine, with emphasis on the sigmoid, rectum, liver, and small intestine areas. For wide scope of treatment, massaage also the pelvic lymphatics, lower spine, solar plexus, pancreas, and stomach.

Schuessler Tissue Salts

For acute constipation sometimes alternating with diarrhea, the remedy of choice is *natrum muriaticum.* For habitual constipation use *kali sulphorica.* For constipation in the elderly *calcorea phosphorica* is suggested. All tissue salts to be taken in 3X potency, three times daily before meals.

Yoga and Deep Breathing

Any of the customary breathing exercises (see reference section) aid in relaxation and promote regularity.

FLATULENCE

SUGGESTED TREATMENT

Acupuncture and Acupressure

Applied nutrition as in the rejuvenating diet. Also take betaine hydrochloric acid, 4 tablets each meal until conditions improve. CV 8 (acupressure only), CV 9, Li 3, Li 4, Li 11, SP 5, SP 6, K 7, ST 36, ST 37

Herbs ***

Western

The most efficient herbs in cases of flatulence are of the carminative type, which are rich in volatile oils and by their action stimulate peristalsis and relax the stomach, thereby helping against gas in the digestive tract:

Angelica *(Angelica archangelica)*
Ginger *(Zingiber officinale)*
In cases of colic accompanied by flatulence, use a combination of

equal parts of:
Caraway *(Carum carvi)*
Camomile *(Matricaria camomila)*
Calamus *(Acornus calamus)*

Chinese

The Chinese herbal philosophy always considers the total health picture of the patient. There is no specific herb formula for flatulence unless it is accompanied by other gastrointestinal disease. In cases of flatulence with no other pathology we recommend the use of Western herbs.

Homeopathy ***

Carbo vegetabilis: The general and most frequently used remedy in cases of flatulence. Use 3X to 6X potency a few times dailiy until condition improves.
Nux vomica: For flatulence associated with constipation.
Camomile: For infantile flatulence and gas-trapping that irritates the infant. Use in 32X potency. The tincture is preferred to globules, three times daily between meals.

Reflexology *

Massage the entire large intestine area: start with ileocecal valve and proceed to ascending, transverse, and descending colon. Emphasize the sigmoid colon area, since it is in the shape of an S, and be sure to massage inward toward the inner aspect of the foot. This reflex is important to those who suffer from intestinal gas. They often get a "gas pocket" or an accumulation of gas in the sigmoid colon. This massage stimulates the gas, which will be either expelled or dissolved.

Schuessler Tissue Salts

Magnesium phosphorica and **calcorea phosphorica:**   use tablets of 3X potency of both remedies. Give one tablet of *magnesium phosphorica* after meals and repeat every half hour until the condition is better. Take one tablet of *calcorea phosphorica* night and morning as a constitutional remedy.

COLITIS AND ULCERATIVE COLITIS

SYMPTOMS

Alternating constipation and diarrhea may indicate the inflammation of the large intestine and may be indicative of an ulcer if blood appears in the diarrhea.

SUGGESTED TREATMENT

Acupuncture and Acupressure ****

B123, LV 2, St 25, ST 36, St 44, CV 4, CV 9, K 5, K 7.
In cases of spastic and ulcerative colitis add Li 4, GB 20, PC 6, Ht 7.*

Applied Nutrition

Drink: Avoid alcohol and milk.

Eat: Bland soups, lightly cooked or steamed vegetables and fruits are permissible. Avocados and bananas are recommended in the raw form. One may eat products of unbleached white flour as well as fine cereals. Special attention should be given to **slippery elm bark** *(Ulmus fulva)*, which has a soothing, nutritive effect on the sensitive, inflamed mucous membrane lining of the gastrointestinal tract.

Avoid anything that can irritate the colon wall by physical or chemical action, by temperature, or by allergic reaction.

Physical irritation might be avoided by excluding high-fiber foods from the diet. Do not eat bran, whole-meal flour, fruit skins, fruit with pips like boysenberry, raw vegetables, nuts, or cooked vegetables high in roughage. The temperature of food and beverages should be medium—i.e., avoid hot coffee, cold beer, or other drinks of extreme temperature.

Be careful of chemical irritants like alcohol, nicotine, vinegar products, strong spices, smelly cheeses, and fried, oily foods.

The main foods causing allergic reactions in the colon are cow's milk products. Avoid coffee and pork products as well. As a substitute, use soya milk or goat's milk. Other suggested foods include eggs, non-fatty meats, liver, fish, and poultry.

Meals should be small in quantity and eaten often, not large, thrice-daily meals. This diet should be followed as long as the inflammation is active; when remission occurs, high fiber should be reintroduced slowly. Heavily processed and allergy-causing foods should be avoided permanently. For an adult of normal weight:

2800 calories	2,000 mg bioflavonoids daily
60 g protein	2 tabl. pituitary nucleoprotein
40 g fat	daily
550 g carbohydrate	10 mg iron
100,000 IU vitamin A	1,800 mg calcium
1,200 IU vitamin D	800 mg potassium
1,200 IU vitamin E	

Aromatherapy

Ylang-ylang *(Unona odorantissima)* is a pleasant herb that may be used as an inhalant or a bath oil. To inhale, use only a drop three times daily. It is a general antiseptic that also relaxes the nervous system. Lavender can be substituted.

Bach Flowers **

Crabapple is recommended for general cleansing. In cases where thoughts are tuned to the past, use **honeysuckle.** If the person is very possessive and feels self-pity, try **chicory.**

Color Therapy

Ruby and blue are the preferred colors for inflamed conditions and are calming.

Herbs ***

Western

Colitis will usually respond to herbal medication combined with appropriate diet. The herbal mixture is:

Wild yam *(Dioscorea villosa)* 33%
Bayberry *(Myrica cerifera)* 22%
Agrimony *(Eupatoria agrimonia)* 11%
Comfrey root *(Symphytum officinale)* 11%
Golden seal *(Hydrastis canadensis)* 11%
Marshmallow root *(Althaea officinalis)* 11%

When stress and anxiety accompany colitis, a nervine herb like **skullcap** *(Scutellaria laterifolia)* or **valerian** *(Valeriana officinalis)* should be taken in addition. A single herb effective in the treatment of colitis with excessive sputum is **squaw vine** *(Mitchella repenis).*

Chinese

Atractylodes Tea *(Yuehpichiashuton).*   This combination consists of:

Ephedra herba 6.0 g
Fibrosum gypsum 8.0 g
Zingiberis rhizoma 3.0 g
Glycyrrhizae radix 2.0 g
Atractylodis alba rhizome 4.0 g
Zizyphi satival fructose 3.0 g

Homeopathy

Podophyllum or **Phosphoric acid** are particularly helpful in 6X potency, three times daily until the acute attack is controlled.

Aloe *(Sucotrine aloes):*   good clinical results in reestablishing physiologic equilibrium; helps where the patient is weak, feeling bowel distress and colic before and during stool. Dose: 6X.

Mercurius *(Quicksilver):*   To be given in no more than 3X potency, when the manifestations are greenish and putrid stool, hiccups, and flatulent distention with stabbing abdominal pain.

Reflexology
Massage large intestine areas, starting at the ileo-cecal and particularly the recto-sigmoid loci. Also press the solar plexus and stomach areas.

Schuessler Tissue Salts
Natrum Muriaticum in 3X to 6X potency is recommended twice daily until condition improves.

HEMORRHOIDS (PILES)

SYMPTOMS

Continual, throbbing pain in the area of the rectum, intensified by sitting in the same position for long periods, may indicate a hemorrhoid condition. A physical examination is simple and conclusive.

SUGGESTED TREATMENT

Acupuncture and Acupressure *

The two major points for treating hemorrhoids are GV 20, located on top of the head, and GV 1, located below the coccyx bone.
Additional points are:
   ST 25 (bilaterally), ST 36, GV 14, BL 21, BL 22, Li 11.

Applied Nutrition
The etiological basis from a nutritional standpoint is the lack of roughage in the diet, also leading to constipation.
Eat: High-roughage food should be introduced to the daily diet—two tablespoons of bran should be taken daily mixed with either yogurt or fruit salad. Make sure to eat the fruits with their skins. Whole grains, cereals, rice, oats, and leafy vegetables should be included.
The RNH Diet is aimed at the prevention of disorders like piles and helps alleviate the symptoms. Puréed or liquefied foods are advisable on the first day. For a typical adult, average weight:

2500 calories	1,000 mg calcium
20 g protein	16 mg iron
125 g fat	10,000 IU vitamin A
212 g carbohydrate	1,000 IU vitamin D

800 IU vitamin E
20 mg vitamin B$_1$
20 mg vitamin B$_2$
20 mg vitamin B$_3$ (niacin)
6,000 mg vitamin C
15 mg zinc

5 mg selenium
100 mg potassium
20 mg vitamin K
Supplements: 8–10 dietary fiber tablets

Aromatherapy

An aromatic bath can be quite helpful. Combine, for one bath, cypress, frankincense, and juniper, in equal parts. For best results, take the bath for ten to fifteen minutes in conjunction with the taking of herbs and homeopathic ointments.

Bach Flowers

Wild oat: Try when frustrated and stiff throughout the body.
Rock water: Prescribed for self-doubt or low self-esteem.

Color Therapy

Focus blue light to the rectal area for fifteen to thirty minutes twice daily. Use color along with other methods of hemorrhoid therapy.

Exercise

The Paula-round muscle exercises are helpful. Lie on your back, bring your legs to a ninety-degree angle, and bend your knees while expelling breath with each motion. Biofeedback can also play a part in these exercises as you learn to sense the anticipated relaxation and so improve on it.

Herbs ***

Western

The most important herbs for piles are astringent, especially those that also tone the vessels involved. **Pilewort** *(Ranunculus ficaria)* is the herb of choice. This can be taken internally as a tea or applied externally as an ointment.
Witch hazel *(Hamamelis virginiana):* In difficult cases, should be combined with **pilewort** either in a tincture or in ointment form.

Chinese

Hemorrhoids tea (Itsuton)   is the general Chinese composition, which combines the following herbs:

Rhei rhizoma 1.0
Angelica sinensis radix 6.0
Scutellariae radix 3.0

Glycyrrhizae radix 2.0
Bupleuri radix 5.0
Cimicifugae rhizoma 1.5

Homeopathy ****

Sulphur: In cases when piles are not bleeding but there is constipation and anal itching, use at 6X potency.
Aloe: When piles protrude with frequent bleeding and diarrhea, use
at 6X potency three times daily until condition improves.
Paeonia: In cases of severe pain and extreme sensitivity to touch,
external application of this ointment may give relief.
Hamamelis: External application of this ointment may give relief.

Reflexology

Hemorrhoids can be relieved by massaging the reflex area to the rectum. This area is located in the back of the leg, along the Achilles
tendon. Start at the back of the leg, level with the ankle bone, and
work your way up a few centimeters. This area is very sensitive and
tender, so a light massage is recommended.

Schuessler Tissue Salts

Calcarea fluorica and *Ferrum phosphorica* in 3X to 6X potency three times
daily until condition improves.

CHOLECYSTITIS (GALLSTONES)

SYMPTOMS

Sharp pains in the abdomen area, usually episodic but severe, are the
first signs of a gallstone condition. The intensity and randomness of
the pain are characteristic of this problem, in contrast to the conditions
described elsewhere in this chapter.

SUGGESTED TREATMENT

Acupuncture and Acupressure **

In all cases of gall bladder disorders the following general formula should
be used:

GB 24, GB 34, GB 36, GB 38, GB 40, GB 43, ST 36 BL 19, BL 48.
For cholecystitis:
GB 25, 38, 40, CV 15, LV 3, CV 12, Li 4.
For gall bladder inflammation:
GB 24, GB 34, GB 40, BL 18, BL 19, ST 36, CV 12.*
Use only eight to ten points at any given session. Combine points from
the general formula and add specific points according to case involved
(whether gallstones or inflammation).

Applied Nutrition

It is most important to detoxify the body, both for prevention of disease and promotion of good health. The three-day metabolic hepatic
detoxification fast will accomplish the cleansing of the organs involved
in the retention of toxins in the body. This diet is very light.
Drink: Low-fat milk. Avoid alcoholic drinks in any form.
Eat: Low-fat food, which is digested easily, after a juice fast of three
days: yogurt, low-fat cheese (white), fish, eggs, whole cereals, fresh
vegetables, fresh fruits. Avoid: fatty-acid foods, fried food, strong-taste
food, butter, nuts, avocado, legumes, chocolate, refined white sugar,
refined white wheat, watermelon, ice cream, vegetables that produce
flatulence.

For an adult of average weight, this is a typical intake:

2000 calories	400 IU vitamin D
75 g protein	400 IU vitamin E
30 g fat	30 mg vitamin B_1
358 g carbohydrate	30 mg vitamin B_2
100 mg calcium	45 mg vitamin B_3
15 mg iron	4,000 mg vitamin C
40,000 IU vitamin A	20 mg vitamin K

Bach Flowers

Wild oat: Take if dissatisfied and no sense of achievement.
Centaury: Recommended for indecisiveness.

Herbs

Western

Herbs may in some cases eliminate small stones with a minimum of
pain. This, however, may take time. A mixture that is believed to do
this is composed of the following herbs:

Marshmallow root *(Althaea offi-cinalis)* 33%
Balmony *(Chelone glabra)* 16%
Fringetree *(Chinanthus virginicus)* 16%

Golden seal *(Hydrastis canadensis)* 16%

This tea should be drunk three times daily.
Cholecystitis requires a mixture that will alleviate pain and reduce the inflammation. The following herbal combination is suggested:

Marshmallow root *(Althaea offi-cinalis)* 33%
Dandelion *(Taraxacum officinalis)* 16%
Fringetree *(Chinanthus virginicus)* 16%

Wahoo *(Euonymus atropupureus)* 16%
Mountain Grape *(Berberis aqui-folim)* 16%

Valerian *(Valeriana officinalis):*   In cases where extreme pain (colic) accompanies this condition, add a nervine herb such as this.

Chinese

Bupleurum and **Cinnamomium tea** *(Tsaihookueichiton):*   The Chinese formula for gallstones, cholecystitis, severe pain, and nausea, composed of:

Bupleuri radix 5.0 grams
Scutellariae radix 2.0 grams
Pinelliae rhizoma 4.0 grams
Ginseng radix 2.0 grams
Cinnamomi ramulus 2.5 grams

Paeoniae lactiflorae radix 2.0 grams
Zingiberis rhizoma 2.0 grams
Zizyphi sativae fructus 2.0 grams
Glycyrrhizae radix 2.0 grams

Major Bupleurum Tea *(Tatsaihooton):*   In cases that also involve pressure in the chest, loss of appetite, hepatitis, hypertension, and the heart. Tea should be drunk three times daily, and, when taken in pill form, according to the suggested prescription. This remedy is composed of the following:

Bupleuri radix 6.0 grams
Scutellariae radix 3.0 grams
Pinelliae rhizoma 4.0 grams
Paeoniae lactiflorae radix 3.0 grams

Aurantii immaturus fructus 2.0 grams
Rhei rhizoma 1.0–2.0 grams
Zizyphi fructus 3.0 grams
Zingiberis rhizoma 4.0 grams

Reflexology

Biliary colic may be relieved by foot massage. Gallstones may be crushed and dissolved by reflexology. Emphasize massage on the reflex area to the gall bladder, which is located just below the reflex area to the liver on the right foot. Massage the liver area as well. For general relief, massage the solar plexus, pancreas, and thoracic spine.

· 2 ·
EAR, NOSE, AND THROAT

AT THE FIRST SIGNS OF ILLNESS

Among the numerous medical specialties, Ear, Nose, and Throat (ENT) is the one we most commonly associate with treatment—either by a doctor or with over-the-counter medications. The eyes are often mentioned along with ENT, but only as they exhibit the familiar symptoms of a cold or an allergy: watering, fatigue, bloodshot. (Inherent problems of the eyes are discussed in Part Nine.)

We should distinguish two quite different manifestations of ENT problems: those that are confined to ear, nose, and throat, and those that are symptomatic of problems originating in another system, such as an allergy or a malignancy in the immune system. The latter will obviously require far more aggressive treatment than the former. Most of this chapter is devoted to simpler, nonsurgical intervention, always bearing in mind the possibility that the ENT symptoms are only the first signs of problems elsewhere.

ENT problems are generally the result of infections (viral, as in the common cold, or bacterial, as in sinusitis); or of allergic reactions (such as hay fever); or of nutritional deficiencies (such as diseases of the gums). But traumas, such as the inhaling of foreign objects, as well as tumors and nerve damage, also can cause ENT problems.

For an illness so common, the "common cold" is often misunderstood. The flu virus, or influenza proper, accounts for only about ten percent of colds. Another eight percent is the result of the parainfluenza virus, and about six percent the respiratory syncytial virus. In contrast, various of the rhinovirus strains (more than one hundred are now known) cause about forty percent of all colds. These viruses are spread by tactile contact of the nose and mouth. Colds are not induced by exposure to cold, damp conditions, although a weakened physical condition may make an individual more susceptible to a viral attack. A normal cold reaches its full strength within two days, with the onset of a scratchy throat, nasal congestion, slight fever, and mild headache. General malaise subsides in a few days, and recovery is rapid and complete. In contrast, the flu usually is characterized by fever, and later complications, such as pneumonia, must be watched carefully.

The sore throat that appears without a cold can be the result of a number of infections of the upper respiratory tract. Streptococcal infection (strep throat) should be considered first; it is clearly identified by obvious redness and some swelling of the throat. Infectious mononucleosis, diphtheria, and scarlet fever are also suspect. Herpes or rubella might be the causative agent if a sore throat is accompanied by a rash. Coughing, hoarseness, soreness in swallowing, and nasal obstructions commonly accompany any type of sore throat.

Laryngitis and pharyngitis manifest some of the above symptoms, though the infection occurs in the larynx or pharynx. Whether bacterial or viral in origin, a persistent infection here should be considered the final stage of an underlying systemic problem that allows this region to be invaded. Various bacteria, such as strep, viruses, the tubercle bacillus, or fungi can all attack these sites.

The lymphoid tissues at the entrance of the pharynx, or the tonsils, can be infected by strep, with resultant fever, chills, and often nausea and vomiting. Tonsilitis is more persistent in children, accompanied often by enlarged lymph nodes.

Stuffiness or obstruction of the nose may be more than a symptom of another infection; they may be primary. Such is the case with acute rhinitis (catarrh), or, more popularly, "a cold in the nose." Again, the rhinovirus is the usual cause of this infection of the mucous membranes of the nasal cavity. Children are particularly susceptible to such attacks. Other types of rhinitis can be caused by sudden environmental changes or by allergies; thus, hay fever. The latter condition can be quite severe when caused by seasonal airborne pollen, but allergies to dust and the like can be equally debilitating.

Nasal polyps may develop from chronic allergies or infections of the nose. Although benign, they can cause nasal obstruction. They should be treated in conjunction with the underlying cause. Recurrent infections may also result in sufficient damage to mucous membranes to cause loss of the sense of smell, which in turn is critical to the sense of taste. Such loss can be partial or even selective. Nosebleeding is likewise the result of damage to the membranes and is usually precipitated by a systemic cause, such as high blood pressure or atherosclerosis—if not by irritation of the nose in sneezing or with other pressure on the nasal passages. (Epistaxis is the technical term for spontaneous nosebleed.)

The four air cavities in the face, the sinuses, are frequently affected by infections of the nose or upper respiratory tract. Sinusitis is aggravated when the fluid in the sinuses is pressed against the face when the head is dropped forward. Sinus pain can be severe, requiring rest and attention to the underlying cause.

The ears are often affected by general head colds or fever, with feelings of pressure and temporary loss of full hearing. Yet there are several problems that can affect the ears alone in the absence of other illness. Diminished hearing is quite common in late middle age through old age. Such loss may be due to degeneration of the ear fluid or a blocking of the three small bones in the inner ear; hearing depends on both the neurological function of this liquid and the conductive function of the bones. Either congenital nerve damage or some sort of trauma can disable this complex system. Proper diagnosis of hearing loss or deafness should include an audiogram to pinpoint which function is failing.

Since the ear system is also responsible for the sense of balance, it is a delicate organ that should be protected from excessive noise and the intrusion of foreign objects. Folk wisdom insists that no object smaller than one's finger should be inserted in the ear (to clear out wax, for example). It is now generally accepted that wax is best removed by massaging the underside of the ear, rather than with swabs or liquid cleaning methods.

A persistent, though intermittent, ringing in the ears, known as tinnitus, is not fully understood in medical practice but may be related to systemic problems such as diabetes. If it is temporary, the patient must learn to compensate. Tinnitus and hearing loss may accompany a more serious syndrome, Ménière's disease, in which attacks of dizziness and nausea can last for a few minutes or for days. Usually one ear only is affected; no cause has been identified.

Behind the ears are air cavities, known as mastoids, that help conduct sound. An infection of these cavities, mastoiditis, is evidenced by tenderness, swelling, and often fevers. Like all ear problems, this condition can be quite painful and requires close attention.

THE COMMON COLD

SYMPTOMS

It may seem superfluous to describe signs of the common cold, but often, in addition to the scratchy throat and nasal stuffiness, there may be more severe inflammation to indicate more than a viral infection. Or there may be severe fever or earaches. Sneezing may or may not accompany the common cold, and if it does it may indicate an allergy rather than a viral infection. Only a qualified physician can properly interpret the many symptoms of ear, nose, and throat conditions mentioned in this chapter.

SUGGESTED TREATMENT

Acupuncture and Acupressure

For common cold with nasal obstruction, rhinitis, chills, fever, and coated tongue:
     GV 16, BL 12, GB 20, LU 7, LI 4, K 4, TAI-YANG, LI 20.
When fever is accompanied by thirst, yellow sputum, and coated tongue:
     GV 14, GB 20, TW 5, LI 4, LU 11.
To both treatments may be added:
     BL 13, LU 1, LU 6.

Applied Nutrition ****

In case of chronic colds it is very useful to check for food allergy with a cytotoxic blood test.

Drink: Avoid dairy products.

Eat: whole grains, cereals, seeds, fish, fresh vegetables and fruits, and a lot of raw garlic. Avoid dairy products, white sugar, white wheat flour, and meat.

An example of a diet for a person of average weight, thirty years old:

1900 calories	1,000 IU vitamin E
40 g protein	50 mg vitamin B_1
80 g fat	50 mg vitamin B_3
255 g carbohydrate	100 mg vitamin B_{12}
4000 mg vitamin C	1,000 mg pantothenic acid
800 mg bioflavonoids	50 mg inositol
50,000 IU vitamin A	800 mg calcium
1,000 IU vitamin D	100 mg phosphorous

400 mg magnesium
50 mg zinc
Thymus nucleoprotein—2 tablets
daily

Adrenal nucleoprotein—2 tablets
daily
Bee products

Aromatherapy

Basil essence: Inhale twice per day when cold is accompanied by depression, hysteria, insomnia, mental fatigue, nervous tension, or epilepsy.

Black pepper: Use as a part of massage oil when cold is accompanied by diarrhea, constipation, dysentery, flatulence, nausea, vomiting, or loss of appetite.

Eucalyptus: Inhale three times a day when cold is accompanied by asthma, bronchitis, catarrh, cough, influenza, sinusitis, throat infections, tuberculosis, or any other respiratory disorder. Continue until improvement is noticed.

Autosuggestion

Colds, the result of a weakened system, can result from mental confusion and feelings of stress and unrest due to work and personal relationships. The affirmation recommended in this case is:

I am a clear thinker. I solve my problems easily and considerately.

Breathing Therapy

Inhale and exhale through the nose deeply ten times at a number of times during the day until improvement is noticed. The respiration should be continuous, connecting inhale to exhale without stopping. If vertigo or dizziness occurs, breathe more slowly. Mentally try to overcome the vertigo/dizziness by imagining yourself exhaling bad feelings from your body.

Color Therapy

Use ultraviolet light over the chest, back, and face for twenty-five minutes twice a day and red light for thirty minutes once a day.

Herbs

Western

The following herbs may be taken separately or in a combined tea in a one-to-one ratio:

Elder flower *(Sambucus nigra)*
Peppermint *(Mentha piperita)*

Yarrow *(Achillea millefolium)*

Drink the tea three to four times daily, or take powdered herbs in capsule form twice daily.

Sea buckthorn *(Hippophe rhamnoids):* Will help reduce fever. Press the berries, skin, and pits; drink juice.

Chinese

Pueraria nasal combination: For stuffy and runny nose.

Yin-Chiao: Eight tablets daily are excellent supplements.

Pinellia and Magnolia combination *(Pan-Hsiahou-Pu-Tang)* is very good for moist, harsh coughs and throat pain:

Pinellia 6 g	Ginger 4 g
Magnolia bark 3 g	Perilla 2 g
Hoelen 5 g	

Homeopathy ****

Camphor: When chill is still present pills (Mother Tincture 0) should be taken every fifteen to twenty minutes until the chills stop.

Aconitum: One to three doses every one to two hours, in 6X potency.

Euphrasia: One dose every two hours, 6X potency.

Sanguinaria: For acrid coryza (head cold) with tight chest and watery mucus, one dose every two hours, 6X potency.

Magnesia muriatica: For loss of smell and tase with colds, six doses every four hours, 12X potency.

Hydrotherapy

In the case of colds soak feet in warm water for ten to fifteen minutes before going to bed. Also, a warm bath with sea salt can be very useful in relieving sinus congestion. To avoid chronic cases, take hot and cold baths or showers in alternation for a few minutes once a day, regularly.

Reflexology **

Press the following for four minutes on both hands three times per day for one month:

1, 2, 5, 16, 20, 52.

Also massage the whole foot with the foot reflexology device, nine minutes each foot, twice a day for three weeks. Continue as a general reinforcement another month, seven minutes each foot once a day.

Scheussler Tissue Salts

Ferrous phosphate and **natrum muriaticum:**   Alternate a tablet of ferrous phosphate (12X) and natrum muriaticum (12X) each hour until condition improves. Continue three times per day for a week.

INFLUENZA

SUGGESTED TREATMENT

Acupuncture/Acupressure **

GV 14, LI 4, LI 11, GB 20, LU 1, BL 13, BL 12, TW 5, ST 36, PC 6. For sore throat add:
LU 11, LU 7, K 6.

Aromatherapy **

Take *eucalyptus* by inhalation twice per day for one week, especially if there is the possibility of complications due to influenza. Also use *lavender 2%* as a part of massage oil.

Applied Nutrition ***

Avoid all dairy products and animal products. Basically, the diet should be similar to that for colds (see page 50).

Autosuggestion

Influenza is caused by an inability to recognize or check negative feelings. The affirmation should be:

> I am thinking and acting positively and with love. I am free from negative influence.

Breathing Therapy

Repeat the same exercises as in breathing therapy for colds, three to four times per day.

Color Therapy

The ultraviolet light lamp should be used all over the upper body for thirty minutes. After massaging the whole upper body with oil, use the red light over the chest, back, neck, and face for another fifteen minutes. Repeat this treatment three times per day till the condition is improved and then continue for another two weeks once per day for twenty minutes.

Herbs ****

Western

Boneset *(Eupatorium perfoliatum):* The herb of choice in infusion (one to two teaspoonfuls of dried herb and leaves), to be drunk hot and at half-hour intervals. Capsules and tinctures are also available. A mixture of **boneset, elder flower, licorice,** and **peppermint** can be taken in tea form, very hot, every two to three hours.
Capsules and tinctures of this are also available.

Chinese

Pueraria combination and **Pinellia and Magnolia** are the formulas of choice.

Homeopathy ***

Bacillinum 30 and **Influenzinum 30:** One dose once a week (separate or in combination) for severe cases; by physician only.
Baptisia: 3X -30 every hour when there is headache, aching limbs, and fever.
Arsenicum album: 3X -30 when you are chilled, restless and anxious, or have diarrhea.
Aconite: 3X in the early stages, especially for children.
Nux vomica: 6X can also be considered in early stages of acute flu.

Hydrotherapy

In addition to hot showers/baths, keep the feet warm by soaking in hot tubs for twenty minutes twice a day. This exercise is of special importance in cold weather.

Reflexology

Massage points 1, 5, 16, 18, 19, 20, 24, 25, 52 for three minutes each. In addition, massage each foot with the foot reflexologer for nine minutes every morning and evening.

Schuessler Tissue Salts

The main remedy for influenza is **natrum muriaticum** six times. Take every hour until the condition improves, then continue the treatment three times per day for another two weeks. If the condition does not improve, take in addition **calcarea phosphorica** 12X and **kali phosphorica** 12X every three hours in alternation (one remedy every three hours) until there is improvement and then continue with **natrum muriaticum** 6X as before.

SORE THROAT

SYMPTOMS

The sore throat of a cold may be only that or may be a streptococcal infection. A lab test is often necessary to determine this for certain, but extreme redness at the back of the mouth and swelling evident at the throat are good signals of a "strep" throat. This bacterial infection, unlike the common virus cold, can be treated effectively with antibiotics.

SUGGESTED TREATMENT

Acupuncture and Acupressure **

Applied nutrition, as in the case of common cold. CV 15, CV 20, CV 21, CV 22, CV 23, GB 44, LI 4, LI 17, LIV 7, SI 7, TW 10, K 2, LU 6, LU 8, ST 12
Ear Points—Lung, Pharynx, Larynx, Kidney

Herbs ****

Western

Garlic or kyolic: in any form.
Balm of Gilead *(Populus gileadensis):*   Very helpful for sore throat conditions. Infuse over two teaspoonfuls of the bud, two ml of tincture three times daily, or two capsules of the powdered herb.
Balm of Gilead and Coltsfoot *(Tussilago farfara):*   Combine well to treat sore throat conditions.
Golden seal *(Hydrastis):*   Another excellent herb for treating sore throat conditions, best taken in capsule form because of its bitter taste.
Oak bark *(Quercus robur):*   In decoction—one teaspoonful of the bark given by itself or together with **Ginger** (zingiberis), taken a half hour before meals, or two to three ml of tincture or two powdered capsules.
Barley: Gargle with cooked barley mixed with lemon a few times daily.
Horseradish *(Armoralia rusticana):*   Grate and mix with honey. May control a hoarse voice and sore throat.

Chinese

Ophiopogon formula *(Mai-Men Tung Tang):*   The formula of choice for sore throat, hoarse voice, and/or dry burning sensation in the throat:

Pinnelia rhizome 5g   Ophiopogon root 10g
Ginseng 2g   Licorice root 2g
Jujube 3g   Rice 5g

Gasping Formula *(Hsiang-Sheng-Po-Tai-Luen):*   For sore throat and hoarseness due to excessive singing and talking.

Forsythia 2.5g
Platycodon 2.5g

Color Therapy

Use blue light for thirty minutes locally on the throat and neck twice daily for three weeks.

Homeopathy **

Aconitum: In the acute stages due to fever and cold use 6X potency three times every hour. If the throat is dry and burning as well as red and swollen, take **Belladonna** 3X hourly.

Apis: If there is edema of membranes and difficulty in swallowing, use three times every hour, 12X potency.

Phytolacca: In cases of severe soreness and herpes of the pharynx, use three times every hour. A gargle of **phytolacca** hourly may also help, 6X potency.

Hydrastis: In chronic cases of sore throat use three times every three to four hours to relieve swelling, aid swallowing, and prevent mucus dropping from the nose to the back of the throat (postnasal drip), 6X potency.

Brom: For hoarseness or scratchiness, use three times every four hours, 6X potency.

Reflexology *

Press the points 10, 16, 20 in both hands and feet for seven minutes each, and point 52 in both hands five minutes each three times per day.

Schuessler Tissue Salts

Ferrum phosphorica   Take 12X twice per day for two weeks in case of sore throat accompanied with inflammation, burning sensations, red throat, dry hoarseness of the throat, or loss of voice.

Kali muriaticum: Take 12X three times per day for two weeks if there is also swelling of glands or tonsils.

Calcarea sulphorica: Take 6X four times per day for a period of three weeks. If there are pains when swallowing or chronic enlarged tonsils, take **Calcarea phosphorica** 12X three times per day for a period of one month.

LARYNGITIS AND PHARYNGITIS

SYMPTOMS

Similar symptoms to sore throat, but persistent. Again, strep should be considered, as this infection can cause damage elsewhere in the body if left unchecked.

SUGGESTED TREATMENT

Applied Nutrition

The same as in the case of common cold *(p. 50)*.

Aromatherapy

For laryngitis accompanied with influenza, asthma, nervous tension, spasmodic cough, and whooping cough, inhale essence of cypress.
For laryngitis accompanied by bronchitis, cattarh, fainting, depression, hysteria, nausea, or migraine, inhale lavender twice a day for one week.

Autosuggestion

The principal emotional cause for this condition is fear of expressing opinions or resentment of authority. The affirmation should be:

I express myself freely and clearly.

Bach Flowers

Heather or **Mimulus:**   if you are fearful about your health.
Gentian: if you are a doubter.

Breathing Therapy

Use treatment recommended for sore throat (p. 56) three times a day.

Color Therapy

Use blue over the chest and throat for thirty minutes, twice a day for two weeks. For the first two days use every four hours until improvement is shown.

Herbs

Western

See Tonsilitis
Antibiotics and Lymph tonics: Should be used.
Red Sage *(Salvia officinalis):*   A gargle is helpful.

Chinese

Pinellia and Magnolia Combination *(Pan-Hsiahou-Pu-Tang):*   See Tonsilitis section for composition.
Pueraria Combination *(Ko-Ken-Tang)*   A second choice.

Homeopathy **

Aconitum: In early stages of acute laryngitis when accompanied by cough, restlessness, and fever. Take three tablets every thirty to forty-five minutes; as conditions improve increase the interval between dosages.
Spongia Tosta: When there is no improvement and when condition is accompanied by hoarseness take three tablets every thirty to forty-five minutes.
Kali bichromium: If condition is accompanied by sticky and thick phlegm and mucus, take three tablets every hour.
Causticum: When the voice is lost from chronic laryngitis, three doses every four hours.
Oxalic acid: For severe laryngitis with pain and a raw sensation, 6X -30.
Phosphorus: When hoarseness worsens in the evening, three doses every three to four hours.
Argentum nitricum: For hysterical or phobic laryngitis (in which a vocal cord may be paralyzed for a few months), take six doses.
Carbo vegetabilis: For painless hoarseness caused by exogenous factors like cold and dampness, take six doses every three hours.
Hepar sulphuris: For hoarseness becoming worse in the morning, singers and public speakers respond well to this remedy. Take three doses.

Hypnotherapy

In case of laryngitis accompanied or caused by stress, hypnotherapy can effectively reduce the stress and the strain on the voice.

Reflexology

Press the following points in both hands three minutes each, twice a day for two weeks:
   1, 5, 6, 16, 20, 52.

Schuessler Tissue Salts

Rest the voice for one week. Then:

Ferrum phosphorica: If laryngitis is a result of strain of vocal cords, fever, or soreness of the larynx, and the voice is hoarse and husky, use 12X every hour until the acute condition is alleviated, then continue the treatment with **ferrum phosphorica** three times a day for two weeks.

Kali muriaticum: If the laryngitis is the result of a cold, accompanied by hoarseness, cough, and white tongue, use 12X, four times a day for two weeks.

Kali phosphorica: If there is hoarseness of voice after nervous strain, tiredness, or general weakness, use 12X, four times a day for two weeks.

TONSILITIS

SYMPTOMS

Enlarged lymph nodes (in the throat area), often with fever and nausea, indicating a strep infection here.

SUGGESTED TREATMENT

Acupuncture and Acupressure **

SI 17, LU 11, LI 4, LI 11 are the main points. Combinations:

1.   LI 4, ST 44, LI 11.
2.   GB 20, BL 10, BL 11, LU 5, LU 11.
3.   For inability to talk: LI 10, LI 17, LI 11, TW 3, ST 40, HT 7.

Ear Points

1.   Throat, tonsils
2.   Helix No 1, No 2, No 3 and posterior auricular veins

Acupuncture only: (2) Bloodletting of two to three drops from two points.

Applied Nutrition **

The same as for sore throat. If antibiotic drugs have been taken, after treatment take one tablet of **lactobaccillus** daily for a week in order to restore the normal intestinal bacteria.

Lactobaccillus should be taken whenever antibiotics have been used in treating an illness.

Aromatherapy

Inhale **bergamot essence** once a day for one week. Do not confuse the bergamot and citrus bergamia (the Rutaceae family) with the herb bergamon (bee balm).

Autosuggestion

Repeat the affirmation twice a day twenty times:

From day to day I am better and healthier in every way.

Breathing Therapy

Use the same technique as in the case of sore throat three times a day for two weeks for acute cases; continue for one month in chronic cases.

Color Therapy

Use blue light on the throat for twenty minutes and inside the open mouth for ten minutes twice a day for two weeks. Also, after the blue light, the yellow light can be used for fifteen minutes twice a day for two weeks.

Herbs ****

Western

Antimicromial and lymphatic tonic herbs will bring best results.
Echinacea, golden seal *(Hydrastis):*   both in decoction.
Myrrh *(Commiphora molmol):*   powder in infusion. Capsules containing these three herbs in 1:1 ratio can be taken twice daily.
Red sage *(Salvia officinalis):*   (**Caution:** Never use during pregnancy.) In infusion or as a gargle combined with **Tormentil** or **Balm of Gilead** *(Populus gileadensis),* three times daily; also in capsule or tincture forms.
Poke root *(Phytolacca auericana):*   Excellent for tonsilitis. (**Caution:** Use only very small amounts because it is a strong emetic and purgative.) In decoction use only ¼ teaspoonful of the root. In tincture form, ½ ml two to three times a day.

Homeopathy ***

Aconitum: At beginning stage three times every hour or **Aconitum + belladonna + camomile** 6X every one to two hours.
Baryta carb: 6X hourly if the right tonsil is affected, or when tonsils are very large with cervical lymph gland enlargement.
Phytolacca: A **phytolacca** gargle may also help.

Baryta muriatica: For chronic enlargement of the scrofolus, with painful swelling, use thirty every eight hours.
Hepar sulphuris: Where purulent infection and abscess occur, 2X - 30.

Reflexology **

Press points 50, 10 and 52 in hands and feet for five minutes, twice a day for two weeks.

Schuessler Tissue Salts

Ferrum phosphorica: In early stages accompanied with fever and vomiting of undigested food, use 12X three times a day for two weeks. For children use 6X.
Kali muriaticum: In the second stage, when the tonsils are swollen and it is difficult to swallow, use 12X twice a day for two weeks. For children use 6X.

RHINITIS (CATTARH)

SYMPTOMS

A "cold in the nose," with stuffiness and catarrh.

SUGGESTED TREATMENT

Acupuncture and Acupressure **

LIV 4, SI 19, LI 4, LI 11, K3, ST 36, ST 40, LU 6, LU 9, BL 23, BL 20, CV 9, CV 17.

Applied Nutrition

Avoid stimulants like coffee, cocoa, tea, white refined sugar, white wheat flour, fried foods, alcohol, and dairy products.
An example of a diet for an average weight person, thirty years old:

2100 calories	500 mg bioflavonoids
70 g protein	50,000 IU vitamin A
100 g fat	1,000 IU vitamin D
230 g carbohydrate	1,000 IU vitamin E
4000 mg vitamin C	50 mg Vitamin B$_1$

50 mg Vitamin B_2 20 mg iron
50 mg Vitamin $\dot{B}_6$ 20 mg zinc
500 mg pantothenic acid   50 mg selenium
600 mg calcium

Aromatherapy

Inhale twice daily for one to three minutes the essence of cedarwood when the catarrh is accompanied by respiratory problems or skin diseases and eucalyptus when the catarrh is accompanied by asthma, bronchitis, coughs, fevers, sinusitis, or urinary tract disorders.

Autosuggestion

The main mental cause for the chronic condition is not being able to solve family problems. The affirmation should be:

"I am solving all my problems with love and peace."

Breathing Therapy

Inhale through the right nostril to the count of four. Stop breathing to the count of two, then exhale through the right nostril to the count of four. Then change in the same way with the left nostril. Repeat this exercise ten times every morning and evening for three weeks.

Color Therapy

Use ultraviolet lamp light all over the nose root and sinuses for thirty minutes twice daily for six weeks. If after three weeks there is no improvement, use the red light in addition once daily for twenty minutes for three weeks.

Herbs

Western

The most effective anticatarrhal herbs have drying action because they are astringent.

Golden seal *(Hydrastis):* For the upper respiratory tract, in infusion three times daily, three to four ml of tincture three times daily, or in capsule form one to two a day. (**CAUTION:** Not to be used by pregnant women.)

Goldenrod *(Solidago virguaria):* Excellent as an infusion (two to three teaspoonfuls of dried herb and leaves). A combination tea of capsules of the above two is very useful.

Garlic or **kyolic** and **onion:** Should be eaten in raw form.

Eyebright *(Euphrasia officinalis):* For nasal catarrh in infusion form (one teaspoonful of dried herb and leaves). This combines well with *Goldenrod* in either tea or capsule form.

Wild indigo *(Baptisia tinctoria)* and **Echinacea:**   Decoction helps if microbial infection is involved.

Chinese

Pueraria combination *(Ko-Ken-Tang)* is the formula of choice:

Common kodzu root-Pueraria 8 g	Cinnamon twigs 3 g
Ma-Huang 4 g	Peony root 3 g
Ginger rhizome 1 g	Licorice root 2 g
Jujube fruit 4 g	

Try *Pueraria Nasal Combination* (Ching-Pi-Tang) for nasal catarrh:

Pueraria combination	Magnolia flowers
Cnidium and rhubarb formula	Coix (Job's tears seeds)
Gypsum	

Ophiopogon combination *(Mai-Men Tung Tang):*   Especially good in the case of sticky sputum.

Homeopathy **

Mercurius Sol: 6X every eight hours is good for those with a general tendency to nasal catarrh, infected throat, or thick and yellow discharge.

Pulsatilla: When it becomes worse at night use 3X to 6X.

Hydrastis: When mucus is present in the throat, 3X every three hours.

Antimonium tartaricum: For chronic catarrh of the larynx, bronchi, and trachea, 6X every six to eight hours.

Reflexology *

In case of nose catarrh, press the following points three minutes each on both hands each morning and evening for one month:
    1, 5, 52, 20.
If the nose catarrh is acute and painful, press these points two minutes each hour until the pain is over, and then continue twice a day for three minutes at each point.

Schuessler Tissue Salts

Kali muriaticum: Use 12X three times per day.

Natrum muriaticum: If the condition is chronic, use 6X twice a day morning and evening, and at noontime take *Kali Muriaticum* 6X for three weeks.

LYMPHADENITIS (SWOLLEN GLANDS)

SUGGESTED TREATMENT

Acupuncture and Acupressure ***

BL 60, LI 13, LI 18, HT 3, LI 10, GB 41, TW 10, TW 13, CV 17, CV 20, CV 21, LI 4
Ear Points: Lung, Pharynx, Larynx, Shen-Men, Internal Secretion, Kidney

Applied Nutrition

See common cold (p. 50)

Aromatherapy

In case of swollen glands in the throat or upper respiratory tract, inhale **bergamot** once daily in combination with **eucalyptus,** bergamot in the morning and eucalyptus in the evening for a period of two weeks.

Autosuggestion

Repeat this affirmation twenty times each morning and evening and every time you use other therapies:

> From day to day and from moment to moment I feel better and healthier in every way.

Color Therapy

Blue all over the swollen glands thirty minutes, three times daily, which can be reinforced by ultraviolet light fifteen minutes after the blue light.

Herbs

See section on Lymph in Section Four, Circulatory System.

Homeopathy **

Bacillinum: For chronic lymphedenitis involving the scrofulus glands the first remedy administered should be **Bacillinum** given in doses of four to five globules of thirty or one hundred once a week or less, by physician only.
Belladonna: In acute cases at onset of glandular swelling, 3X hourly.
Baryta: 6X every hour.
Arum triphyllum: For submaxillary gland swelling, 6X every two to three hours.

Hydrotherapy

A hot-water bottle or hot towel on the swollen glands can reduce pain and help the glands. The patient should stay in a warm room and rest in bed until improvement begins.

Reflexology **

A secondary treatment for swollen glands is reflexology. Press these points of the hands and feet, according to the location of the glands in the throat, mouth, or nose for three minutes twice a day for three weeks:

1, 10, 50, 45, 43, 44, 52

Schuessler Tissue Salts

Where inflammation is the cause, take the following remedies together three times daily for two weeks, one tablet each:

Ferrum phosphorica 12X
Silica 6X
Calcarea Phosphorica 12X
Natrum muriaticum 12X

EPISTAXIS (NOSEBLEED)

SUGGESTED TREATMENT

Acupressure and Acupuncture
Press:

ST 3, BL 10, LI 4, LI 7, GV 12, GV 14.
Lie down or sit to avoid recurring hemorrhage. Keep head high or tilted back. A sterile cotton plug will help stop the bleeding. Ice also helps. Points are:

LI 4, GV 23, LI 20, ST 3, K 3, Bl 15, BL 64.
Ear Points: Adrenal, Appex 1–3, Forehead, Internal nose, Lung.

Applied Nutrition **

Bleeding from the nose can be caused in many ways, such as by external trauma, nose picking, nasal infections, or drying nasal mucosa, or it may be a secondary symptom of blood dyscrasias, hypertension, hemorrhagic disease, nasal tumors, or infectious disease, such as measles or rheumatic fever. If the bleeding is due to an external cause, the diet should be normal, healthy food with the Master formula. First-aid treatment should be local. Sit up with head tipped downward for a few minutes until the bleeding is stopped. If the bleeding continues, press the area for five to ten minutes. After the bleeding stops, a cotton plug moistened with wheat-germ oil should be placed in the nose for a few hours.

Aromatherapy

Inhale cypress essence every hour until the bleeding is stopped; continue by inhaling the essence of frankincense once per day for two weeks.

Autosuggestion

Repeat this affirmation twenty times every morning and evening:

I am calm and relaxed in every way.

Breathing Therapy

After the bleeding is stopped by other therapies, breathe deeply in and out through the nostrils: *in* to the count of four, stop to the count of two, *out* to the count of eight, then repeat ten times. Do this exercise three times per day.

Color Therapy

Apply blue over the nose for thirty minutes every two hours until the condition improves; continue twice per day for another three weeks.

Herbs *

Western

Witch hazel *(Hamamelis virginiana):* Place a plug of cotton wool soaked in distilled **witch hazel** into the nostril.

Homeopathy ****

Millefolium: The general remedy of choice. Use thirty every twenty to thirty minutes.
Arnica: If the nosebleed is the result of being hit, use thirty every ten to fifteen minutes.
Bryonia: For nosebleed occurring in the morning, 3X every fifteen minutes, or three times daily as a prophylactic.
Carbo vegetabilis: For older people with recurrent bleeding, 6X every eight hours.

Reflexology ***

Press the following points for five minutes each in the hand until the bleeding is stopped. Continue treatment in hands and feet twice per day for another month:
    1, 5, 52.

Schuessler Tissue Salts

Ferrum phosphorica: Use 12X every thirty minutes until the bleeding is stopped and then continue with **ferrum phosphorica** 12X three times a day for three weeks.

ALLERGIC RHINITIS (HAY FEVER)

SUGGESTED TREATMENT

Acupuncture and Acupressure **

CV 17, CV 20, GV 16, GV 23, LI 4, LI 19, LI 20, LIV 8, K 9, BL 10, BL 11, BL 12, ST 36, SI 3, Yin-Tang
Ear points: Lung, Kidney, Allergy

Applied Nutrition ****

As in most cases of allergy, it is very important to find out by a cyto-toxic blood test the foods, dust, or pollen causing the allergy and to avoid contact with them. The diet and example of foods should be the same as in the case of colds.

Aromatherapy

Inhale eucalyptus essence twice per day until the condition improves and then continue with this remedy for two weeks twice per day. Also apply as a massage oil the essence of rose 2% on the nose and neck before using color therapy.

Autosuggestion

The main mental cause of hay fever is emotional stress and fear. The affirmation for this condition should be:

   I am at peace and in love with my life.

Breathing Therapy

Breathe in and out through the right nostril by pressing your hand on the left nostril, then reverse. Repeat this exercise ten times each morning and evening. If the nose is congested, start the exercise with reflexology or acupressure until the air passages are open.

Color Therapy

Use blue light for thirty minutes all over the face three times a day, and ultraviolet on the nose and in the nostrils for twenty minutes.

Continue this treatment until you are congestion-free and the nose is clear again. If there is cough, then apply ultraviolet light in the (open) mouth and on the neck and chest for thirty minutes twice a day.

Herbs ***

Western

Ephedera: The choice for allergic reactions. Decoction of one and a half to two teaspoonfuls should be drunk three times daily. Also three to four ml three times daily of tincture, or powdered capsules can be taken.

Try also **Combination Tea:**

Elder flowers 40%   Eyebright 20%
Ephedera 20%   Golden seal 20%

or capsules twice daily.

Red clover *(Trifolium pratense)*   is claimed to build resistance to allergies. Infusion of one to three teaspoonfuls of dried herb and leaves three times daily.

Licorice *(Glycyrrhyza glabra):*   Reputed to build resistance. Decoction of ½ teaspoonful of dried herb or two to three ml of tincture twice daily.

Chinese

Ma-Huang Combination *(Ma-Huang-Tang)* is recommended:

Ma-Huang herb 5 g   Licorice root 1.5 g
Cinnamon twigs 4 g   Apricot seeds 5 g

Minor Blue Dragon Combination *(Hsiao-Ching-Lung-Tang):*   Try if there is copious nasal drainage:

Ma-Huang 3 g   Wild ginger root (Asarun) 3 g
Peony root 3 g   Schizandra fruit 3 g
Ginger rhizome 3 g   Cinnamon twigs 3 g
Licorice root 3 g   Pinellia rhizome 6 g

or

Pueraria Nasal Combination
(Ching-Pi-Tang)

Homeopathy ***

Chrome alum: The general remedy, three times every four hours.
Teucrium: 1X to 6X is helpful when the allergen is grass.
Mixed pollen: Can be potentized at your homeopathic pharmacy and should be taken in late summer and early autumn.
Sabadilla: 3X-30 every eight hours for two weeks before and after hay fever season as a preventative.

Reflexology **

Press the following points for three minutes each every four hours until the condition improves:

1, 3, 5, 6, 16, 20, 52.

Also use the foot reflexologer device twice a day for nine minutes on each foot.

Schuessler Tissue Salts

Magnesium phosphorica: 12X every hour.
Natrum Muriatica: When there is also a craving for salty foods take 12X every second hour in alteration with **magnesium phosphorica** 12X. Use the remedies every hour until the condition improves and then continue the treatment with **natrum muriaticum** 12X three times a day for another two weeks.

SINUSITIS

SYMPTOMS

Pain, often severe, when the head is bowed—and even when upright—across the eyebrows and bridge of the nose.

SUGGESTED TREATMENT

Acupuncture and Acupressure ***

LI 20, B1 2, BL 7, GB 20, GB 30, LI 4, LIV 2, LU 7, BL 13, ST 3, ST 36.
Ear points: Adrenal, Forehead, Internal nose, Lung.

Applied Nutrition

This is similar to the diet in the case of colds.

Drink: For best results, start with three days juice fasting and gradually introduce the diet. An example of a diet for a person of average weight, thirty years old:

1900 calories	100 mg vitamin B_{12}
50 g protein	1,500 mg pantothenic acid
70 g fat	150 mg vitamin B_{15} (panganic
268 g carbohydrate	acid)
4000 mg vitamin C	100 mg calcium
500 mg bioflavonoids	560 mg magnesium
50,000 IU vitamin A	100 mg phosphorus
1,000 IU vitamin D	50 mg iron
1,000 IU vitamin E	2 mg copper
50 mg vitamin B_1	15 mg. zinc
50 mg vitamin B_2	50 mg potassium
50 mg vitamin B_3	Adrenal nucleoproteins
50 mg vitamin B_6	Thymus nucleoproteins

Aromatherapy

Inhale eucalyptus essence twice per day for three weeks and massage with lavender essence two times in vegetable oil. The lavender can be used with the color therapy twice a day.

Autosuggestion

The principal mental problem in this condition is quarrels and bad feelings toward someone close, especially business partners, children, or spouses. The affirmation should be:

Everybody loves and cares for me. I love all my family and friends.

Breathing Therapy

Use the same exercises as in the case of colds twice per day and after the air passages are open by means of other therapies. Continue this exercise a month after improvement.

Color Therapy

In acute or chronic cases, use the color blue locally twice per day for thirty minutes; use yellow after the blue for five minutes twice a day in combination with blue.

Continue this treatment one month after improvement. Before applying the treatment use massage oil on all the nose and sinus areas.

Herbs ****

Western

Echinacea, goldenrod *(Solidago virginiana)*   are very helpful.
Golden seal *(Hydrastis)* and **Marshmallow leaf** *(Althea officinalis):*   are also antimicrobial and anti-inflammatory. A mixture of these four herbs can be made into capsules (two a day), tincture (three to five ml, three times daily), or decoction.
Garlic or **kyolic:**   Should be taken regularly.
Eucalyptus: Oil can be inhaled or sniffed.
Pine *(Pynus silvestris):*   Tincture 203 ml twice daily, or infuse ½ teaspoonful of twigs.
Blueberries, carrots, and **cucumbers:**   Juice is also recommended.

Homeopathy *

Ignatia 6X and **thuya** 3X are preferred.

Reflexology **

Press all points number 1, four to six times per day, on every finger or toe, for five minutes. Also press point 52 in both hands for seven minutes each.

Schuessler Tissue Salts

Ferrum phosphorica: In the case of painful sinusitis accompanied by fever, flushed face, and rapid pulse, use 12X every hour until the condition improves.
Kali muriaticum: In case of thick white mucus discharge, which gives the feeling of stuffing the head, use 6X every hour until the condition improves.
Natrum muriaticum: In case of nasal obstruction with water discharge accompanied by loss of smell or inflammation in the sinus area, use 6X every hour until the condition improves.
Silica: In case of a chronic condition, with thick discharge of mucus, ulceration of mucus membranes, or chronic nasal catarrh, use 12X every hour until the condition improves.
In all cases, after improvement continue treatment with the same remedy three times per day for one month.

NASAL POLYPS

SUGGESTED TREATMENT

Acupuncture and Acupressure **
For nonmalignant nasal mucus membrane polyps:
  LI 19, LI 20, GB 28, K 3, LU 7, GV 14, GV 15, GV 24, GV 25, GV 26, BL 38.

Applied Nutrition
Use the same diet as in the case of colds; (p. 50).

Aromatherapy
Use basil essence 2% as part of massage oil before the color therapy.

Autosuggestion
Repeat the following affirmation twenty times morning and evening:

> From day to day I am better and healthier in every part of my nose and face.

Breathing Therapy
Use the same technique as in colds three to four times per day, ten breathings each exercise.

Color Therapy
Use locally over the face and nose after massaging with oil: blue and ultraviolet in alternation for twenty minutes each, three times per day.

Herbs ***

Western
Rhatany *(Krameria triandra)* and *Blood root (Sanguinaria canadensis):* In 1:1 ratio, may be used twice daily for long duration.
Thuya *(Thuya occidentalis):* Fluid extract can be used to paint polyps very gently twice a day with a very fine brush.

Homeopathy ***

Teucrium: Use local snuff or paint with **teucrium** (mother tincture).
Thuya: Thirty every six hours is the remedy of choice; *Thuya* tincture can be painted twice daily.
Phosphorus: For bleeding polyps, take 3X every six to eight hours.

Reflexology ***

Press the following points four to six times per day for three minutes each for one week after the improvement of this condition (decrease or vanishing of the tumor or abscess):

1, 3, 5, 6, 20, 52.

Also massage the entire feet with a foot reflexologer device twice per day, nine minutes on each foot for one month after improvement of the condition.

Schuessler Tissue Salts

Silica and **kali muriaticum:**   In alternation every hour use **silica** 12X and **kali muriaticum** 12X for the first two days, then continue twice per day with the same treatment.

EAR INFECTION AND EARACHE

SUGGESTED TREATMENT

Acupuncture and Accupressure ***

TW 17, TW 20, GB 11, GB 20, ST 6, ST 7, BL 23, K 3, K 7, LI 4, LI 11, SI 3, SI 19, ST 36.

Applied Nutrition **

For best results against inflammation it is very useful to start with juice fasting for three days. On the first day after fasting, 50% of the diet; 75% on the second day; and the full diet thereafter.

An example of a diet for a person of average weight, thirty years old:

2300 calories	1000 IU vitamin D
70 g protein	600 mg calcium chelated
100 g fat	300 mg magnesium
280 g carbohydrate	100 mg phosphorous
3,000 mg vitamin C	20 mg zinc
25,000 IU vitamin A	

Aromatherapy

Use the essence of basil in vegetable oil in 2% concentration, around and back of the ear, twice a day for three weeks.

Autosuggestion

The main emotional cause of an earache is the fear of hearing unpleasant things. In this case, repeat the following affirmation twenty times every two hours until the pain is over:

I love to listen, and I hear with love and please everything is said.

Repeat the following affirmation twenty times each morning and evening for one month:

From day to day I can hear and feel better and better.

Color Therapy

For widespread infection use the colors blue and green alternately, fifteen minutes each, on both ears. In the case of earache use blue and violet the same way.

Herbs ****

Western

Echinacea: in decoction, tincture, or powdered capsules
Garlic or **kyolic:** for the infection
Wild indigo *(Baptisia tinctoria):*   in decoction (one teaspoonful), tincture (two ml), or powdered capsules.
Golden seal *(Hydrastis):*   powder, if there is catarrh and lymphatic swelling.
Elder *(Sambucus nigra):*   in infusion, if there is catarrh, or tincture, powder, or juice from berries.
Cleavers *(Galium aparnine)* and **goldenrod** *(Solidago virgauria):*   other herbs to be used depending on nose and throat involvement.
Lobelia: two drops of tincture
Camomile: infusion
Mullein oil *(Verbascum thapsus)*

Chinese

Pueraria Combination *(Ko-Ken-Tang):*   Formula of choice

Pueraria (Kodzu root) 8 g	Cinnamon twigs 3 g
Ma-Huang 4 g	Peony root 3 g
Ginger rhizome 1 g	Licorice root 2 g
Jujube fruit 4 g	

Bupleurum and **Schizonpeta** *(Shih-Wei-Pai-Tu-San):*   For chronic cases with little secretion.

Homeopathy **

For earache, use the A.B.C. formula—**aconite, belladonna, camomile**—six doses each hour.
Pulsatilla: Add three doses hourly after A.B.C. if there is catarrh and darting pain.

Plantago: Two drops of tincture are also recommended.
Mercurius sol: If there is excessive pus and discharge, take six doses every eight hours.

Hydrotherapy

Apply hot and cold towels soaked in water alternately on the painful ear—the hot towel for one minute and the cold one for a few seconds.

Hypnotherapy

Hypnotherapy is effective in controlling all types of pain, but remember that reducing pain does *not* solve the underlying problem. Self-hypnosis should be done in combination with other therapy.

Reflexology *

In almost every case of otitis (ear infection) in the middle, internal, and external ear, press each for three minutes each hour until the pain subsides:
9, 52, 55.
Repeat this treatment every four hours for four days after the acute pain is over. Continue for another two weeks, twice per day.

Schuessler Tissue Salts

Kali phosphorica: In case of otitis accompanied by discharge from the ear use 6X every thirty minutes until the discharge stops. Then take **ferrum phosphorica** 12X alternating with magnesium 6X every six hours for another two to four weeks after all symptoms are gone.
Ferrum phosphorica and **magnesium:**   For an earache take **ferrum phosphorica** 6X and **magnesium** 6X every hour until pain ceases; continue with the same remedies for another two to four weeks.
Calcarea phosphorica: For pain around the ear, take 12X every thirty minutes; when the pain stops, continue with **ferrum phosphorica** 12X every morning and evening for another week.

DEAFNESS AND HEARING DISORDERS

SUGGESTED TREATMENT

Acupuncture and Acupressure ****

The following modalities are mainly helpful in hearing difficulties that stem from hysteria, difficulties in perception because of nervous or psychological causes, and Ménière's Disease. A chronic illness of the whole body also may cause hearing problems.

Physiological and not organic causes respond best to Acupuncture/
Acupressure.
Massage or Acupuncture points:
BL 23, B1 47, GB 20, GB 25, TW 17, TW 21, GB 2, GV 15, SI 19, LIV
2, ST 40, K 3, BL 60, TW 3.
Ear points: Ear, Inner ear, Neurogate, Kidney, Occiput, Endocrine

Applied Nutrition

Use the same diet and fasting as in the case of otitis. An example of
diet for a person of average weight, thirty years old:

2300 calories	300 mg folic acid
70 g protein	50 mg niacinamid
100 g fat	Hypothalamus extract nucleopro-
280 g carbohydrate	teins
2000 mg vitamin C	500 mg calcium
500 mg bioflavonoids	50 mg phosphorus
50,000 IU vitamin A	10 mg iron
1,000 IU vitamin D	100 mcg chromium
1,000 IU vitamin E	2 mg copper
50 mg vitamin B_1	50 mg zinc
50 mg vitamin B_2	50 mg potassium
100 mg vitamin B_6	50 mcg iodine
500 mcg vitamin B_{12}	100 mcg selenium
1000 mg pantothenic acid	

Aromatherapy

Use lavender essence as 5% of the massage oil.

Autosuggestion

The mental cause might be things you do not want to hear, feelings of
rejection from those around you, feelings of stress while talking, feelings of being unable to communicate on the same level with your peers.
The affirmation should be:

> I listen with love and understanding to those around me, I love to listen
> (to my friends and family).

Repeat one or more of those affirmations twenty times each, twice a
day for one month.

Color Therapy

Use blue light in combination with indigo locally twenty minutes each
twice a day for three weeks. Before treatment use massage oil on the
ears and the surrounding area.

Herbs ***

Western

Elder flowers *(Sambucus nigra):* If the deafness is caused by accumulation of catarrh in the middle ear, use in infusion three times daily to remove the catarrh, or **Euphrasia officinalis** two to three times daily. Use two to four ml of tincture or two capsules of the powder.

Garlic: as an herb, food supplement, or in capsule form (**kyolic,** too) is often helpful, as is **Echynacea** and powdered **golden seal** *(Hydrastis).*

Mullein *(Verbascum thapsus)* and **poke root** *(phytolacca americana):* are also helpful.

Chinese

Pueraria Combination *(Ko-Ken-Tang):* In cases where deafness is caused by catarrh and suppuration:

Pueraria 8 g	Cinnamon twigs 3 g
Ma-huang 4 g	Peony root 3 g
Ginger rhizome 1 g	Licorice root 2 g
Jujube fruit 4 g	

Rehmannia eight formula *(Pa-wei-ti-huang-wan),* for the elderly hard-of-hearing:

Yam *(Dioscorea)* 4 g	Chinese foxglove roots and rhi-
Asiatic cornelian cherry fruit 4 g	zome *(Rehmannia)* 8 g
Alisma 3 g	Wolfsbane *(Aconite)* 1 g
Cinnamon twigs 1 g	Peony bark 3 g

Homeopathy ***

Pure olive oil: to remove wax and discharge from ear, drops should be placed in the ear two to three nights in a row, then the ear cleared with a syringe.

Plantago tincture or **Verbascum** and **Thapsus** are good alternatives.

Mercurium sol: For deafness stemming from a block in the Eustachian tube, use 6X every three hours.

Phosphorus: 6X or 30 every eight hours is the choice for the elderly.

Calcarea carbonica: 30 daily is best for children.

Reflexology *

Press the following points three minutes every four hours each until the condition is improved:

9, 52, 12.

In addition, massage both feet with a reflexology roller twice a day for seven minutes each.

Schuessler Tissue Salts

In many cases these remedies can be of great value.

Ferrum phosphorica: Use 6X three times a day for two weeks, and continue with **Kali muriaticum:**   6X three times a day for another two weeks.

LOSS OF SMELL

SUGGESTED TREATMENT

Acupuncture and Acupressure **
LI 4, LI 20

Applied Nutrition
The same as in colds (p. 50).

Aromatherapy
The same as in colds.

Autosuggestion
The affirmation is:

> Every day my physical and mental functions improve more and more in every way.

Breathing Therapy
Use the same technique as in the case of colds, four times a day for one month.

Color Therapy
The same as in colds (p. 51).

Herbs ***

Chinese

Bupleurum and **Schizonepeta:**   Use to clear catarrh.

Homeopathy ****

Sanguinaria: For loss of smell and taste during catarrh, use three doses every four to six hours.

Ammonium muriaticum: For loss of smell accompanied by cough and blocked nose, use 3X every four to six hours.

Reflexology
The same as for colds (p. 51).

Schuessler Tissue Salts ****

Magnesium phosphorica: If a cold is not involved, use 12X every two hours each day until the condition improves; continue for another three weeks.

MÉNIÈRE'S DISEASE

SYMPTOMS

Dizziness or nausea resulting from an infection in one ear, in most cases.

SUGGESTED TREATMENT

Acupuncture and Acupressure ****

This condition of aural vertigo calls for reduction of water and salt intake at time of attack.
Main points:
   GB 20, LIV 3, TW 17, SI 19, PC 6, ST 36, CV 12, K 3.
Ear points: Neurogate, Sympathetic, Kidney, Occiput, Adrenal, and Heart.
Two to four points should be treated at a time, applying pressure six to eight times.

Applied Nutrition **

Drink: Start with three days of juice fasting and gradually continue with the recommended diet. Avoid coffee and alcohol.
Eat: Avoid salt, tobacco, and fried food.
An example of a diet for a person of average weight, thirty years old:

2200 calories	2000 mg vitamin C
60 g protein	50 mg B_1
100 g fat	50 mg B_2
265 g carbohydrate	50 mg B_6

700 mg nicotinic acid	1000 mg calcium
2000 mg pantothenic acid	300 mg magnesium
200 mg B_{15}	15 mg iron
25,000 IU vitamin A	20 mg zinc
1,000 IU vitamin D	100 mcg selenium
800 IU vitamin E	

Aromatherapy

Use the essence of **lavender** 2% blended with **camomile** 2% in massage oil. (**CAUTION:** Do not use during pregnancy.)

Autosuggestion

Three times a day repeat the affirmation twenty times:

From day to day I'm better in every way.

Color Therapy

Use blue and violet one after the other for twenty minutes each, twice a day, for one month, on both ears.

Herbs **

Western

For tinnitus, two herbs are effective:

Black cohosh *(Dimicifuga racemosa):* in decoction two to three times daily or in tincture three times a day. Two capsules of the crushed root a day are also good.

Golden seal *(Hydrastis):* infusion, tincture, or capsules. A capsule containing both herbs in one-to-one ratio is recommended twice daily after meals. (**CAUTION:** Avoid golden seal during pregnancy.)

Chinese

Atractylodes and Hoelen Combination *(Ling-kuei-chu-kan-tang):*

Hoelen 6 g
Cinnamon twigs 4 g
Licorice root 2 g
Paichu (white atractylodes rhizome) 3 g

Homeopathy ***

If worse after sleeping,
Lachesis: 6X every four to six hours.
China: 3X every four to six hours, or
Salycylic acid 30.

Reflexology **

Press the following points for three minutes each three times per day:
  3, 9, 20, 21, 18, 24, 52.
It is also important to massage the feet three times a day, nine minutes each.
In case of vertigo, press point 52 on each hand for six minutes until the vertigo is gone.

Schuessler Tissue Salts **

Ferrum phosphorica: 12X
Natrum sulphorica: 6X
Magnesium: 12X
One tablet each three times per day for three weeks.

MASTOIDITIS

SYMPTOMS

Tenderness and swelling behind the ears; occasional fever.

SUGGESTED TREATMENT

Acupuncture and Acupressure ***

There are two formulas. First:
  GB 2, GB 20, GB 21, LI 4, LI 11, SI 14, SI 15, SI 17, ST 19, SP 2, TW 3, TW 17, TW 21, ST 5, ST 6, ST 36.
(This is good if there is also difficulty in hearing.)
Second:
  GB 2, GB 12, GB 20, GB 21, LI 4, LI 11, SI 14, SI 15, SI 19, SP 2, TW 3, TW 17, TW 21, BL 10, BL 60, K 3, ST 6, ST 36

Applied Nutrition

As in most cases of ear problems, it is recommended that you start with three days of juice fasting and then introduce the diet gradually. An example for a person of average weight, thirty years old:

2300 calories   Master Formula
70 g protein   3000 mg vitamin C
100 g fat   1000 mg biofavonoids
280 g carbohydrate   25,000 IU vitamin A

1000 IU vitamin D

200 mg vitamin B_{12}

1000 mg calcium chelated

400 mg magnesium chelated

100 mg phosphorous chelated

15 mg zinc

15 mg iron

Aromatherapy

Massage the ear and its surroundings with the essence of **hyssop** 10% in a massage oil, twice a day for one month. (**CAUTION:** Do not use the hyssop essence in cases where epilepsy is present.)

Autosuggestion

The mental reason for mastoiditis might be an inner fight between the wish to listen to what is happening around you and an unwillingness to face the truth. The affirmation should be:

I listen with love and self-confidence. Everything I hear improves my situation.

Color Therapy

Use the blue light on both ears for thirty minutes twice a day for two weeks.

Herbs ****

Western

This condition is treated similarly to boil and abscess therapy, to help drain the lymph gland.

Echinacea: A superb anti-inflammatory anti-microbial, in a decoction of two to three spoonfuls of root or as seven to twelve ml of tincture, three times daily.

Wild indigo *(Baptisia tinctoria):*   Another lymphatic helper. Use one half to one part of root in decoction, or two to three ml of tincture, three times a day.

Pasque flower *(Pulsatilla anemone):*   Can also be used in decoction of one half to one teaspoonful of the dried herb. (**CAUTION:** The *fresh* plant is dangerous.)

These three plants combine well in powder form and capsules.

Chinese

Bupleurum and Schizonepeta *(Shi-wei-pai-tu-tang):*

Bupleurum 3g

Platycodon 3 g

Ginger rhizome 1 g

Hoelen 3 g

Siler root 2 g

Angelica root 2 g

Schionpeta 1 g   Cnidium 3 g
Licorice root 1 g   Cherry bark 1 g

Pueraria Combination *(Ko-ken-tang)* is a second choice.

Homeopathy **

Belladonna: At early stage, try 3X every two to three hours.
Silica: When more advanced, take 6X every six hours.
Asarum europum: 6X is good if there is a ringing, plugged sensation or catarrh.

Reflexology *

In early cases of acute or chronic mastoiditis, reflexology can be a good addition to the treatment. Press the following points six times per day for three minutes each:
   1 (the sinus, to avoid complications), 9, 52, 18, 19.
Continue for two months.

Schuessler Tissue Salts

The following remedies can be used for chronic mastoiditis:

Ferrum phosphorica 12X
Kali phosphorica 6X
Natrum sulphorica 6X

Take all these remedies three times per day until your condition improves.

TINNITUS (RINGING IN THE EARS)

SUGGESTED TREATMENT

Acupuncture and Acupressure ****

   GB 2, GB 20, TW 17, TW 21, LI 4, LI 11, GV 15, TW 3, TW 5, CV 23, K 3, LIV 2, Bl 23.
For tinnitus after infectious disease:
   ST 7, GV 20, GB 20, TW 18, HT 7, ST 36.
Ear points: Ear, Inner ear, Neurogate, Kidney, Occiput, Endocrine.

Applied Nutrition
As in the case of ear infection.

Aromatherapy

Use the essence of basil, as in the case of ear infection. Combine with color therapy for best results.

Autosuggestion

The mental cause for this condition might be your inability to talk with those around you at the same level of knowledge. The affirmation should be repeated twenty times, three times a day for one month:

> *I am satisfied with my knowledge and cleverness.*

Bach Flowers

Mimulus: to help counteract the fear of attacks.

Breathing Therapy

Take 175 deep breaths continuously every hour until the condition improves.

Color Therapy

Use blue for thirty minutes on the affected ear each morning and evening followed by indigo for ten minutes.

Herbs ***

Western

Black cohosh *(Cimicifuga racemosa):*   in decoction two to three times daily, three ml of tincture, or two capsules of the crushed root.
Golden seal *(Hydrastis):*   in infusion, tincture, or capsules.
(**CAUTION:** Avoid golden seal in pregnancy.)
These two herbs may be taken in a combined capsule (1:1), twice a day after meals.

Chinese

Coptis and Rhubarb Combination *(San-huang-hsieh-hsin-tang):*   For tinnitus due to hypertension.

Golden thread rhizome *(Coptis)*
1 g
Skullcuproot *(Scute)* 1 g
Rhubarb rhizome 1 g

Major bupleurum: Recommended for the obese.
Rehmannia eight: Choice for the elderly.

Homeopathy **

China: 6X -30X recommended when the ringing is pronounced.
Hydrastis: 3X every four to six hours in the case of infection.
Aurum: 3X - 30X when hypertension, depression, or piercing pain is involved.

Reflexology *

Press the following points on both hands and feet for five minutes every four hours until the condition improves:

1, 9, 12, 52.

Schuessler Tissue Salts

Kali phosphorica: Use 12X every hour until the condition improves and continue with *ferrum phosphorica* 6X and *kali phosphorica* 12X three times per day for two weeks.

· 3 ·

THE RESPIRATORY SYSTEM

The close working relationship between the heart and the lungs is dramatically underscored in the very serious illness, congestion, or congestive heart failure in the extreme case. ("Congestion" is also popularly used to describe fluids in the nose, ears, or throat in a head cold. This is treated in Part II.) When fluid accumulates excessively in the lungs (pulmonary edema, edema being the excess of fluid), the normal exchange of oxygen and blood in the lungs is interfered with. The ventricles of the heart fail to receive sufficient oxygen and so fail to pump adequate supplies of blood to other tissues of the body. Edema in the legs is one sign of a central congestion problem. Many of the clinical manifestations of heart failure result from excessive accumulation of fluid. Prevention of edema is a primary health concern, to preserve the vital supply of oxygen.

Air may also be interfered with by the closing of the bronchial tubes. This may occur in asthma and bronchitis, but when the bronchial walls become distended, hardened, and progressively weakened the condition is described as emphysema. Chronic infections and hereditary factors may play a role in the course of this disease, but typically it is associated with smoking and air pollution. This is obviously a life-threatening condition.

Equally serious is the inflammation of the lungs known as pneumonia. This is often the final stage in a series of other problems, but it can also occur suddenly as a result of coryza ("cold in the head") or other common respiratory problems. The onset of pneumonia is usually identifiable by sudden chills, rapid rise in temperature, and very fast heartbeat. The stethoscope is the common diagnostic tool, but patients may exhibit obvious symptoms: palpitations, agonizing chest pains, pleurisy, coughing up blood or pinkish mucus, and great difficulty breathing.

When the air passages are blocked due to chronic inflammation of the bronchial tubes or to temporary secretions of mucus the condition is less serious because it can be temporarily alleviated and usually reversed. Various forms of bronchitis are treated in a wide variety of ways.

Blockage of air passages at specific times of the day or night, during definite seasons of the year, and with life-threatening intensity is known as asthma. Although asthma is classified as an allergic disease, its cause is not easily identified from patient to patient. It was once regarded as largely psychosomatic in origin, since half of all cases begin before age ten and are usually accompanied by feelings of panic. Hypersensitivity to various pollens, etc., accounts for only a third of asthmatic attacks. After age thirty there is less than a one in six chance of becoming asthmatic. Whooping cough and coughing blood are conditions that often accompany asthma, although they have their own causes and treatments. General difficulty in breathing (dyspnea) may be related to asthma but usually is not episodic.

A completely distinct class of illnesses, lung abscesses, also have a wide variety of causes and manifestations. A lung abscess may result from an infection, a parasite, or a fungus; it may be the manifestation of an aneurysm, or weakening of the lung wall; it may be in the form of a cyst or other damage to the wall from a foreign substance (e.g., an occupational disease such as silicosis); or it may be a malignancy, primary or metastatic—the spread of a tumor from another site. The defense mechanisms of the lung can be undermined by alcohol, smoking, drugs, or previous illness. Difficulty in breathing, not easily identified as asthma or bronchitis, is one clue that some sort of abscess may be present in the lungs.

The lungs are surrounded by a two-layer membrane consisting of muscles, fibers, blood vessels, and connective tissue. It is not surprising, therefore, that pleurisy, the disorder of this membrane, the pleura, has so many manifestations. Inflammation or infection of the pleura can result in sharp, stabbing pain, as in a muscle pull, or in a weakening condition in which breathing is constricted. The healing process may be long because of the relative size of the lungs and their surrounding membranes.

The lungs are so large because they manage, in a simple yet marvelous way, the essential exchange of air and blood that makes life possible. Each of the two lungs contain a membrane (the "alveolar") that divides the lung. To one side of the membrane blood is pumped from the heart: blood that has given up its oxygen in its journey through the body. To the other side of the membrane, through the bronchi—tubes connecting the lung to the respiratory tract—comes air, with its precious oxygen. The lung instills new oxygen into the blood, which returns to the heart to be pumped out again to replenish all the tissues of the body—and, of course, the brain. The lung maintains its shape by continually receiving air at atmospheric pressure, while the space between it and the surrounding pleura is just below that pressure. One can see how each cough or change in breathing pattern may signify a change in health condition. One can see also how the diagnosis of an illness involving this delicate system must take the entire condition of the person into consideration.

HEAD CONGESTION

SYMPTOMS

Difficulty in breathing, tightness in the chest, feeling of fluids throughout the body.

SUGGESTED TREATMENT

Acupuncture and Acupressure **

BL 13, BL 15, BL 20, BL 23, GV 14, ST 40, LU 1, LU 7, CV 22, LI 4, LI 20, Yin-tang (GV 24.5).
Moxa may be applied mainly to:
BL 13, 15, 20, 23, LU 7.

Applied Nutrition ****

It is important to start with the three-day cleansing juice fast, followed by the rejuvenating diet. Since the cause may be an allergy to food or to a chemical substance, a diet containing different types of food is recommended. Rotate diet every four days.
Drink: Eliminate dairy products and alcohol.
Eat: Eliminate dairy products, white sugar, white wheat flour, red meats, and fried foods.
An example of a diet for a person of average weight, thirty years old:

2200 calories
50 g protein
80 g fat
320 g carbohydrate
2000 mg vitamin C
600 mg calcium
400 mg magnesium

300 mg bioflavonoids
100 mg pantothenic acid
50 mg vitamin B_1
50 mg vitamin B_2
50 mg vitamin B_7
50 mg vitamin B_{12}

Autosuggestion

The mental states that can cause congestion of the lungs are confusion, disorder of thinking, and oversensitivity. Repeat the following thirty times, once per day for a month:

I am free. I am at peace with my mind and my body.

Color Therapy

Red light fifteen minutes on chest and back, once per day, for one month.

Herbs ***

Western

The following herbs are expectorants and anti-inflammatories:

Coltsfoot *(Tussilago farfara)*:   An excellent expectorant with anticatarrhal action. Being also an antispasmodic, it is the herb of choice, in the form of an infusion of one to two tablespoons of the dried leaves, three times daily.

Lobelia: Very good when congestion and fever combine. As a relaxant it is also recommended for those who suffer from hypertension.

Mullein *(Verbascum thapsus)*:   Reduces inflammation and helps the mucous membranes as well as being an expectorant. An infusion tea of ***mullein, lobelia,*** and ***coltsfoot*** combines well and may be taken two to three times daily.

Chinese

Minor Blue Dragon Combination *(Hsiao-ching-lung-tang)*:   A superb formula (though not suited for people of fragile health or with night sweats) for congestion with headache, cough, and sputum.

Pinellia 6 g
Ma-huang *(Ephedera)* 3 g
Paeonia 3 g
Cinnamon 3 g

Asarum 3 g
Licorice 3 g
Schizandra 3 g

Homeopathy ****

Aconite: The remedy of choice within the first twenty-four hours of onset. May be taken in 3X to 6X every thirty minutes. If the condition does not improve, try *Sulphur* 30c every two hours.
Veratrum viride: In case of pneumonia along with congestion, 3X every one to two hours, this is the remedy of choice.

Reflexology **

Press the following points in the feet or hands for three minutes each. Commence at the left side and continue with the right hand or foot, every morning and evening:
   1, 16, 18, 19, 24, 25, 21, 22.

Schuessler Tissue Salts

Ferrum Phosphorica: The first choice, especially when accompanied by inflammation, catarrhal fever, or congestion of nasal membranes.
Kali muriaticum: When accompanied by thick, white, tenacious phlegm, catarrhs of the head, white or gray-coated tongue.
Natrum muriaticum: When accompanied by transparent discharges, a salty taste, loss of sense of smell, or anemia.
Calcarea phosphorica: For chronic states.

EMPHYSEMA

SYMPTOMS

Extreme difficulty in breathing, related directly to bronchial tubes; lack of sufficient oxygen uptake to walk upstairs.

SUGGESTED TREATMENT

Acupuncture and Acupressure **

Bl 12, BL 13, BL 22, BL 20, BL 23, LU 1, LU 5, LU 9, K3.
Ear points: Lungs, Shen-Men, Sympathetic, Adrenal, Occiput.

Applied Nutrition ****

As in bronchitis and asthma, it is of the utmost importance to find out if an allergy is the source. So it is recommended to check for allergies through blood tests (cytotoxic test).

The diet, master formula, and supplements should be as in asthma diet therapy.

Aromatherapy *

The main aromatherapy essence is **eucalyptus** extract *(Eucalyptus globulus)*, which can be used either in the massage oil (2%) or by inhalation, twice per day for three weeks.

Autosuggestion

The primary mental reason for emphysema is suppressed hate toward one's parents or the persons responsible for one's growth and education in early childhood.

The affirmation should be:

> *I am at peace and love.*
> *I love myself and the world around me.*
> *I love myself and my family.*

Color Therapy ***

Use red and orange alternately for ten minutes each on chest and back twice per day for six weeks. Before applying the colors, rub the chest and back with massage oil for the first three weeks.

Herbs ****

Western

Elecampane *(Inula helenium)*: To remove phelgm and mucus. To prepare, pour a cup of cold water onto one teaspoonful of chopped root. Let stand for nine to ten hours. Heat and drink very hot two to three times daily. Tincture—2 ml three times daily.

Comfrey root *(Symphyton officinalis)*: For clearing sputum. Drink in decoction or take three to five ml three times daily in tincture form.

Chinese

Ma-huang Combination *(Ma-huang-tang)*:

Ma-huang 5g	Licorice root 1.5 g
Cinnamon 4g	Apricot seeds 5 g

Pinellia and Magnolia Combination (Pan-Hsia-Hou-Pv-Tang): For emphysema accompanied by weak digestion, nausea and vomiting.

Pinellia rhizome 6 g	Perilla leaves 2 g
Hoelen 5 g	Ginger rhizome 4 g
Magnolia bark 3 g	

Homeopathy **

Lobelia: The remedy of choice three times every three to four hours.

Hypnotherapy
As in most cases where an allergy factor is involved, the release from stress and phobias is very important.

Reflexology **
Press the following points for five minutes each, five to ten times per day in both hands and feet. In order of the severity of the point to be pressed:
16, 18, 19, 20, 21, 24, 25, 52.

Schuessler Tissue Salts

Ferrum phosphorica: As in most cases of respiratory problems, this tissue salt is very useful here. Take six twice per day for three weeks.
Natrum muriaticum: Take for chronic cases.

PNEUMONIA

SYMPTOMS

Sudden chills, rise in temperature, irregular or fast heartbeat, difficult breathing, chest pains, coughing blood.

SUGGESTED TREATMENT

Acupuncture and Acupressure *

GV 14, GV 20, LI 4, TW 5, BL 12, BL 13, BL 23, LU 1, LU 5, LU 9, CV 17, K 3.

Applied Nutrition **

Drink: Vegetable juices, fresh water, and herb tea.
Eat: The macrobiotic diet, containing 70% whole rice, 20% lightly cooked or lightly steamed vegetables, 5% fresh salad and 5% seeds, is highly recommended. An example of a daily diet for an average-weight person, thirty years old:

1800 calories

40 g protein

60 g fat

275 g carbohydrate

Take every hour:

1000 mg. vitamin C, up to 8 g
200 mg. bioflavanoids, up to
1600 mg.

Take Daily:

50,000 IU vitamin A
1,000 IU vitamin D

800 IU vitamin E

Nuceloproteins

Adrenal extract
Thymus extract

Lung extract

Enzymes and Digestive Acids

100 mg Betaine hydrochloric
acids and enzymes

Bee products

Pollen, on spoon daily
Bee propolis, 150 mg. three times
daily

Honey with crushed fresh garlic,
one spoon every hour until the
acute phase is over.

Aromatherapy *

Use the extract oil of **camphor** 2% or a massage oil all over the chest,
back, and throat, once per day for three weeks.

Autosuggestion

The primary mental causes of pneumonia are depression, feelings of
deprivation, and a tendency for suicidal activities. The affirmation should
be:

> *I am free and healthy.*
> *I take life with joy and love.*
> *I am taking life with love and happiness*

Color Therapy

Use red light over the chest, back, and throat for thirty minutes each
day for one month.

Herbs ****

Western

Giant Solomon seal: An infusion is helpful. A poultice from this plant can be applied two to three times daily.

Hyssop *(Hyssopus)*:   Infusion four times daily or two to four drops of tincture is also good, along with **Garlic, Boneset,** and **Mullein.**

Chinese

Pueraria Combination *(Ko-ken-tang):*

Pueraria 8g	Jujube 4 g
Ma-Huang 4g	Licorice 2g
Cinnamon 3g	Ginger 1 g
Paeony 3 g	

Other formulas are:
Pinellia and Magnolia Combination and **Minor Blue Dragon Combination.**

Homeopathy **

Aconitum: In *acute* state use 3X each hour or
ABC Formula: 6X every one to two hours.
Arsenicum album: For those who are anxious or fidgety 6X every one to two hours.
Bacillinum: 30 once a week, but do not repeat if there is no improvement.
Hepar: 6 every three to four hours, effective when there is purulent mucus.

Reflexology *

It is very important in acute cases to press the points on both hands for one minute each, every hour, to reinforce the lungs, the vitality of the respiratory circulation, and the autonomic nervous system:

2, 16, 18, 19, 24, 25, 52.

In chronic cases press the same points twice daily for three minutes each.

Schuessler Tissue Salts

Kali sulphorica: Take 12X in alternation with **calcarea sulphorica,** six every thirty minutes until the acute phase is over and the fever is back to normal.

Ferrum phosphorica: Continue with 3X and **calcarea sulphorica** 12X morning and evening for another two weeks.
Silica: 12X, continue for another month.

BRONCHITIS

SYMPTOMS

Mild but irritating problem of mucus in bronchial tubes.

SUGGESTED TREATMENT

Acupuncture and Acupressure **

For bronchitis with excess phlegm:
BL 23, B1 47, B1 13, B1 15, LU 1, LU 4–7, LU 9, CV 14, CV 17, SP 6.

Applied Nutrition ****

In most cases it is recommended that you start the treatment with three days of fasting and the rejuvenating diet. Introduce food gradually: 50% the first day and 75% the second.
Drink: Avoid dairy products.
Eat: Fresh vegetables, fresh fruits, seeds, whole grains, cereals, small amounts of fish, and vegetable oils. Avoid all dairy products, fatty meats, poultry, fried food. It is very important to examine yourself for food allergy by the cytotoxics test. Also check your mineral balance and possible toxic trace metals such as lead.

An example of a daily diet for a person of average weight, thirty years old:

2,100 calories
50 g protein
80 g fat
295 g carbohydrate
the master formula of vitamins and chelated minerals and:
3,000 mg vitamin C
25,000 IU vitamin A
1,000 IU vitamin D

400 IU vitamin E
2,000 mg pantothenic acid
1,000 mg lecithin
4 tablets of adrenal extract (nucleoproteins)
120 mg betaine hydrochloric enzymes at each meal
1,000 mg calcium
600 mg magnesium
20 mg zinc

Aromatherapy **

Use as a massage oil of **basil** essence 2% on the upper body, especially the chest and back if depression, hysteria, nervous tension, chronic colds, insomnia, or mental fatigue is involved.
Camphor should be used when there is fever, heart failure, hypotension, rheumatism, ulcers, constipation—as a massage oil or by inhalation.

Augosuggestion

In most cases of respiratory problems, early childhood has a strong effect, usually involving negative relationships in the family.
The autosuggestion should be repeated twenty times every morning and evening and also every time there are respiratory problems:

> *Peace and love: Everybody loves me. I love myself.*

Breathing Therapy

In most cases of respiration difficulties it is very important to practice breathing. The most efficient exercises are those done rhythmically:
Breathe in (inhale) to the count of four; hold in (stop breathing) to the count of two; breathe out (exhale) to the count of eight; hold out (stop breathing) to the count of two. Repeat this exercise ten times each morning and evening and when there are breathing difficulties during the day. The technique of "rebirthing" is very useful but should be done under the supervision of a qualified "rebirther." The technique is to inhale and exhale continuously and rythmically, connecting the inhale to the exhale without stopping for one hour. Do this daily for ten days, then once per week for ten weeks.

Color Therapy *

Use red light twenty minutes on the chest and back once or twice per day for a period of two to four months. If you have a chronic condition, it is beneficial to oil the chest and back. Before using the red light use ultraviolet all over the body for twenty minutes once per day for four months.

Herbs ***

Western

The best herbs are pectorals (expectorants) and demulcent, to help clear phlegm and sputum and at the same time soothe the membranes and inflamed bronchial tissues; antimicrobial and anti-inflammatory herbs; and herbs to help the lymphatic system to clear congestion and drain swollen lymph nodes. These are:

Coltsfoot *(Tussilago farfara)* or **angelica root:**   teas in decoction form.
White horehound *(Marrubium vulgare):*   in infusion.
Comfrey root *(Symphytum officinale):*   in decoction.
Garlic *(Allium Sativum):*   pills or raw.
Echinacea: in decoction.
Capsules of **garlic, parsley,** and **echinacea,** taken twice daily, half an hour after meals, are effective.
Eucalyptus: as a tea, recommended for children.
Icelandic moss *(Cetaria islandica):*   in decoction, recommended for children.
Cleavers *(Galium aparine):*   A prime herb for lymph drainage. Combines well with **echinacea** and **poke root** *(Phytolacca Americana).*

Chinese

Chinese herbalists prescribe formulas for two types of bronchitis: moist cough and harsh cough.
Blue Dragon: This famous combination was mentioned before for cough and sputum and is excellent when there is a persistent cough accompanied by much watery sputum, congestion, and a full chest.
Minor Bupleurum Combination *(Hsiao-Chai-Hu-Tang):*   when there is also a slight fever, cough, and sticky yellow mucus and phlegm.

Bupleurum 7 g	Jujube 3 g
Scute 3 g	Licorice 2 g
Pinellia 5 g	Ginger 4 g
Ginseng 3 g	

Ophiopogon Combination *(Mai-Men Tung Tang):*   Excellent for those with small, sticky sputum and dry throat—a "harsh cough." It is good for both adults and infants with bronchial asthma.

Pinellia rhizome 5 g	Ophiopogon root 10 g
Ginseng root 2 g	Licorice root 2 g
Jujube Fruit 3 g	Rice 5 g

Homeopathy **

Aconitum: In the early onset, 3X every forty-five minutes to one hour is recommended, or
ABC Formula: Consisting of **aconitum, bryonia,** and **camomile,** six, 3X to 6X daily.
Ipecac: 3X every hour in cases of nausea.

Hypnotherapy

In most cases this is very useful when done with a qualified hypnotherapist.

Reflexology *
Press the following for three minutes each on each hand; continue pressing those points until the respiration is back to normal.
  1–16, 18, 19, 24, 25, 52.

Schuessler Tissue Salts

Ferrum phosphorica: 6X; should be continued twenty-four hours.
Kali muriaticum: If symptoms lessen and conditions improve, every two hours.
In chronic cases take:
Kali sulphorica: 6X for six days, and then
Calcarea phosphorica: 6X for six days and then
Silica: 6X for six days.
Take each every two hours six times per day, five tablets each time.

PERTUSSIS (WHOOPING COUGH) AND HEMOPTYSIS (COUGHING BLOOD)

SUGGESTED TREATMENT

Acupuncture and Acupressure ***
The main points for general cough are:
BL 13, BL 15, Bl 23, BL 47, LU 1, LU 7, SP 6, SP 9, CV 14, CV 17, CV 20.
Ear points: Adrenal, Lungs, Pharynx and Larynx.
For whooping cough the points are:
PC 6, LI 4, GV 14, GV 12, LU 9, and ST 40.
  Ear points: Bronchi, Lungs, Stop Wheezing, Neurogate, Sympathetic.
  Treat only two to three points at a time, one ear one day and the other the next.
For hemoptysis the points are:
LU 10, LU 5, PC 5, HT 7, LU 9, PC 8, BL 13, GV 14.
Another point combination is: CV 5, LIV 14, TW 5, K2, and LU 7.

Applied Nutrition

Drink: Avoid dairy products.
Eat: Avoid all stimulants in food like white sugar, refined wheat, and dairy products.

An example of a diet for a person of average weight, thirty years old:

2200 calories	and the master formula, and
50 g protein	1500 mg vitamin C
80 g fat	1000 mg pantothenic acid
320 g carbohydrates	200 mg adrenal extract

In most cases of respiratory problems the combination of **honey** and crushed **garlic** is very helpful. Take six spoons of honey and six garlic cloves, crush together, and let interact for six hours. Take one spoon every four hours during the day until the cough disappears.

Aromatherapy *

In case of a cough persisting beyond a day, use **benzoin**—one drop on the tongue, once per day for the first two weeks. **Black pepper** is recommended in cough complicated by fever, influenza, or nausea. **Cardamon** is best for a cough accompanied by headache, mental fatigue, or loss of appetite. Use the black pepper or the cardamon separately by inhaling the odors of the essence, or take one drop of each essence on the tongue once per day for one week.

Autosuggestion

The reason for coughs from the subconscious mind are: nervousness, bad feelings about oneself, feelings of annoyance. Repeat the following affirmation twenty times each morning and evening:

> *I express myself in a peaceful way. I speak with love. I love myself.*

Color Therapy

First use ultraviolet light all over the body for twenty minutes, and then apply red light over the chest and between shoulders for thirty minutes each day for a period of three weeks.

Herbs ****

Western

Thyme *(Thymus vulgaris)*:   Makes an excellent tea and bath in treatment of cough. It is mainly helpful in cases of dry or spasmodic cough. Make an infusion over one to two teaspoons of leaves of the chopped herb (fresh or dry). Drink two to three times daily. To make a **thyme bath,** one liter of boiling water to five or six tablespoons of the herb (dry or fresh); let stand for fifteen to twenty minutes, strain, and add to bath. The herb can also be put into a nylon stocking and left in the bath tub.

Coltsfoot *(Tussilago fargara)*:   A superb herb for treatment for coughs, it combines well with **mullein** *(Verbascum thapsus)* and **licorice** *(Glycyrrhiza glabra)*—an effective infusion to be drunk three times daily.

Sundew *(Drosera)*:   Whooping cough may lead to complications and is best treated by this herb and **mouse ear** *(Pillosella officinarum)*, which is the specific herb for this condition. An infusion of these herbs may include **coltsfoot** *(Tussilago farfara)* and **white horehound** *(Marrubium vulgare)*, taken two to three times daily.

Comfrey *(Symphytum officinale)* and **Elecampane** *(Inula helenium)*:   Should be considered as infusions when coughing blood and with a dry throat.

Chinese ****

Minor Blue Dragon Combination *(Hsiao-Ching-Lung-Tang)*:   For congestion. (**CAUTION:** *Not recommended for patients in weakened condition.*)

Ma-Huang Combination: Good for severe coughs and may be given to children.

Ma-Huang (Ephedera) 5g
Cinnamon twigs 4g
Licorice 1.5g
Apricot seeds 5g

Tang Kuei and Gelatin Combination *(Chiung-Kuei-Chiao-Ai-Tang)*:   For hemoptysis with anemia.

Tang Kuei 4.5 g	Rehmannia roots 6 g
Cnidium 3 g	Licorice root 3 g
Peony root 4.5 g	Mugwort Leaves *(Artemisia vulgaris)* 3 g
Gelatin 3 g	

Homeopathy **

Aconitum: For a short, irritating cough with sudden onset 3X every three hours and

ABC Formula (aconitum, belladonna, camomile):   In 6X, may be taken every hour.

Ipecac: Use 3X to 6X for a rattling cough that becomes worse at night.

Drosera: Those who are near the sick should take 6X nightly and upon rising as preventive measures.

Coquel: 12X or 30c every four to six hours is the remedy of choice to stop this cough.

Acalypha indica: For dry cough with hemoptysis use 3X to 6X every half hour.

Ipecac: For hemoptysis and nausea, 3X every twenty to thirty minutes is recommended.

Reflexology *

Press the following points in the feet or hands for two minutes each and use a foot reflexologer for five minutes on each foot every one to two hours, until improvement is noticed:

1, 16, 18, 19, 24, 25, 21, 22, 52.

Schuessler Tissue Salts

Ferrum phosphorica: 6X at the first stage of a cough and for the inflammatory symptoms accompanying a cough.

Kali muriaticum: 6X in cases of loud, spasmodic coughs accompanied by white or grayish-white coated tongue.

Magnesium phosphorica: 6X for a spasmodic, noisy cough; such a cough is also relieved by hot drinks.

Kali sulphorica: 6X for the late stage of an inflammatory cough, which is always worse in a warm room or in the evening.

ASTHMA

SYMPTOMS

Difficulty breathing, usually at night or during exercise, often with life-threatening sessions of gasping for air.

SUGGESTED TREATMENT

Acupuncture and Acupressure **

LU 1, LU 7, LU 9, LU 4, LU 6, GV 15, BL 13, BL 15, CV 22, CV 12, CV 17, LI 4.
Moxa three times (Cones) or five to ten minutes
Moxa roll (not in summer) on LU 6, BL 13, BL 15.
Ear points: Lung, Shen-Men, Internal Secretion, Asthma Points.

Applied Nutrition ****

As in bronchitis, the attacks may be due to some allergen in the air like pollen from plants, animal hair, bird feathers, or from various foods such as wheat flour, white sugar, dairy products, eggs, fish, berries, spices, chocolate, spinach, buckwheat, food colorings, food preservatives, etc. The list of food that may cause an attack is very long; therefore, it is of utmost importance to have a blood test (C.T.T.) and a mineral-trace elements analysis.

Drink: Avoid dairy products.

Eat: Diet should be very light; fresh vegetables, fresh fruits, seeds, whole grains, cereals, and grilled low-fat meats only after checking against the possibility of an allergy factor in the blood. Exclude all allergy-causing foods as well as dairy products, white sugar, processed foods.

An example of a daily diet for a person of average weight, thirty years old:

2100 calories	1,000 IU vitamin D
50 g protein	800 IU vitamin E
80 g fat	2,000 mg pantothenic acid
295 g carbohydrate	Chelation Minerals
Master formula and:	1,000 mg calcium
3000 mg vitamin C	600 mg magnesium
50,000 IU vitamin A (during attacks only 25,000 IU)	20 mg zinc

Nuceloproteins

4 tablets of adrenal glands	2 tablets of ribonucleic acid
2 tablets of thymus glands	2 tablets of hypothalamus

Enzymes and Digestive Acids

120 mg betaine hydrocloric acid (three tablets with each protein meal)	100 mg bile extract
	50 mg pepsin
	100 mg lipase
140 mg pancreatin	100 mg papain

Bee Products—not to be used in case of an allergy

Bee pollen, 25 g daily	garlic, one spoon every four
Bee propolis, 10 g daily	hours
Bee honey with crushed fresh	

Cell Therapy

Thymus extract injection once per day for three weeks.	Adrenal extract injection once per day for three weeks.

Aromatherapy *

There are many aromatic essences to treat asthma. The most efficient method is to use them as a 1%–2% extract in a massage oil, or inhaled directly in the lungs once per day for a period of two to three weeks. For massage oil use the following extracts:

Benzoin   1% in cases accompanied by cough, arthritis, skin irritation.

Cypress   2% in cases accompanied by diarrhea, influenza, liver disorders, nervous tension.

For inhalation use the following extracts:

Eucalyptus   in cases accompanied by influenza, colds, fevers, sinusitis, hay fever, migraines, bronchitis, catarrh, or any other respiratory disorder.

Autosuggestion

The mental cause for asthma is oversensitivity toward family, especially parents, from not being allowed as a child to express one's feelings. The affirmations should be taped—twenty times each—on a cassette and played back each morning and evening for three months. The affirmations should be:

> *I am free.*
> *I take responsibility for my own life.*
> *I love myself as I am.*
> *I accept myself as I am.*
> *From day to day I am healthier and stronger in every way.*
> *I breathe easily and smoothly.*
> *My lungs and respiratory system are healthy and strong.*
> *I receive all the air I need.*
> *I receive all the love I need.*
> *I overcome all my difficulties.*

After repeating each of these affirmations twenty times on the cassette, repeat each one after the other until one side is full (thirty minutes). Copy this side on the other so that the cassette is always ready to be listened to.

Bach Flowers

Larch: for those who feel they are failures.
Mimulus: for fear of future.
Mustard: for sadness.
Holly: for hate and jealousy.

Breathing Therapy ****

Use the same technique for breathing as in case of bronchitis, including rebirthing.

In cases of an attack, exhale all the air you can while breathing; after six to ten minutes of this you will immediately feel it is much easier to breathe.

Practice this method of breathing (exhaling as much as you can) twice per day for two months, twenty exhalations each time.

Color Therapy

Use red light for twenty minutes on chest and back after aromatherapy. Follow with yellow, orange, and blue on chest and back for another ten minutes total.

Ultraviolet is a good addition to the previous colors, another five minutes. The total time is about thirty-five to forty minutes twice per day for a period of four to five months.

Herbs

Western

Grindelia *(Grindelia camporum)*:   For asthma with spasm, in infusion (also combined with **lobelia**).

Sundew *(Drosera)*: Also good for this condition. Infusion three times daily.

When excess sputum is present use or add:

Comfrey root: decoction and

Ginger *(Zingiber)*, or the excellent **Coltsfoot** *(Tussilago fargara)*:   infusion, capsules, or tincture.

Icelandic moss *(Icelandica)*:   For children, in a decoction.

Ephedra: For those with allergies, in a decoction.

Valerian, hops *(Humulus lupulus)*:   For nervous people.

Lime blossom *(Tilia europea)*:   For asthma accompanied by heart disorders, this and other heart tonics are important.

Chinese

Minor Bupleurum Formula: The formula of choice (See Cough).

Ma-Huang Combination *(Ma-Huang-Tang)*:   for childhood asthma and bronchial asthma.

Uma-Huang 5 g	Licorice root 1.5 g
Cinnamon twigs 4 g	Apricot seeds 5 g

Homeopathy **

Phosphorus: 6X when breathing is wheezy and worrisome.
Arsenicum album: 3X every six to eight hours for those who improve with heat.
Cuprum metalicum: 6X or **Ipecac** − 3 for those vomiting after an attack.

Hypnotherapy

As in bronchitis, hypnotherapy is very effective in a period of three to ten treatments, when the primary cause is psychosomatic.

Reflexology **

Press each point for three minutes every morning and evening. At times of an attack use reflexology as first aid in addition to acupressure. Press 1, 2, 16, 52, 20, 21, 18, 19, 24, 25 on hands and feet. The most important points are 2, 16, 52, 20, and they should be treated until the breathing difficulties disappear.

Schuessler Tissue Salts

The following tissue salts should be given every fifteen to thirty minutes until the attack is over:
Ferrum phosphorica: 12X and
Magnesium phosphorica: 6X in alternation. Continue this treatment for three days after the attack is over. Then continue with **Natrum sulphorica:** 12X morning and evening for four weeks, followed by **Calcarea phosphorica:** 6X for another four weeks. These remedies are especially efficient for children who suffer asthmatic attacks and wheeze at every change of weather.

LUNG ABSCESS

SUGGESTED TREATMENT

Acupuncture and Acupressure **
LIV 2, BL 65, BL 13, GV 10, BL 38, LI 4, LI 11, ST 36, SP 10.

Applied Nutrition

Drink: Avoid alcoholic beverages and coffee.
Eat: Diet should be low in foods containing purines such as meats, eggs, poultry, and seafood.

An example of a daily diet for an average-weight person, thirty years old:

2300 calories	100 mg Vitamin B_6
40 g protein	50 mg niacinamid
80 g fat	500 mg pantothenic acid
355 g carbohydrate	100 mg folic acid
Master Formula and also:	50 mg vitamin B_{15} (panaganic
5000 mg vitamin C	acid)
800 mg bioflavonoids	600 mg calcium
100 mg vitamin B_1	100 mg phosphorous
100 mg Vitamin B_2	500 mg magnesium

Aromatherapy *
Use **bergamot citrus bergamia** extract by inhalation twice per day for two weeks.

Autosuggestion
The mental cause for lung abscesses might be family problems with feelings of revenge.
Repeat the following affirmation twenty-five times each morning and evening for one month:

I am at love and peace.
My thoughts are positive and good.

Color Therapy
Use the color orange in alternation with red for fifteen minutes each twice per day for one month.

Herbs

Western ****
Anti-inflamatory herbs are used, including:
Echinacea *(Angustifolia)*:   in decoction two to three times daily.
Marshmallow *(Althea officinalis)*:   in decoction form.
Wild indigo *(Baptisia tinctoria)*:   in decoction with **echinacea.**

Chinese ****
Bupleurum and Schizonepeta Formula *(Shih-Wei-Pai-Tu-Tang)*:   Formula of choice. This is a general treatment for boils, abscess, and carbuncles and will help the lung abscess as well.

Bupleurum 3 g	Ginger rhizome 1 g
Platycodon 3 g	Hoelen 3 g

Siler root 2 g

Angelica root 2 g

Schizonepeta 1 g

Licorice root 1 g

Cnidium 3 g

Cherry bark 1 g

Homeopathy ****

Aconitum: Use 3X every hour for those hot and restless.

Hepar: For pus, use 6X every two to three hours.

Capsicum: With copious and putrid mucus try 3X every two to four hours.

Reflexology *

Reflex the following points three minutes each point three times per day:

16, 20, 21, 18, 19, 24, 25, 52.

Schuessler Tissue Salts

Take in alternation

Ferrum phosphorica: 12X and

Calcarea sulphorica: 6X every hour.

One tissue salt for a few day until the pain is over; then continue with **ferrum phosphorica** each morning and **Calcarea sulphorica** each evening for two months. Then continue with

Silica: 6X until the abscess disappears.

DYSPNEA

SYMPTOMS

Less acute difficulty in breathing.

SUGGESTED TREATMENT

Acupuncture and Acupressure ****

PC 6, CV 12, LI 4, LU 1, LU 7, TW 5, BL 13, BL 15, BL 22, K 7.

Aromatherapy **

In case of dyspnea use as a massage oil 1% of the essence of **camphor** when the symptoms or diseases in addition to dyspnea are heart failure, tuberculosis, flatulence, hypotension, ulcers.

Use **hyssop** in cases of dyspnea accompanied by asthma, bronchitis, cough, fever, catarrh, hypertension.

Autosuggestion

The primal mental cause of dyspnea is fear of not having enough air, due to previous phobias in early childhood. Repeat the following affirmations twenty times each morning and evening for three months:

> *I am completely free.*
> *I am responsible for my own life.*

Color Therapy

(see attached yellow top on p. 183)

Herbs

Western ***

Pill-Bearing Spurge *(Euphorbia pilulifera)*:   In infusion three times daily will help dyspnea.
Grindelia and **mouse ear:**   Other antispasmodic herbs that are also helpful.
This condition should be treated with regard to other symptoms like asthma and bronchitis.

Chinese ***

Minor Blue Dragon Combination: See Cough. For congestion, short breathing (dyspnea), asthma and stridor.

Homeopathy **

Bromium: For difficult inspiration, use 3X every fifteen to thirty minutes.
Valeriana: For dyspnea aggravated by nervous causes, use 6X.
Lachesis: For dyspnea relieved in open air, use 6X.

Hypnotherapy

Hypnotherapy is very important in cases where the dyspnea is due to psychosomatic origin.

Reflexology

In cases of dyspnea stimulate all points of the lung, blood circulation, spleen, liver, and heart at the following pressure points in both hands and feet for three minutes each point twice per day for two months:
1, 16, 20, 21, 18, 19, 24, 25, 52.

Also reflex the whole feet with the foot-massager device for nine minutes each foot.

Schuessler Tissue Salts

Ferrum phosphorica: 6X
Magnesium phosphorica: 3X
Kali muriaticum: 12X
Take one of these tablets twice per day for two months.

PLEURISY

SYMPTOMS

Sharp pains in the chest and upper back, often with problems in breathing.

SUGGESTED TREATMENT

Acupuncture and Acupressure **

BL 12, BL 13, BL 14, BL 15, BL 17, LIV 3, LIV 13, LIV 14, HT 3, ST 36, GV 14, TW 6, GB 34.
For hydrothorax:
CV 6, SP 6, BL 13, 15, 18, ST 36.
Ear points: adrenal, lungs, subcortex.

Applied Nutrition

Drink: Four to eight glasses of plain water per day, fresh juices and herb tea.
Eat: Diet should be light and rich in vegetables, fruits, seeds, and whole grains.
An example of a diet for an average-weight person, thirty years old:

1900 calories	600 mg calcium
70 g protein	300 mg magnesium
60 g fat	3000 mg vitamin C
270 g carbohydrate	400 mg bioflavanoids
Master formula and also:	1500 mg pantothenic acid

Aromatherapy

Use **camphor** essence 2% in a massage oil base once per day for a period of three weeks.

If the pain is very severe, use **camphor** oil twice per day together with the color therapy.

Autosuggestion

In case of pleurisy repeat the following affirmation.

> *My chest is strong and healthy.*
> *I am strong and healthy.*

Color Therapy

Use in alternation the following colors after oiling the chest with massage oil containing aromatherapy (see Aromatherapy for Pleurisy):
Red light for twenty minutes, then blue for fifteen minutes, and green for another ten minutes

Do this treatment once or twice daily according to the severity of the case, for three weeks. After three weeks continue without oil for another two weeks.

Herbs

Western ****

Pleurisy root *(Asclepias tuberosa)*:   As its name indicates, this is very useful, and an infusion can be drunk two or three times daily. Two ml of tincture is also good.

Comfrey foot *(Symphytum officinale)*:   Valuable as a decoction, as are **boneset** *(Duratorium perfoliatum)* in infusion and **garlic.**

Chinese ****

Ginseng and Astragalus *(Pu-Chuang-I-Chi-Tang)*:   For pleurisy or pleuritis, the formula of choice. This formula is for those who are weak, tired, and have gastrointestinal disorders.

Ginseng root 4 g	Bupleurum 1 g
Chinese angelica 3 g	Cimicifuga 0.5 g
Licorice root 1.5 g	Astragalus 4 g
Paichu 4 g	Ginger rhizome 0.5 g
Mandarin orange peel 2 g	

Other formulas include:
Ophiopogon Combination: in case of excessive thick sputum, **Minor Bupleurum formula,** and **Bupleurum and Cinnamon Combination.**

Homeopathy ***

Aconitum: At earliest stage, use 3X every hour.
Sulphur: When movement causes pain, use 3X to 6X every two hours.
Hepar sulphuris: For chronic pleurisy with much mucus use 6X every four to six hours.
Apis: For hydrothorax, use 3X every two hours.

Hypnotherapy

This system is useful to control the pains in a natural way. Also, the affirmations are better suggested under hypnosis.

Reflexology *

In case of pleurisy the most important points to press are:
    52, 16, 20, 51.
Press each point for five minutes on left and right hand while patient is lying down. Continue the treatment on both feet on points:
    16, 20, 21, 51
Repeat the treatment every hour until the symptoms are gone, and after that continue twice per day at the same points.

Schuessler Tissue Salts

Ferrum phosphorica: 6X followed by **kali muriaticum:** 12X
These two remedies should be taken separately, one each hour in alternation.

· 4 ·
THE CIRCULATORY SYSTEM

Heart disease is the leading cause of death in the industrialized nations. Together with coma, also a circulatory disease, it accounts for more than one half of all deaths in the United States.

Heart disease is of course, not the same as heart attack (or myocardial infarction). Heart disease includes all the problems of the circulatory system, the most prominent of which is arteriosclerosis.

It is well recognized that the hardening and obstruction of the arteries is by far the major cause of heart attacks. But the arteries are more than simple pipes; they consist of a fibrous outer layer, a layer of muscles and elastic fibers that act like pumps for the circulating blood, and an inner coating ("intima") that absorbs nutrients from the bloodstream and passes them through to the tissues. Therefore, arteriosclerosis may be the general name for diseases of the arteries, but atherosclerosis is the name we have given to problems of the intima in the major arteries. These are the problems we associate with the buildup of cholesterol at damaged sites, leading to blockage of a major source of oxygen to the heart.

The major artery, the aorta, begins to show fatty streaks at puberty, and this normal deterioration continues to about age thirty. Meanwhile, the buildup of plaque—raised lesions often containing lipids (fats, especially low-density lipoprotein, or LDL)—appears, apparently as a function of diet and/or lack of exercise. In this century autopsies have shown that this second kind of atherosclerosis has become more intense with each passing year, inviting the conclusion that this is indeed a disease of modern civilization. Accumulations of calcium and other minerals at critical sites in the aorta may also cause atherosclerosis.

The risk factors in heart disease are more important as a whole than any single factor in predicting the possibility of the disease. There are eight major factors of varying importance: (1) family history; (2) emotional stress; (3) obesity; (4) physical inactivity; (5) high blood cholesterol; (6) diabetes mellitus; (7) smoking; and (8) hypertension.

Hypertension, or high blood pressure, is measured by two figures, separated by a slash, such as 120/80, a normal reading. The upper reading, or first figure, records the present level of load on the heart, which may vary from day to day depending on emotional factors, dietary changes, and so forth. The second figure represents an underlying condition of the heart. If hypertension cannot be shown to be the result of another condition (liver, drugs, adrenal dysfunction), then it is called primary, or essential, hypertension. A reading over 160/95 is considered prima facie evidence of the disease. Symptoms commonly include headache, dizziness, palpitations, blurred vision, and fatigue. Although there is some debate over the importance of each preventive measure, it is generally agreed that exercise, dietary control of sodium, fats, and cholesterol, and stress reduction are helpful for most people with hypertension and in atherosclerosis.

Various diseases or pains follow from problems in the basic circulatory system. Poor circulation in general may cause soreness, numbness, or coldness in the arms and legs. If there is prolonged blockage of blood flow, there is risk of loss of activity or infection. Pains in the chest (angina pectoris) and palpitations (strong feeling of heartbeat) are often the result of heart weakness of one kind or another. Anemia signifies reduced blood flow or inadequate production of red blood cells. Varicose veins typically occur in women, with changes in hormonal activity from puberty to menopause. In men, the occurrence of the disease may involve hereditary factors as well as circulatory deficiencies.

The circulatory system is matched throughout the body by the lymphatic system, which carries the main actors in the immune, or self-defense, system from site to site. (The other main component of the immune system is blood cells—see Part Eight.) This "phantom" system has some five to six hundred gateways, or "nodes," situated along its length, to filter out foreign bodies and in general remove the threats to health the immune system is designed to seek out and destroy. The lymph nodes may themselves become the sites of illness, through infection or allergic reactions. These are also the sites of autoimmune diseases, in which the body strikes out at itself as if it were an enemy.

If a heart attack occurs, a patient can expect to go through several months of recovery in which a whole new category of problems appears. This "post-M.I." period may occasion pains in the left arm and shoulder, chest and fever pains unlike angina pectoris, and emotional stresses. The patient may also experience hypotension, or low blood pressure, as well as weakness of the heart due to destruction of heart muscle.

The circulatory system represents the greatest single area in which the individual can take responsibility for his or her health.

HYPERTENSION (HIGH BLOOD PRESSURE)

SYMPTOMS

Usually unseen and unfelt, measurable only by a blood pressure test, but a general run-down condition is common.

SUGGESTED TREATMENT

Acupuncture and Acupressure
GB-20, LI 11, ST 36, LIV 3, BL 15, BL 22.
Also massage ST 9.
(**CAUTION:** If blood pressure exceeds 200/100, do not do acupressure at all.)
For headache and dizziness, add:
   LIV 2, GV 34, Taiyang.
For fullness of chest, nausea, and vomiting, add: PC 6, ST 40, SP 9.

Applied Nutrition ★★★★

Drink: Dairy products. Avoid alcohol.
Eat: Dairy products (low-fat cheese, yogurt), fish, whole-wheat bread without natran, green vegetables, vegetable oils rich in unsaturated lipids, whole rice. Avoid nuts, meats, chocolate, white-sugar products, or any flatulence-causing foods or foods containing saturated fatty acids, such as meat, poultry, butter, etc.

The recommended diet example for an average-weight person, thirty years old:

1700 calories	40 g fat
100 g protein	235 g carbohydrate

In addition to the basic vitamin/mineral formula:

500 IU vitamin A	600 IU vitamin E
400 IU vitamin D	4000 mg vitamin C

100 mg vitamin B_{15}	50 mg niacinamide
50 mg vitamin B_1	1000 mg pantothenic acid
50 mg vitamin B_2	300 mcg folic acid
100 mg vitamin B_6	100 mcg biotin
500 mcg vitamin B_{12}	

Add the following minerals in the form of amino acid minerals chelated. They are important in cardiovascular disorders:

500 mg calcium	50 mg zinc
100 mg phosphorus	90 mg potassium
15 mg iron	30 mg manganese
200 mcg chromium	200 mcg iodine
200 mg magnesium	100 mcg selenium
3 mg copper	50 mcg molybdenum

Aromatherapy *

Use two drops of each oil for three to four weeks: **hyssop** *(Hyssopus officinalis)*, **lavender** *(Lavendula officinalis)*, **marjoram** *(Origanum marjorana)*, **melissa** *(Melissa officinalis)*. This aromatherapy oil can be used for massage oil all over the body or for inhaling. Oils may also be used in a bath, each one of them separately.

Autosuggestion

Repeat the affirmation at least twice per day, ten times:

I am relaxed, happy, and enjoy life as it is.

Bach Flowers

Agrimony: for the alcoholic person.
Willow: for those resentful and bitter toward life.
Walnut: for one in a transition period.

Biofeedback ***

Use a self-treatment biofeedback device that teaches you to relax by indicating when you are in stress or unrelaxed. In this way anyone can control his or her tension and lower his or her blood pressure.

Color Therapy **

Apply the color green three times per day for twenty minutes all over the body for at least thirty days.

The effect of green is to balance the system and is primarily a nerve sedative.

Herbs

Western ****

Lime blossom *(Tilia europea)*:   For treating hypertension associated with arteriosclerosis and anxiety, take an infusion. Pour one cup of boiling water onto one teaspoonful of the dried flowers; leave to infuse ten minutes, filter, and drink.

Hawthorn berries *(Crataegus)*, **lime blossom** *(Tilia europea)*, and **Yarrow** *(achillea)*:   A mixture of all, in equal parts, may prove effective.

Garlic: Eat for a few months **(kyolic** O.K.**)**, or take two **garlic** and **parsley** capsules three times daily.

Chinese ****

Siler and Platycodon Formula *(Sang-Feng-Tung-Shen-San)*: For hypertension accompanied by obesity and constipation.

Chinese angelica root 1.2 g	Ma-Huang *(Ephedera)* 1.2 g
Cnidium 1.2 g	Paichu (White atractylodes rhizome) 2.0 g
Peony root 1.2 g	
Gardenia fruit 1.2 g	Rhubarb rhizome 1.5 g
Ginger rhizome 1.2 g	Field mint 1.2 g
Forsythia fruit 1.2 g	Platycodon (balloon flower root) 2.0 g
Siler root 3.0 g	
Licorice root 2.0 g	Skullcap root (scute) 2.0 g
Chinchieh herb *(Schizonepeta)* 1.2 g	Gypsum 2.0 g
Nitrous sulfate 1.5 g	Talc 3.0 g

Rehmannia Eight Formula: For older people with hypertension, fatigue, frequent nightly micturition, and kidney atrophy or nephritis.

Yam *(dioscorea)* 4.0 g	Chinese foxglove *(rehmmania)* 8.0 g
Cornus 4.0 g	Aconite root 1.0 g
Hoelen 3.0 g	Tree paeony bark 3.0 g
Cinnamon twigs 1.0 g	

Homeopathy **

Thyroidinum: 12X (prepared from thyroid gland) is a good assistant in a wide variety of hypertension cases.

Nux vomica: 6X for intermittent arterial hypertension.

Crataegus: A nutritional cardiac helper; use five drops of the mother tincture.

Hypnotherapy **

In cases of hypertension hypnotherapy is very useful if there is an emotional factor causing stress or tension.

Reflexology *

Press in the hands or feet the following points for two minutes, beginning with the left hand, then right hand, then left foot, then right foot, morning and evening:

52 (hands only), 1, 2, 3, 18, 19, 20, 21, 22, 24, 25.

After that massage your feet twice a day with reflexology roller for five minutes each foot.

Schuessler Tissue Salts **

Kali phosphorica and **calcarea phosphorica:**   Use 6X potency twice a day.

ARTERIOSCLEROSIS AND ATHEROSCLEROSIS

SUGGESTED TREATMENT

Acupuncture and Acupressure **

BL 15, BL 17, BL 18, BL 23, ST 9, ST 36, CV 12, LIV 2, LIV 3, LI 4, LI 11, GV 13, GV 14.

Applied Nutrition ****

Drink: Avoid alcohol and coffee.

Eat: Avoid any kind of saturated fatty acids, cigarettes, refined sugar, and table salt. In the first three days use the fasting program, and then continue with the health diet given in the beginning. An example of a diet for a person of average weight, thirty years old:

1900 calories	200 IU vitamin E if high blood
50 g protein	pressure
60 g fat—mainly polyunsaturated	4,000 mg vitamin C
fatty acids	300 mg vitamin B_{15} (pangamic
290 g carbohydrates	acid)
12,000 IU vitamin A	6,000 mg lecithin
400 IU vitamin D	200 mg raw heart glandular tab-
800 IU vitamin E if normal blood	lets
pressure	100 mg free amino acids

Aromatherapy

Use the essence of **juniper** oil 2% as a massage oil in case of skin disorders and arteriosclerosis, and use the essence of **rosemary** oil 2% as a massage oil when there are nerve problems of any nature together with arteriosclerosis.

Autosuggestion

Mentally caused due to fear of death. Mentally repeat the autosuggestion twenty times, three times per day:

I love myself—unconditionally.

Bach Flowers

Agrimony: for anxious people
Scleranthus: for alternating moods
Mimulus: for fear of being alone
Chicory, heather: for mental congestion

Chelation Therapy ****

For most of the circulation disorders this approach is very efficient, either intravenously or through the digestive system as tablets. Take the following amino minerals chelated:

Calcium 600 mg	Zinc 35 mg
Magnesium 425 mg	Manganese 90 mcg
Phosphorous 186 mg	Copper 2 mg
Potassium 42 mg	Chromium 35 mg
Iron 18 mg	Selenium 50 mcg
Sulphur (L-cysteine) 6 mg	Molybdenum 15 mcg
Iodine (kelp) 15 mg	

Color Therapy

The best colors for arteriosclerosis are yellow and violet. Use orange all over the body and apply locally on the chest area. Apply these colors for twenty minutes for one week. Then skip one week and continue every other week to apply color therapy by using lamp treatment with the colors mentioned above.

Herbs ***

Western

Lime blossom *(Tilia europea)* and **garlic** (raw or in capsules):   These most effective herbs are antiatheromatic and help to both prevent and get rid of cholesterol deposits. **Lime blossom** combined with **hawthorn berries** *(Crataegus)* and/or **mistletoe** *(Viscum album)* and a tea of this mixture in 1:1 ratio (or two parts of **lime blossom)** is recommended two to three times daily. Two capsules a day after meals can be made of these crushed herbs.
Artichoke: As a tea, pour one cup of *cold* water over one and a half

to two tablespoons of dried leaves. Decoction: Boil one minute, let stand five minutes, strain. Drink three cups daily.

Chinese

Coptis and Rhubarb Combination *(San-Huang-Hsieh-Hsin-Tang)*: The formula of choice in cases of arteriosclerosis (and hypertension).

Coptis Rhizome 7 g Rhubarb Rhizome 7 g
Scute 7 g

Homeopathy **

Phosphoricum: 3X every six to eight hours

Reflexology

Press twice per day for five minutes each point of the foot and hand:
    11, 13, 17, 18, 19, 21, 24, 25, 52.
It is also recommended to massage the whole foot once a day for five minutes as a regular practice.

Schuessler Tissue Salts **

Calcarea fluorica 6X, **ferrum phosphorica** 6X, and **natrum muriaticum** 6X: Use the combination three times per day, three tablets each.

POOR CIRCULATION AND CHILBLAINS

SYMPTOMS

Chilblains are a particular case of poor circulation in combination with exposure to cold temperature without actual freezing of the tissues. Sometimes the cold red skin becomes ulcerative or hemorrhagic lesions. The treatment is generally similar to that for poor circulation. In case of accompanied ulcers or hemmorhagic lesions, local and external treatment should be applied.

SUGGESTED TREATMENT

Acupuncture and Acupressure ****

BL: 14, BL 15, BL 23, BL 25, ST 12, CU 14, TH 4, LI 4, HT 7, ST 36, SP 6

Applied Nutrition ***

In case of anemia and poor circulation it is very important to include in the diet enough proteins in addition to iron, B_{12}, zinc, pilic acid, B_2, B_6, and vitamins A,D, and E.

Drink: Avoid coffee and all stimulants.

Eat: Avoid salt in food, saturated fatty acids, and all stimulants.

An example of a diet for an adult of average weight:

1900 calories	800 IU vitamin E
100 g protein	3,000 IU vitamin C
40 g fat	20 mg vitamin B_1
285 g carbohydrate	20 mg vitamin B_3
Master formula and:	20 mg vitamin B_6
1000 mg calcium	100 Mcg vitamin B_{12}
20 mg iron	200 mg vitamin B_{15} (pangamic
20,000 IU vitamin A	acid)
1,000 IU vitamin D	

Aromatherapy ***

Camomile-rosemary-camphor: Use **camomile** in case of anemia as a bath oil or as a massage oil. It also can be used by inhalation in bath oil. Use 2% of this essence.

For massage oil use also 2% of this essence in a vegetable oil and massage the whole body for twenty to thirty minutes each day for a period of three weeks.

In case of poor circulation, a lymph drainage massage oil can be the treatment. It can also be helped by using **camomile** oil essence 1% if poor circulation is present with anemia, burns, depression, rheumatism.

If there is poor circulation with skin problems, ulcers, wounds, heart failure, or hypotension, use **camphor** 1% in a massage oil for two weeks.

If there is poor circulation with asthma, arteriosclerosis, fainting spells, liver ailments, migraine, or nervous disorders, use **rosemary** as a massage oil 2% every day for a period of three weeks, twenty minutes each day.

Autosuggestion

Repeat the following sentence twenty times per day:

I love life and life loves me in every way.

Color Therapy **

Use red light on the torso with the face upward fifteen to twenty minutes and the same on the back, and follow with ultraviolet.

Herbs

Western

Cayenne *(Capsicum minimum)*:   Infusion for fifteen minutes
Ginger *(Zingiber vulgaris)*:   Infusion of fresh root for fifteen minutes or a decoction of dried root (chop root, bring to boil, simmer for ten minutes).
Prickly ash *(Zanthoxylum americanum)*:   Either bark or berries. Infusion of bark for fifteen minutes three times daily.

A good combination for poor peripheral circulation and chilblains:

Prickly ash (bark) 3 parts   Infuse for ten to fifteen minutes.
Hawthorn berries 3 parts   Drink three times daily.
Ginger 1 part

Chinese ***

Tang-Kuei, Evodia and Ginger Combination *(Tang-Kuei-Szu-Ni-Chia-Wu-Chu-Yu-Sheng-Chiang-Tang)*:   This formula is indicated for those with chilblains, tendency towards anemia, cold extremities.

Tang-Kuei 3 g   Asarum 2 g
Cinnamon twigs 3 g   Akebia 3 g
Peony root 3 g   Jujube fruit 5 g
Licorice root 2 g   Evodia fruit 2 g
Ginger rhizome 4 g

Tang-Kuei and Paeonia Formula *(Tang-Kuei-Shao-Yao-San)*:   This formula is indicated to those who are anemic with chills or chilblains, having dark color around eyes, suffering from dizziness or thirst. There may be pain or chills in the lower abdomen.

Tang-Kuei 3 g   Paichu. (white atractylodes rhi-
Cnidium 3 g   zome) 4 g
Peony root 4 g   Hoelen 4 g
Alisma 4 g

Vitality Combination: A general Chinese herbal formula to aid blood circulation for those suffering from cold extremeties, diarrhea, and dizziness.

Peony Root 3 g   Paichu 3 g
Ginger rhizome 3 g   Aconite 1 g
Hoelen 5 g

Homeopathy **

Carbo vegetabilis: 6X every eight hours is good for those with poor circulation, blue and ice-cold hands and feet that often are very wet.
Pulsatilla: 3X every eight hours, mostly for women and girls (blond) who suffer from chilblains and delayed menses.
Tamus: Ointment may be applied locally morning and night at onset of chilblains.
Rhus tox: 3X every six hours. Should be taken when there are inflamed chilblains with burning sensation. **Rhus** ointment should be applied.

Hydrotherapy **

Once a day do hot and cold showers for five to fifteen seconds each, alternating, four to six times. Use soft hairbrush to rub entire body toward heart.

Reflexology ****

In case of poor circulation and anemia it is important to press points for five minutes twice daily and continue with reflexology all over the feet and hands as a general massage for one hour:
16 lungs, 18 heart, 19 spleen, 24 liver, 25 gall bladder.

Schuessler Tissue Salts *

Ferrum phosphorica: 6X. Take one tablet in the morning.
Calcarea phosphorica: 6X. Take one tablet in the evening.
Natrum muriaticum: Add to above in case of anemia, one tablet at noontime.

THROMBOSIS AND PHLEBITIS

SUGGESTED TREATMENT

Acupuncture and Acupressure **

Because thrombosis is a cause of death we only consider the preventive measures. The best approach is to keep the circulatory system at peak and thus avoid this problem.
UB 14, UB 23, PC 6, ST 36, UB 11, SP 6.
For acute phlebitis:
GV 4, GV 12, GV 14, GV 20 and local points.

Applied Nutrition ***

Drink: Low-fat milk. Avoid whole milk and coffee.
Eat: Yogurt, green vegetables, vegetable oils, fresh fruits, whole rice, wheat grain bread free of salts. In this disease as well as all other cardiovascular disorders it is important to avoid table salts, fried food, saturated fatty acids, spicy foods, canned food, meat, fish, ice cream, butter, chocolate, dried fruits, nuts, and eggs.

It is recommended to use the juice fasting for three days and use the diet of:

30% vegetables
40% whole rice
10% fruits
5% low-fat fish
5% low-fat dairy products
10% whole cereals other than the whole rice
In addition, use vegetable oils and vegetable salts and drink at least four to ten cups of purified water per day.

An example of a diet for person of average weight, thirty years old:

1700 calories
50 g protein
70 g fat
220 g carbohydrate
Master formula and amino minerals chelated
500 mg calcium
380 mg magnesium
100 mg potassium
15 mg iron
15 mg zinc
10 mg manganese
30 mg chromium

Aromatherapy ***

For thrombosis or phlebitis and pulmonary disorders, liver disorders, diabetes, kidney stone disorders, and nervous disorders use the massage oil 2% of **juniper** all over the body, especially in the places of the thrombosis or phlebitis once per day for about fifteen minutes for two weeks. For thrombosis or phlebitis and rheumatism, asthma, bronchitis, gall stones, hypotension use **rosemary** as a massage oil 1% all over the body for thirty minutes daily for three weeks. It can also be used in the bath in combination with **juniper** (1% of each essence).
Note: It is important to remember that the aromatherapy as a massage is for prevention or for minor pain of phlebitis. When there is a thrombosis precaution must be taken not to move the thrombosis in the direction of the heart or lungs.

Autosuggestion

Repeat the following sentence twenty times each morning and evening:

> From day to day my blood circulation is stronger and healthier in every way.

Color Therapy *

Use red and yellow all over the body in general, thirty minutes per day for six days, then rest six days. Continue alternating. Use red locally to the part of the body affected.

Herbs

Western ****

In cases of local pain and inflamation of leg phlebitis it is best to apply external lotions, ointments, and poultices. The best plants are:

Arnica *(Arnica montana)*   **Marigold** *(Calendula)*
Comfrey *(Symphytum officinale)*

Chinese ****

Coptis and Rhubarb Combination *(San-Huang-Hsieh-Hsin-Tang)*: For those suffering arteriosclerosis and hypertension and prone to thrombosis and phlebitis.

Coptis rhizome 1 g
Scute 1 g
Rhubarb 1 g

Homeopathy

Hamamelis: For simple acute inflamation use 3X every hour.
Pulsatilla: For phlebitis after child delivery use 3X every hour and apply **hamamelis** ointment locally.
Bothrops lanciolatus: 6X or **lachesis** 200 are recommended (Materia Medica).

Reflexology **

In cases of thrombosis and phlebitis it is important to press and massage the whole foot or hand in addition to the specific location of the thrombosis or phlebitis. For foot thrombosis:
    point 34 in the atlas of reflexology.
In any case, to reinforce the vitality it is very important to massage:
    point 18 heart.

Schuessler Tissue Salts *

Kali phosphorica: 12X for thrombosis and mental depression, nervous tension, headaches.
Calcarea phosphorica: 12X for thrombosis and indigestion, very low vitality, anemia.
Calcarea fluorica: 12X for thrombosis and apatic relaxation, muscular weakness, poor blood circulation, skin cracks, tooth problems.

HEART WEAKNESS (PALPITATIONS)

SUGGESTED TREATMENT

Acupuncture and Acupressure ***

PC 4, PC 6, HT 7, BL 14, BL 15, Bl 39
For chronic heart palpitations use moxa on these points.
For acute cases massage on PC 4, PC 6, HT 7 for best results.

Applied Nutrition **

Drink: Four to six cups of distilled water per day. Avoid stimulating drinks like coffee, tea, or alcohol.
Eat: Whole rice well cooked or other whole cereals, fresh vegetables, unheated seeds, fresh bananas, fresh apples, fresh watermelons and melons. Avoid any stimulating food like white sugar, refined food, or saturated fatty acids, as this condition might occur due to allergy to foods, medicines, or particles in the air as well as other causes. Special attention should be given to finding the cause of palpitation. The nutrition should be enriched with a combination of chelated minerals.
An example of a diet for a person of average weight:

1800 calories	60 g fat
50 g protein	265 g carbohydrate

The following supplements are in addition to the master formula:

5000 IU vitamin A	600 mg calcium, chelated minerals
400 IU vitamin D	
400 IU vitamin E	300 mg magnesium, chelated minerals
30 mg B_1	
30 mg B_2	100 mg potassium, chelated minerals
30 mg niacin	
50 mcg B_{12}	10 mg iron, chelated minerals
1000 mg vitamin C	20 mg zinc, chelated minerals

10 mg Manganese, chelated min-   100 mg chromium, chelated
erals   minerals

Aromatherapy *
The following essences can be used as a massage oil or in the daily
bath:
Lavender for palpitation accompanied by asthma, bronchitis, depression, earaches, flatulence, headache.
Melissa for palpitation accompanied by fever, allergies, general colds,
hypertension, vertigo, vomiting.
Ylang-ylang for palpitation accompanied by frigidity, impotence, skin
problems, nervous tension.

Autosuggestion
This condition is due to fear of new events and fear of failure. Repeat
this suggestion to yourself at least ten times daily.

> *I love myself and accept new events calmly and relaxedly.*

Bach Flowers

Aspen: For palpitation in person with fears and anxieties of unknown origin.
Olive: When person is also physically and mentally exhausted.
Rescue remedy: For traumatic situations, to stablize emotions, ease
fear and panic. Place four drops of rescue remedy into a quarter glass
of water. Sip at three- to five-minute intervals as long as needed.

Color Therapy **
The color blue should be applied to the heart region for a time of ten
to thirty minutes per day until you feel more relaxed.

Herbs

Western
For nervous tachycardia due to stress and anxiety use this mixture:

Motherwort *(Leonorus cardiaca)* 2
Mistletoe *(Viscum alba)* 1
Valerian *(Valeriana officinalis)* 1
Hawthorn berries *(Crataegus):* Add to above mixture when hypertension and other heart problems are involved. The tea should be taken
two to three times daily. To prepare the infusion, pour a cup of boiling
water onto one to two teaspoonfuls of the mixture. Leave to infuse for

twenty minutes. Filter and drink. In tincture form: two to three ml of the mixture two to three times daily.

Chinese

Ginseng and Tang-Kuei Formula *(Jen-Sheng-Tang-Shao-San)*: Should be used when palpitations are accompanied by cold feet, dizziness, stiff shoulders, and anemia.

Chinese angelica root (Tang-Kuei) 3 g	Paichu rhizome (white atractylodes) 3 g.
Cndium 2.5 g.	Hoelen (China root) 3 g.
Peony root 3 g.	Ginseng root 3 g.
Alisma 3 g.	Licorice root 1 g.
Cinnamon twigs 1.5 g.	

Atractylodes and Hoelen Combination *(Ling-Kuei-Chu-Kan-Tang)*: For headaches, dizziness, severe palpitations.

Hoelen 6 g.	Licorice root 2 g.
Cinnamon twigs 4 g.	Paichu 3 g.

Homeopathy ****

Palpitation is a symptom of most heart disorders. Here we consider it as the major complaint.

Spigelia: The treatment of choice; 3X every two hours.

Lachesis: For palpitations at minimal excitement, 6X every two hours.

Nux vomica: When there is indigestion, flatulence after eating, and constipation, 3X is recommended every two hours.

Reflexology ***

Press for one to four minutes in the left hand and foot under the small finger. Point number 18 and point number 52 in right and left hands for autonomic nervous system. For two minutes, every day, in the morning and evening. Start each point for one minute per day and increase the time gradually to optional therapy time.

Schuessler Tissue Salts ***

For the strengthening of the heart nerves and supplying nutrition to the nerves use the following tissue salts three times per day.

Kali phosphorica: 6X potency, especially if the palpitation is accompanied by general tension of the body.

Magnesium phosphorica: 4X. A valuable nerve nutrient that acts well with **Kali phosphorica.** It helps steady nerves.

Calcarea phosphorica: 6X—this tissue salt is needed to increase the general nutrition of the nerves and the heart function.

ANGINA PECTORIS

SYMPTOMS

Severe chest pain, unrelated to exercise in most cases—difficulty breathing without tightening of chest muscles.

SUGGESTED TREATMENT

Acupuncture and Acupressure

CV 14, CV 17, PC 6, BL 15, BL 14, HT 5.

Applied Nutrition ****

As this condition causes difficulties in supplying oxygen to the heart, we should go onto the rejuvenating diet and the basic vitamins/minerals formula.

An example of a diet for an adult of average weight:

2100 calories	600 IU vitamin E
60 g protein	3,000 mg vitamin C
50 g fat	200 mg vitamin B_{15}
353 g carbohydrate	4,000 mg lecithin
10,000 IU vitamin A	140 mg raw heart glandular tablets
400 IU vitamin D	lets

Also minerals in the form of amino acid chelated minerals:

750 mg calcium	20 mg zinc
375 mg magnesium	94 mcg manganese
186 mg phosphorus	1 mg copper
42 mg potassium	35 mg chromium
20 mg iron	50 mcg selenium
6 mg sulphur (L-cysteine)	10 mcg molybdenum
.15 mg iodine (kelp)	

Aromatherapy **

Use **camphor** oil, very small quantity (about 1% of camphor in a base of vegetable oil), then apply external massage on the chest and back region.

Autosuggestion

Repeat the affirmation:

I breathe all the air I need for perfect health.

Bach Flowers *

Rescue Remedy: Four drops into a quarter glass of water, to be sipped every two to five minutes.

Color Therapy **

Apply yellow and red locally on the heart region for thirty minutes three times per day for ten to fifteen days.

Herbs

Western ****

Hawthorn berries *(Crataegus oxyacanthoides):*   To increase blood rich in oxygen to the heart through the coronary artieries, use on a regular basis.

Lime blossom *(Tilia europea);*   To help reduce cholesterol deposits. A basic combination tea is:

Hawthorn Berries *(Crataegus)* 3 parts	Lime blossom *(Tilia europea)* 2 parts
Motherwort *(Leonorus cardiaca)* 2 parts	Lily of the valley *(Convalaria magalis)* 1 part

In infusion add one teaspoonfull of mixture to a boiling cup of water; cover cup for twenty minutes, filter, and drink two to three times daily.

Mistletoe *(Viscum alba):*   Add one part when hypertension is also there.

Chinese ***

Bupleurum and Dragon Bone Combination (Chai-Hu-Chia-Lung-Ku-Li-Tang):

Bupleurum (hare's ear root) 5 g	Cinnamon twigs 3 g
Pinellia rhizome 4 g	Oyster shell 2.5 g
Skullcap root *(Scute)* 2.5 g	Hoelen 3 g
Jujube fruit 2.5 g	Rhubarb rhizome 1 g
Ginger root 2.5 g	Dragon bone 2.5 g
Ginseng root 2.5 g	

Homeopathy **

Black widow spider *(Lactodectus mactans* 30) or
Night-blooming cereus *(Cactus grandiflorus):*   One pilule every two to three minutes until pain decreases.

Reflexology *

Massage the whole foot base. Bathe feet for five minutes. Pay special attention to:

   kidney 21, heart 18, galbl. 25, liver 24, pancreas 22.

Then press in both hands and feet one minute each point two times per day.

   18, 19, 21, 22, 26, 52.

Schuessler Tissue Salts **

Magnesium phosphorica: 6X during and before the attack.
Kali phosphorica: 6X night and morning to be given between the attacks.

POST-MYOCARDIAL INFARCTION (HEART ATTACK)

SUGGESTED TREATMENT

Applied Nutrition ****

In case of post-M.I. it is recommended to eat properly a restricted diet, avoiding all unnatural foods.

Drink: Low-fat milk, pure water, mineral water, soda, pure juice of fruits or vegetables, herb teas. Avoid tea, cocoa, alcohol.

Eat: Green fresh vegetables, fresh fruits, whole grains, cereals, seeds, sea fish (salt-water fish), dairy products (yogurt, low-fat white cheese), half a tablet per day of master formula, camomile (one tablet per day), multi-amino-minerals chelated. Avoid cigarettes, all types of meat, poultry, and canned meats, fried food, saturated fatty acids, white sugar and foods containing white sugar, white wheat flour and food containing white wheat flour, table salt, all types of spices, artificial flavorings, artificial colorings, artificial preservatives in foods, canned food, and any type of processed food.

   The diet should be as near to the rejuvenating diet as possible. Also take the master vitamins and minerals formula and take 25,000 IU of beta-carotin as vitamin A and 400 IV vitamin E.

Autosuggestion **

The main causes of heart problems are emotional conflicts, lack of joy and happiness, rejection of love life, feeling of pressure and strain.
Repeat the following thirty times twice per day:

I accept myself joyfully. I accept all of life. I love myself and my way of life.

Bach Flowers

Rock rose: for panicky people
Heather and rock water: for overanxiousness
Olive: for physical exhaustion
Hornbeam: for mental exhaustion

Chelation Therapy ***

In post-M.I. the chelation therapy can be very useful in an intravascularly injected form but must be performed under the supervision of a qualified physician.

Herbs

Western

Garlic and parsley: Capsules two times, three times daily (**kyolic** O.K.)

Chinese **

Bupleurum and Dragon Bone Combination *(Chai-Hu-Chiang-Lung-Ku-Mu-Li-Tang):*

Bupleurum root 5 g	Cinnamon twigs 3 g
Pinnellia rhizome 4 g	Oyster shell 2.5 g
Scute root 2.5 g	Hoelen 3 g
Jujube fruit 2.5 g	Rhubarb rhizome 1 g
Ginseng root 2.5 g	Dragon bone 2.5 g

HYPOTENSION

SUGGESTED TREATMENT

*Acupuncture and Acupressure ****
GV 25, LIV 3, PC 6, ST 9, GV 26, LI 11, ST 36

*Applied Nutrition ***
The diet in hypotension should be rich in proteins, minerals, and vitamins of the B complex especially. An example of a diet for a patient of average weight, thirty years old:

2500 calories   70 g fat
70 g protein   398 g carbohydrate

Basic minerals/vitamins formula, and you may add salt to your food.

Aromatherapy **

Massage with 2% of **rosemary** essence oil in vegetable oil base. To be
used in all hypotension accompanied by reduction or loss of nerve
function such as paralysis, loss of speech, hysteria, epilepsy, debility,
apathy, doubts, and confusion.
Camphor: Two drops inhaled or in massage oil 1% in case of hypotension accompanied by heart failure, extreme shock, cardial disease, or infections like typhoid or pneumonia, or any condition with a
cold body.

Autosuggestion

Low blood pressure is mainly, from the point of view of the mind, a
state of fear, phobias of all kind, stress, and indecision. So the affirmation should be:

> *I am sure of myself, I am strong and healthy. I can do it now. I am*
> *protected and secure.*

Color Therapy *

The combination of green and yellow stimulates the heart and raises
the blood pressure. Apply this combination twice per day for fifteen
minutes for two weeks.

Herbs

Western ***

American and Asiatic ginseng: In tea form, place one half teaspoon of shredded root in one cup of water. Bring to boil for one and
one half minutes. Let stand twenty minutes. Drink once or twice daily.
In powder form, mix one gram (3/100 oz.) pulverized root in two or
three tablespoons of water. Take two or three times daily. Ginseng
should be taken on a regular basis if there is any degree of debility
present.
Oats *(Avena sativa)*, **kola** *(Cola vera)*, or **rosemary** *(Rosmarinus officin-*
alis):   In case of stress and nervous exhaustion, one should use nervine tonics.
To enjoy a **rosemary** bath, pour one half liter of water over fifty g.
Let stand for fifteen minutes. Strain the liquid and add it to the bath

water. Bathe at 33 to 35 degrees C (95°F) for no longer than ten minutes, *only* in the daytime. Rest for half an hour.

Chinese

Ginseng and Astragalus Combination *(Pu-Chung-I-Chi-Tang):* Indicated for those with tendency towards anemia, fatigue, and gastric disorders.

Astragalus 4 g	Tang-Kuei 3 g
Ginseng 4 g	Cimicifuga 1 g
Licorice 1.5 g	Ginger 2 g
Atractylodes 4 g	Jujube 2 g

Tang-Kuei and Paeonia Formula *(Tang-Kuei-Shao-Yad-San):* Effective for women with chills. It improves blood circulation and is a body tonic.

Homeopathy

Crataegus, oleander, and laurocrasis: Use 6X - 30C.
Broom *(Sarothamnus scoparius)*, **hawthorn berries** *(Crataegus)*, and **kola** *(Cola vera):* Combination may be drunk as an infusion. **CAUTION:** Broom is contraindicated in pregnancy and hypertension.

Hypnotherapy

As in hypertension, this condition, when caused by a constant mental state, can be wonderfully helped with hypnotherapy treatment by removing all the underlying fears, phobias, and stress.

Reflexology ***

In reflexology we treat the same points as in hypertension because the main treatment is to balance the body and its activities, so we treat all parts related to the heart, autonomic nervous system, kidneys, pituitary and hypopis, spleen, liver, and gall bladder. The points according to the atlas of reflexology are:
    52 (hands only), 1, 2, 3, 18, 19, 20, 21, 24, 25
for two minutes each point. Start with the hands and continue with the feet. Also massage both feet with the reflexology roller for nine minutes twice a day.

Schuessler Tissue Salts *

Natrum muriaticum, ferrum phosphorica, calcarea fluorica: Use 3X to 6X potency three times per day after meal.

VARICOSE VEINS

SUGGESTED TREATMENT

Acupuncture and Acupressure **
SP 5, SP 11, BL 38, ST 32, ST 36, CV 1.
May be pressed for ten minutes daily. Cannot help aesthetically, only prevents the situation from worsening.

Applied Nutrition ****
In this diet it is very important to avoid constipation. Therefore use the same diet as in constipation (see applied nutrition in constipation).
In case of ulcers use in addition to diet in constipation and master formula:

Vitamin E till 1,000 IU per day   Vitamin C till 5,000 mg per day
Vitamin A till 50,000 IU per day   Calcium 1,200 mg per day
Vitamin D till 1,000 IU per day

Aromatherapy *
Use **cypress** as an essence of 2% in a massage oil. This essence is especially good for women because of its properties. Also it can be very useful while massaging with this oil in the Lymph Drainage Massage system. Once per day for thirty minutes.

Autosuggestion
Repeat the following affirmation twenty times each morning and evening:

> From day to day all my tissues are becoming stronger and stronger in every way.

Color Therapy
Use red and yellow all over the affected area for thirty minutes once per day. In cases of ulcers in the legs use blue light radiation for thirty minutes followed by ultraviolet for forty-five minutes, every day for ten to sixty days.

Herbs

Western ***

Cayenne (Capsicum minimum), **ginger** (Zingiberis officinalis), **Rue** (Ruta gravelones), **Prickly ash** (Zanthoxylum americanum): To increase leg and peripheral circulation, teas and tinctures are best. These teas are

made as infusion and can be taken three times daily for a few weeks.
Buckwheat *(Fagopyrum esculentum)*, **hawthorn berries** *(Crataegus)*, and **Horsechestnut** *(Aesculus hippocastanum):* Important to tonify the blood vessels.
Yarrow *(Achillea)* and **dandelion** *(Taraxacum):* Diuretics, required in case of water retention—edema of ankles. The following mixture tries to take care of all these problems:

Hawthorn berries 3 parts   Yarrow 2 parts
Horsechestnut 3 parts   Ginger 1 part
Prickly ash bark 2 parts

Use two teaspoonfuls of the mixture. Infuse for fifteen minutes. Drink three times daily.

Homeopathy *

Hamamelis: Tincture or lotion may be applied locally at night. Hamamelis 3X every three hours when veins are affected.
Pulsatilla: 3X is recommended every eight hours after child delivery.
Carbo vegetabilis: When constipated and with poor circulation.
In cases of ulcers of varicose veins:
Mercurius sol: If accompanied by infection, pus, and foul-smelling discharge.
Lachesis: Blue color in area mainly on *left* side.

Lymph Drainage Massage
Before applying lymph drainage massage, the diet for this condition should be followed for at least one month. Also, it must be applied with extreme caution in case of a thrombose in the veins of the legs, as they might move to the heart and cause an M.I. Consult, a licensed physician before applying this massage. This is a very special deep massage. With the thumb press firmly and deeply, always in the direction of the blood flow in the veins. Repeat this deep massage for about twenty minutes to each vein, always in the same direction. Try to put the vein in place and move the blood into the heart. While massaging the whole leg—always in the direction of the heart. Use the whole open hands on the leg in a circular motion. Start from the feet and work toward the upper leg and thigh.

Reflexology *
In cases of varicose veins and ulcers reflexology can do much by massaging the whole feet or hands and pressing the following points three

times per day for five minutes each point after massaging the whole feet:
   18, 19, 24, 25, 21, 22, 34, 26.

Schuessler Tissue Salts

Calcarea fluorica: 6X when the veins are dilated, or when there is a tendency to varicose ulcerations or bluish discoloration of the tissues or muscular weakness.
Ferrum phosphorica: 6X for inflammation of the veins, red streaks following the course of vein, throbbing pain along a vein. Can be used as alternative to calcarea fluorica. Also good for those suffering from inflammation and those who are advanced in years.
Magnesium phosphorica: 6X for severe, acute, cramplike, spasmodic pains. Also for those suffering from flatulence or neuralgia.

LYMPHATIC DISORDERS

SYMPTOMS

Swollen glands, dizziness, or headache, and overall weakness.

SUGGESTED TREATMENT

Acupuncture and Acupressure **

In adenopathy and all glandular diseases where there appears swelling use:
BL 19, BL 60, LI 13, HT 3, LI 4, SP 6, ST 36, PC 4, TW 6, TW 10, LI 11.
In some cases of lymph vessel and node inflation bleed:
PC 3.
For axillary lymph problems add:
GB 22, GB 40.
For burning sensation of lymph nodes add:
PC 7, LIV 3.
For inflammation of lymph nodes in neck add
LI 10, GB 41, TW 10.
For inflammation of groin add:
SP 11, ST 30.
For congestion and inflammation of female genitalia add:
K 2, K 10.

Applied Nutrition ****

In all cases of inflammation affecting the lymphatic glands and system the cleansing diet is very important.

Drink: Avoid dairy products such as cream and milk, alcohol, beer, coffee, tea, and cocoa.

Eat: Avoid red meats, white meats, greasy, fatty foods, dairy products such as cheese, butter, and yogurt, vinegar, pickles, white sugar and products containing sugar, white wheat flour and products containing wheat flour, artificial additives, preservatives, colorings.

It is recommended to use the three-day cleansing juice while fasting and rejuvenating diet after fasting. The following is an example of a diet for an adult of average weight:

1900 calories	800 IU vitamin E
50 g protein	5,000 IU vitamin C
60 g fat	3,000 mg lecithin
290 g carbohydrate	B complex
25,000 IU vitamin A	Multi-minerals in amino minerals
400 IU vitamin D	chelated form

Aromatherapy **

Apply the aromatherapy as an odor only for two minutes twice daily for a period of one week and also apply locally as a massage oil once a day for a period of two weeks.

Benzoin 2%:   Apply in case of lymphatic inflammation accompanied by skin irritation or skin wounds.

Camomile 2%:   Use in case of lymphatic inflammation accompanied by fever and anemia.

Camphor 1%:   Use in case of lymphatic inflammation accompanied by general pains, burns, heart failure.

Lavender 2%:   Use in case of lymphatic inflammation accompanied by diarrhea, colic, nervous tension, hypertension, headache, earache, fainting.

Autosuggestion

The main mental cause is lack of joy and feelings of unwelcome. In this case repeat the following affirmations twenty times each morning and evening:

> *My world is filled with joy, and I love myself. I am welcome and wanted in this world.*

Color Therapy *

Apply locally ultraviolet for thirty minutes twice daily for a period of twelve days. It is advised to apply massage oil or aromatherapy oil on the glands affected before applying the color therapy. Do not massage the infected areas.

Herbs

Western

The main herbs used for lymphatic drainage and cleansing are:

Golden seal *(Hydrastis)*   Poke root *(Phytolacca americana)*
Echinacea   Cleavers *(Galium aparine)*
Marigold *(Calendula)*

Teas of each or a mixture can be taken three times daily.

Chinese **

Besides the lancing procedure in case of lymphadenitis, chinese herbology recommends the following formula:

Bupleurum and Schizonepeta Formula *(Shih-Wei-Pai-Tu-San):* Indicated in presence of lymphadenitis, chronic inflammations, furnucles, and anthrax.

Bupleurum (hare's ear root) 3 g   Tang-kuei 2 g
Platycodon (baloon flower root)   Schizonepeta 1 g
3 g   Licorice root 1 g
Ginger rhizome 1 g   Cnidium 3 g
Hoelen 1 g   Pseudocerasi bark (cherry bark)
Siler root 2 g   3 g

Homeopathy **

Belladonna: In case of acute stages and at the onset of glandular swelling use 3X daily every one to two hours.
Baryta carb: 6X hourly; can be taken if belladonna has not been very effective in twenty-four to forty-eight hours.
Arum triphyllum: For submaxillary gland swelling 6X every two to four hours.
Mercurius sol: In cases of suppuration in inguinal glands, 6X four to six times daily.
Silicea: After drainage and evacuation of gland use 6X four to six times daily.
Calendula or **Aloe:**   externally, lotions may be applied.

Reflexology **

The reflexology treatment is very important in improving the blood and lymphatic circulation and in this way healing inflammations af-

fecting the lymphatic glands. Press the following points for three minutes each morning and evening on the hands:

18, 19, 24, 25.

Also massage the whole foot twice a day, the sole and upper parts of
the foot. Stimulate by massage the lymphatic reflex points all along the
left and right ankle junction. Press your fingers into the reflex points
of the lymphatic system. Using your thumb and fingers, stretch the
skin from heel toward the toes, using moderate pressure. Also massage
and stretch the affected parts of the body presented in the reflexology
point of the foot.

Schuessler Tissue Salts *

Use the following salts twice a day:

Calcarea fluorica: In the cases of lymphatic inflammation accompanied by poor circulation.

Calcarea sulphorica: In cases of lymphatic inflammation by skin
ailments and wounds that are slow to heal.

Ferrum phosphorica: In cases of lymphatic inflammation accompanied by respiratory ailments, sore throat, or bleeding.

· 5 ·

PAIN AND
NEUROLOGICAL
DISORDERS

There are many pain-sensitive structures of the head: the tissues covering the cranium, specific cranial nerves (fifth, ninth, and tenth primarily), and the upper cervical nerves. When there is some sort of stimulation or pressure in these areas a common headache is likely to result. The vast majority of headaches are easily understood by the sufferer as the result of an immediate cause (being in the sun too long, overindulgence, emotional tension, excessive noise, etc.). They respond quickly to aspirin or similar pain relievers. Only in the last few years has the mechanism of aspirin been understood: This and other drugs inhibit the action of neurotransmitters, the prostaglandins and prostacyclins that carry pain messages to the brain.

Headaches may also, but far less frequently, be a sign of serious illness: systemic infections, severe hypertension, eye problems, digestive or respiratory malfunctions. When headaches occur chronically the masking of the pain with painkillers is, of course, treating the symptoms and not the cause.

One type of chronic headache, migraine, probably is unrelated to any disease state other than circulation in the head itself. It is believed that the pain of migraine results from dilation of the arteries of the scalp (dura). Flashes of light, distorted vision, and other unusual aspects of migraine are attributed to constriction of the blood vessels within the cerebrum ("intracerebral vasoconstriction"). Women between the ages of ten and thirty are by far the most frequent sufferers of these headaches. Migraine also tends to run in families but usually recedes after age fifty.

The neurotransmitters are only one class of chemical substances transported in the blood in response to any sort of injury or trauma. The most overt act of the immune system, which we will discuss directly in Part Eight, is to rush "defense troops" such as lymphocytes and thrombocytes to an injured area. For example, when you fall and skin your knee the capillaries in the area become more permeable to allow these chemicals to surround the "foreign" intrusion. Thus the area swells with liquids and becomes red. The healing process begins with the formation of scar tissue with the help of fibroblasts carried in the bloodstream. Accordingly, the better the blood flow the faster and sounder the healing process.

Traumas of this kind are easier to understand than pains within the body—the most common of which are back pains. Lower back pain, in particular, can come on suddenly and be completely debilitating. There are diseases and structural problems of the spine that can lead to acute or chronic back pain, such as disk abnormalities or curvature of the spine. "Throwing the back out" from improper lifting or other strain can also be treated from a structural standpoint. But typical, sporadic lower back pain is usually more elusive. It may be local—an irritation of nerve endings via anything from a blast of cold air to doing sit-ups improperly. Or it may be from a distant source—"referred" pain—like the pelvis or abdomen. When such pain emanates from a root disease or other malady to a wide area, it is called "radicular." Finally, muscular spasms often accompany back pain as a protective mechanism of the body—and these often require extreme measures, such as traction.

Sciatica is a form of pain originating at the base of the spine but extending from the buttocks to the toes—the length of the sciatic nerve. Once considered the result of rupture of a disk or of osteoarthritis of the lower spine, it is now frequently encountered in sports medicine with overdevelopment of the posterior muscles. In either case, the result is compression of the sciatic nerve at the base of the spine, with spasmodic pain lasting for several months. The pain can be acute in the case of a ruptured intervertebral disk.

All the major joints of the body—ankles, knees, hips, elbows, and shoulders—share common maladies that are as elusive in causation as back pain. Muscles, ligaments, tendons, and bones are all suspect. Various structural tests—Is the pain localized? Can the joint be twisted? etc.—will usually determine the underlying problem. Rheumatoid arthritis, isolated infections, and calcium deposition are as likely to be responsible as overuse or injuries in sports. The role of the neurotransmitters in causing inflammation as a reaction to trauma is important in all joint problems.

Far less frequent neurological problems, but far more serious, are facial neuralgia, epilepsy, and parkinsonism.

The trigeminal nerve controls the chewing process and accordingly the major facial muscles. Although it is not known why this nerve occasionally is the subject of stabbing pains, sometimes leading to facial paralysis, most victims experience sensitive areas around the mouth and nose.

Convulsions or seizures of epilepsy affect one of every two hundred people, in varying degrees. In children, a good portion of such episodes can be traced to some sort of brain damage. In adult onset there are few specific causes that have been identified, although infections and toxic agents are often associated with the disease.

Parkinson's is a disease of the central nervous system characterized by tremor, muscular rigidity, and weakness. Symptoms resembling parkinsonism result frequently from poisoning or overdoses of tranquilizers. The disease is not confined to the older population but must be carefully diagnosed at any age. Outbreaks of the disease have coincided with epidemics of encephalitis (1919–1924) and are now a matter of great concern because of the increased use of psychoactive drugs in our society.

HEADACHES AND MIGRAINE HEADACHES

SUGGESTED TREATMENT

Acupuncture and Acupressure ****
For general headaches, massage these points:
   GV 24, GV 20, GV 19, GV 16, UB 7, UB 4, UB 10, GB 21, UB 13, LI 4, LI 11.
For lateral temporal pain:
   GB 7, TW 20, GB 12.
Acupuncture points
For whole-head headache:
   GV 20, GB 20, GV 16, LI 4, UB 40, UB 60.
Vertex headache:
   GV 20, GB 20, K 1, LIV 3, K 3, LI 4.
Frontal headache:
   LI 4, ST 36, ST 8, GV 23, Yin Tang, UB 2.

Occipital headache:
  GB 20, UB 60, SI 3.
Parietal headache:
  GV 20, SI 3, UB 67, LIV 3.
Headache from tiredness:
  CV 6, ST 36.
Headache with dizziness:
  LI 17, UB 12, UB 60, CV 4, TW 1.
Migraine with vomiting, fullness of chest, and vertigo:
  GB 20, Tai-yang, GV 20, LIV 3, GB 8, TW 3, CV 12, ST 40, PC 6.
Ear points: subcortex, forehead, occiput, kidneys, pancreas, gall bladder, and points of tenderness in ears.

Applied Nutrition ***

Commence the diet with three days of juice fasting. Then continue with the "rejuvenating diet" below. A cytotoxic blood test is very important to test for allergic reactions. An example of a diet for a person of average weight, thirty years old:

2400 calories
50 g protein
100 g fat
325 g carbohydrate
Master Formula of vitamins and
minerals and also:
3,000 mg vitamin C
1,500 mg bioflavanoids
25,000 IU vitamin A
1,000 IU vitamin D

1,000 IU vitamin E
B_{50} complex (one tablet per day)
2,000 mg calcium
800 mg magnesium
15 mg iron
100 mcg chromium
50 mg zinc
50 mcg iodine
100 mcg selenium

Enzyme Formula

150 mg betaine hydrochloric acid
150 mg pancreatin
150 mg bile extract

75 mg pepsin
120 mg lipase
120 mg papain

Nucleoprotein Formula

50 mg pituitary extract
50 mg adrenal extract
50 mg thymus extract

50 mg pancreas extract
50 mg kidney extract
50 mg RNA extract

General Supplements

2,400 mg lecithin
3,000 mg brewer's yeast

800 mg alfalfa

Aromatherapy
Taken internally twice per day, five tablets of brown sugar containing the following extracts:

Camomile 8x   Marjoram 4x
Lavender 4x   Mint 4x

Autosuggestion **
Reduce stress wherever possible—see Part Ten. This type of meditation is often helpful. Repeat the following affirmations twenty times, recording them on a cassette. Then listen to the tape twice a day:

> *From day to day I am more relaxed, happier, and healthier.*
> *I love myself unconditionally.*
> *From day to day I enjoy more peace, love, joy, relaxation, and health.*
> *I am well, and in my world all is well.*
> *I relax into the flow of life and let life flow through me with ease.*
> *I am flexible, open, and accepting. I welcome other viewpoints, too.*
> *From day to day I feel better and better in every way.*
> *From day to day I am better and better in every way.*

Color therapy
Radiate the following colors twice a day, one after the other, locally:

Blue—thirty minutes
Violet—fifteen minutes

Herbs

Western **
Balm *(Melissa officinalis)*, **Lavender** *(Lavendula)*, **Meadowsweet** *(Filipendula ulmaria)*:   For headaches resulting from gastro intestinal disorders. Infusion (three to four times daily) or capsules/tincture.
Rhubarb, balmony, or **cascara:**   Add if there is constipation.
Valerian, Skullcap *(Scutelaria)*, **Passiflora:**   Add for headaches due to nervous tension.
Lavender: bath is a good relaxant.
Lavender, rosemary, marjoram, or **peppermint:**   Local massage with oil.
Other useful single herbs for headache:
Blue flag *(Iris versicolor)*: a tincture dose of ten drops to half a cup of water is helpful for right supraorbital headache accompanied by nausea and vomiting.
Wood betony *(Betonica officinalis)*:   Eases neuralgic-type headache. Infusion, tincture, capsules.

For migraine attack:
Black willow *(Salix nigra):* in decoction
Wood betony
Jamaican dogwood *(Piscidia erythrina):* In decoction for migraine accompanied by insomnia or dysmenorrhea.
Black horehound *(Ballota nigra):* For nausea and vomiting. Combines well with **meadowsweet** and **camomile** in infusion. **Damiana, kola, sarsaparilla, ginseng:** Recommended when migraine is due to fatigue, lassitude, and general debility.

Chinese **

Cnidium and Tea Formula: For common cold, headache, women's habitual headache caused by occluded blood.
Bupleurum and Paeony Formula: For vertigo, "flushing-up", menoxenia, heavy head.
Gambir Formula: For headache due to hypertension.
Evodia Combination: For severe paroximal headache with vomiting.
Hoelen Five-Herb Formula: For headache with thirst and oliguria.
Ma-Huang, Asarum, and Aconite Combination: For headache with chills in old and emaciated people.
Cinnamon and Ginseng Combination: For headache due to gastrointestinal weakness, gastroptosis.

Homeopathy ****

Pulsatilla: 3 to 30X for periodic throbbing headache associated with indigestion of fatty foods. Condition improves outdoors and worsens lying down.
Ignatia: 6X to 7X daily for bandlike pressure headache across the forehead accompanied by nausea and dizziness.
Arnica: 3X to 6X in short intervals for bruised-like ache worsened by movement of frontal region.
Aconitum: 1X to 3X at onset of headache.
Belladonna: 3X to 30X for burning, throbbing ache.
Iris: For right-sided headache with vomiting.
Gronoine: For throbbing pain intensified by heat or exposure to sun.
Nux vomica: 3X to 30X for splitting headache after eating with nausea and vomiting.
Gelsemium: For right-sided headache over eye or temple intensified by movement and noise.
For migraine:
Lycopodium: For right-eye pain, nausea, and dizziness, worse in

afternoon and evening. This remedy is complemented well by **chele-donium,** and they can follow each other at 1X to 2X every two hours.
Spigelia: For left-sided pain due to fatigue and general debility.
Phell: 3 every four hours for intense pain at top of head, burning temples and sinuses, tearing, and intolerance to light and sound.

Hydrotherapy
Very often a few glasses of water or juice, taken early, will reduce headache pain. For long-term problems, try alternating hot and cold showers once a day. This improves blood circulation and in many cases eliminates or reduces headaches.

Reflexology **
Press the following points every hour until pain is over. Then continue with the same treatment until one month after the headache or migraine is over. For three minutes each point:

1—sinuses-in each finger, 6—eye, 7—temple, 9—ear, 12—spine, 24—liver, 52—autonomic nervous system, 55—general pain—in each finger.

Schuessler Tissue Salts
Take five tablets of each of the following every half hour until the pain is over:

Ferrum phosphorica: 6X   **Kali phosphorica:** 6X

After the attack is over take five tablets of each of the following twice a day for one month after all symptoms are over:

Ferrum phosphorica: 12X   **Silica:** 6X
Kali phosphorica: 12X   **Magnesia phosp:** 12X
Natrum muriaticum: 6X   **Natrum sulphorica:** 6X

MUSCULAR ATROPHY

SUGGESTED TREATMENT

In these disorders a combination of as many therapies as can be done is very important. Also, the mental state should be taken into consideration. The patient should stay calm and relaxed. Meditation is a good exercise for these disorders. The cure of these disorders is very difficult but can be helped. The treatment is very long and sometimes for life.

Acupuncture ***
Spinal muscular atrophy:
    GB 20, GV 14, GV 6, GV 7, GV 4, HT 3, GB 30

For dystonia musculorum:
GB 20, GV 16, CV 12, LIV 3, KI.
In general:
GB 34, GB 39, SP 6, ST 36, TW 5, GV 4, LI 4 in tonification, GV 20.

Applied Nutrition *

Take the same diet therapy as in the "General Treatment of Immune Disorders."
Also take 5,000 mg brewer's yeast divided during the day into six portions.

Autosuggestion

Repeat the same cassette with affirmations as in the case of "General Treatment of Immune Disorders."

Color Therapy

Radiate the following colors one after the other, twice per day, all over the body:

Red—thirty minutes   Yellow—thirty minutes
Orange—thirty minutes   Green—five minutes

Herbs

Chinese

Rehmannia Eight Formula: For sensory paralysis, numbness, weakness of the legs and feet.
Astragalus Combination: As a general tonic.

Homeopathy

Iodum: 3X, every 6 hours with fever.
Arsenicum album: 3X, every 6 hours for wasting of muscles and paralysis.
Sarsaparila: 6X, every 9 hours for skin in folds.
Abrut: 30, every 4 hours for general marasmus, legs most wasted, from below upward.

Reflexology **

Massage the whole feet and hands three times per day, ten minutes each foot and hand.
Press the following points three times per day until condition improves. Then continue twice per day, three minutes each point:

2—pituitary, 3—cerebrum, 4—cerebellum, 11—parathyroid, 12—spine, 13—thyroid, 16—lung, 17—solar plexus, 18—heart, 20—adrenal gland, 21—kidney, 22—pancreas, 24—liver, 35—sciatic, 51—thymus, 52—autonomic nervous system.

Schuessler Tissue Salts
Take the following remedies one after the other:

Calcarea phosphorica: 3X in the first week, 6X in the second week, 12X in the third week.
Kali phosphorica: 6X
Calcarea fluorica: 6X

Ferrum phosphorica: 12X
Kali muriaticum: 12X
Silica: 12X
Natrum phosphorica: 6X with undigested foods.

LOCAL TRAUMA

SUGGESTED TREATMENT

The trauma should get immediate first-aid treatment and, if needed, further treatment by conventional methods.

Acupuncture ****
Local points.

Applied Nutrition
The same diet as in headache.

Aromatherapy
Take internally five tablets of the following extracts on brown sugar tablets every hour until pain is over:

Camomile 12X
Rosemary 4X

Anise 4X

Autosuggestion
The same as in headache.

Color Therapy
Radiate the colors one after the other until pain is over:

Blue—thirty minutes

Violet—fifteen minutes

External Treatment
Also apply wheat-germ oil on the trauma externally.

Homeopathy ***

Arnica: 3 every thirteen to thirty minutes.

Thuya: 3–30.
Rhus tox: For muscular bruise.

Hypnotherapy

Hypnotherapy is very effective in reducing any pain in the body.

Reflexology

To relieve any pain in the body press the following points every hour until pain is over:

52—autonomic nervous system   55—general pain

Schuessler Tissue Salts

Take every half hour the following remedies until pain is over, five tablets of each:

Ferrum phosphorica: 12X
Kali phosphorica: 12X   **Natrum muriaticum:** 12X

BACK PAIN (UPPER AND LOWER BACK)

SUGGESTED TREATMENT

Applied Nutrition

Take the same diet therapy as in the headache diet.

Aromatherapy

Massage the whole back daily with vegetable oil as a base for the following extracts: **camomile** 12%, **geranium** 6%, **lavender** 6%.

Autosuggestion ***

Repeat the same as in headache.

Color Therapy

Radiate the following colors three times per day until condition of pain is over:

blue—thirty minutes   orange—ten minutes
yellow—fifteen minutes   green—five minutes.

Hypnotherapy **

Can alleviate the pain and stiffness of the back.

Reflexology

Press the following points every hour until pain is over, five minutes each point:

12–spine–press in the most painful place, 52–autonomic nervous system, 55–general pains

Schuessler Tissue Salts

Take every half hour the following remedies until pain is over:

Ferrum phosphorica 12X   **Natrum muriaticum** 12X
Calcarea phosphorica 6X   **Kali phosphorica** 12X

SCIATIC PAIN

SUGGESTED TREATMENT

Acupuncture/Acupressure ****
UB 40, UB 60, GB 30, GB 34, GV 4, LI 4

Applied Nutrition
Take the same diet therapy as in headache diet therapy.

Aromatherapy
Massage with the following extracts in vegetable oil base daily before the color therapy: **pine** 12%, **camomile** 8%, **marjoram** 4%.

Autosuggestion
Repeat the same cassette as in the headache treatment.

Color Therapy
Radiate the following colors twice per day locally:

red—fifteen minutes   green—ten minutes.
violet—twenty minutes

Hypnotherapy
Hypnotherapy is very useful in all cases of pain control.

Homeopathy ****
Colocoynth: 6X when worse in cold and damp weather.
Gelsemium: 6X to 12X when worse when resting at night.

Reflexology ****

Press every hour five minutes each point until pain is over:

34–leg, lower leg, 35–sciatic–7 minutes each foot, 12–spine, 52–autonomic nervous system, 55–general pain.

Schuessler Tissue Salts

Take the following remedies every hour until pain is over. Then continue twice per day with the same remedies until three weeks after pain is over:

Ferrum phosphorica 12X   **Kali phosphorica** 6X
Kali muriaticum 6X   **Calcarea phosphorica** 6X

LARGE JOINT PAIN

SUGGESTED TREATMENT

Acupuncture/Acupressure ****
Elbow: LI 4, LI 10, LI 11, ST 37, TW 10
Shoulder: LI 15, TW 14, LI 4, GB 21
Neck: SI 3, GV 14, GB 21, UB 60
Hip: GB 30, GB 34
Ankle: ST 41, SP 5, K 3, UB 60, UB 62
Wrist: LI 4, TW 4, PC 7, SI 5, LU 7

Applied Nutrition
The same diet therapy as in headache.

Aromatherapy **
Massage locally the painful area before the color therapy daily with the extracts of **camomile** 16%, **lavender** 4%, **eucalyptus** 4%.

Autosuggestion
The same as for headache.

Color Therapy
Radiate the following colors three times per day locally on the painful area:

blue—thirty minutes   violet—fifteen minutes.
green—fifteen minutes

Hypnotherapy
The same as for headache.

Homeopathy
Arnica, Rhus, Tox, Ruta: 6X 3 to 6 times daily until pain disappears.

Reflexology ***
Press the following points for any pain in the joints every hour for five minutes each point until pain is over.
For pain control of: leg, knee, hip, lower back, toes, press the following points:

12–spine–lower part; 34–leg, knee, hip; 35–sciatic; 52–autonomic nervous system; 55–general pain

For pain control of: wrist, hand, elbow, shoulder, neck, fingers, press the following points:

12–spine–upper part, 52–autonomic nervous system, 55–general pain, 24–liver, 18–heart

Schuessler Tissue Salts
Take the following remedies for any joint pain in the body, five tablets of each remedy every hour until condition improves:

Ferrum phosphorica 12X   **Natrum phosphorica** 6X
Kali phosphorica 12X   **Calcarea phosphorica** 6X
Kali muriaticum 12X   **Silica** 6X

FACIAL NEURALGIA AND PARALYSIS

SUGGESTED TREATMENT

Acupuncture **
ST 36, ST 3, ST 4, ST 5, ST 6, ST 7, ST 8, LI 4, LI 20, SI 19, GB 20, TW 17, TW 23, TW 5, GB 41, GV 20. Tai-yang, Yin-tang.
Use Moxa but not in face and eyes.
Ear points: Face, Adrenal, Shen-men, Neurogate.

Applied Nutrition
Take the same diet therapy as in the headache treatment diet therapy.

Aromatherapy *

Take internally for facial neuralgia on brown sugar tablets, twice per day, five tablets: **camomile** 18% and **geranium** 6%. Massage the whole affected area with the following extracts daily in vegetable oil base: **basil** 12%, **juniper** 4%, **lavender** 8%. Use in every case of paralysis in which the nerves are not damaged or destroyed.

Autosuggestion **

The same as in headache treatment.

Color Therapy

In facial neuralgia radiate the colors twice per day: blue, fifteen minutes; violet, ten minutes; green, 10 minutes. In paralysis radiate the colors twice per day: red, thirty minutes; yellow, fifteen minutes; orange, ten minutes; green, five minutes.

Herbs

Western

Damiana: A good nerve tonic and muscular tonic.

Ginseng: In tea or elixir or capsules

Masterwort *(Imperatoria ostruthium):*   One ounce of powdered root in a pint of boiling water; steep a few minutes. Drink half a cup two or three times daily.

Chinese

Pueraria Combination: In the initial stage of the disease, especially after a cold.

Cinnamon and Aconite Combination: For external weakness conformation.

Siler and Chiang-Huo Combination: At the numbness conformation.

Astragalus and Cinnamon Five Combination and **Astragalus and Vitrex Combination:**   Both are indicated for the symptoms of pale complexion and generalized edema in women.

Smilax and Akebia Combination: For syphilitic facial paralysis.

Ma-Huang and Ginseng Combination: Use during the lingering period following an acute episode of the disease with no symptoms other than paralysis.

Homeopathy ***

Aconite: 3, every hour—when from cold, at first.
Caustic: 6, every 2 hours—when from cold, if it does not yield soon.

Kali Chloricum: 3 every 2 hours—when there is tenderness of the part affected.
Graphaitis: 6 every 4 hours—with swelling.

Hypnotherapy
The same as in headache treatment.

Reflexology
Press the same points as in the headache treatment.

Schuessler Tissue Salts
Ferrum phosphorica 12X, **natrum phosphorica** 12X, **Silica** 6X: For facial neuralgia take five tablets every hour.
Kali phosphorica 30X, **kali phosphorica** 12X, **kali muriaticum** 12 X, **calcarea phosphorica** 12X, **silica** 6X: For paralysis take three times per day.

EPILEPSY

SYMPTOMS

Episodic convulsions, including loss of consciousness and physical control.

SUGGESTED TREATMENT

Let the patient lie down comfortably. Do not try to stop the attack. Tight clothing can be loosened; the patient should be turned to the side to allow excess saliva to flow freely.
Do not try to open the patient's mouth or to force anything between the teeth. The patient should rest after the attack.

Acupuncture and Acupressure **
Acupressure or shiatsu may be used to reduce the frequency and shorten duration of attacks of true epilepsy. First press:
   GV 20, GV 21, GV 19, UB 10, GB 20.
To relax and stop spasms of extremities:
   UB 63, UB 13, UB 15, UB 22, UB 23.

To relieve chills of attack:
  LI 11, ST 36, SP 6.
Use pressure and Moxa together.
In case of constipation add:
  ST 25, CV 12.
Acupuncture points:
  GV 16, GB 20, GV 26, GV 14, M-BW-29 (Yao Qi).
For petit mal add:
  PC 6, HT 7, GV 24.
For psychomotor-type epilepsy add:
  PC 5, CV 12, HT 7.
For focal epilepsy add:
  LiV 3, LI 4.
To relax muscles add:
  GB 34, SP 6.
Between seizures:
  CV 4, K 3 needling or moxa.

Applied Nutrition
The same diet therapy as in headache.

Aromatherapy
Take the following extract internally on brown sugar base, five tablets twice per day: **thyme** 12%, **juniper** 4%, **lavender** 4%.

Autosuggestion
As in headache therapy.

Color Therapy
Radiate the following colors one after the other daily: violet, thirty minutes; indigo, fifteen minutes; blue, ten minutes.

Herbs

Western ***
Hyssop *(Hyssopus officinalis):* Infusion for petit mal.
Skullcap *(Scutelaria laterifolia):* Infusion for epileptic seizures.
Caroba *(Yacaranda caroba, Bigonia caroba):* Has soothing effect on nervous system.
Lycopodium *(Calvatum):* As an internal remedy, the ground spores are mixed with lactose as follows: ten parts of spore powder to ninety parts lactose. Make decoction by boiling an ounce of the mixture with

one pint of water for fifteen minutes. Dosage: one tablespoon three times daily.

Mistletoe *(Viscum album):*   The leaves in infusion for convulsions.

Chinese ***

Gentiana Combination: "For reducing liver fire," according to Chinese traditional principles.

Replenishing the Left Yin Pills *(Chuo-Kuei-Wan):*   For dizziness, night sweats, tinnitus, and epilepsy.

Six Major Herb Combination: For epilepsy accompanied by sputum, vomiting, fullness of chest. (Damp phlegm accumulation, according to T. C. M.)

Bupleurum and Cinnamon: For epileptic seizures.

*Homeopathy ***

For recent epilepsy:

Kali Cyanatum: 3 every eight hours for falling, violent convulsions, and dyspnea.

Belladonna: 1X to 3X four times for young children.

Kali Bromium: 30 every eight hours when at menstrual period.

For chronic epilepsy:

Bufo: 6 every eight hours.

Plumbum Metalicum: 30 twice daily for constipation, cachexia

Absinthium: 3 every eight hours for petit mal

Stramonium: 3 every six hours for epilepsy caused by fright and for stammering.

Hypnotherapy

As in headache therapy.

*Reflexology ***

Press the following points twice per day, five minutes each point:

2–pituitary, 3–cerebrum, 4–cerebellum, 12–spine, 52–autonomic nervous system

Schuessler Tissue Salts

Take the following remedies three times per day, five tablets each:

Kali muriaticum: 12X
Silica: 12X

Calcarea Phosphorica: 6X

PARKINSON'S DISEASE

SYMPTOMS

Tremor and rigidity of muscles, with other problems of the central nervous system usually associated with drug abuse. Inability to stop nervous shaking, loss of muscle control, general weakness.

SUGGESTED TREATMENT

By using natural methods we can reduce the problem, but it is very hard to cure this disease.

Acupuncture *

GV 14, K 3, LIV 3, SP 6, LiV 2, UB 18.
Ear points: Brain stem, Shen-men, Occiput, Subcortex, Liver.
For Parkinson's Paralysis Agitans:
   GV 20, GV 21, GB 20, CV 23

Applied Nutrition

Commence the diet with three days juice fasting. Then continue with the rejuvenating diet therapy.
Drink: Avoid any stimulants, alcohol, beer, wine, coffee.
Eat: Avoid any stimulants, refined or processed foods, smoking, etc.
The diet therapy is the same as in headache treatment.

Autosuggestion

The same as for headache.

Color Therapy

Radiate the following colors twice per day until condition improves: orange, fifteen minutes; green, thirty minutes.

Herbs

Western

Passion flower (*Passiflora*):   Infusion

Chinese

Minor Rhubarb Combination with **Paeonia and Licorice Combination:**   Taken three to four times with an ordinary dose of **magnolia bark,** this formula will stop tremors and relax muscle stiffness.

The quantity of rhubarb is adjusted according to the condition of bowel movement.

Bupleurum Formula with **Paeonia and Licorice Combination** plus **magnolia:**   This combination is for persons with irritability, debilitating anxiety, and insomnia.

Homeopathy **

Anthimonium Tartaricum: six every two hours for trembling of head and paralytic hands tremor.

Reflexology *

Press three times per day the following points, three minutes each point:

2–pituitary, 3–cerebrum, 4–cerebellum, 12–spine, 20–adrenal, 21–kidney, 24–liver, 52–autonomic nervous system.

Schuessler Tissue Salts

Take the following remedies three times per day until condition improves, five tablets each:

Silica: 12X   **Kali muriaticum:** 6X
Ferrum phosphorica: 6X   **Calcarea phosphorica:** 6X

· 6 ·
THE SKIN SYSTEM

The skin system is, to use a modern cliché, our interface with the world.
It has greater diagnostic importance than we usually give it. Under the
eyes and hands of a careful physician, the skin tells much about systemic conditions and our general state of health. The skin is also of
great psychological importance: It tells much about our youthfulness
and vigor, and when the skin exhibits inherent problems it may rob us
of self-confidence.

There are seven general types of skin defects, in order of seriousness:
(1) macules—colored spots; (2) papules—small raised areas of the skin;
(3) nodules—subcutaneous, larger elevations of the skin; (4) vesicles—
fluid forming under the skin; (5) pustules—openings in the elevated
areas, suggesting infection; (6) scaling and crusting—the result of tissues throwing off unwanted matter; and (7) ulcers—rupture of the
layers of skin. Scars may form as a final stage in any of the above skin
disruptions, as the end result of inflammation. Wounds, burns, and
cuts may trigger one or several of these stages.

The face is of primary concern to most people, but many skin disorders are most evident in other parts of the body. Psoriasis usually
affects the scalp, elbows, knees, back, and buttocks, yet it is popularly
perceived as a facial problem. Because of its persistence and appearance—scales and nodules over large areas—psoriasis is a major concern for many people. Approximately three percent of the white population is affected, primarily in youth and middle age. Although no
specific causes have been determined, it appears that psoriasis is partly

hereditary, partly the result of other local traumas, climate, or psycho-somatic factors.

Eczema and urticaria likewise affect hands and feet more than the face, but any appearance of these conditions on the face is likely to be much more traumatic to the individual. Many causal factors have been suggested: allergies, specifically to eggs, shellfish, nuts, and various fruits; insect bites; drugs. Both conditions are characteristically chronic and are marked by inflammation, crusting, persistent reddening, and often ulceration.

With acne we come to the true "teenager's syndrome," involving as many as eighty percent of young people. The sebaceous glands in the face are the largest and most active in the body. Acne is an inflammation of these glands by rapid changes in puberty. Contributing factors are allergies to such common fast foods as chocolate, sodas, nuts, milk (in large quantities), and sugar. Attempts to remove or reduce these lesions by pinching and applying medications usually result in further aggravation of the condition. Acne also appears to worsen in the winter and during periods of psychological stress. Contact dermatitis is closely related to acne but may appear chronically at other parts of the body.

When bacterial infection occurs in any of the above conditions the result is either a boil or a series of boils, often known as carbuncles. These pustules increase alarmingly in size and eventually erupt in natural progression. Their size is such that scars often result.

Warts are similarly threatening in appearance, though benign. The common tumors appear on hands and are easily treated. On the neck and face warts are annoying but short-lived. Venereal warts should be distinguished from various venereal diseases, in that they have no known etiology and are easily cured. In general, however, warts are contagious.

Impetigo is a common bacterial infection, highly contagious in infants and young children. It may spread explosively but is dangerous only in adults, and then only due to the possibility of ulcers or warts.

The very word "herpes" is enough to raise fears or apprehension, yet type II is the only one that is spread by genital contact, in the form of a large virus. Type I often appears on the mouth and is transitory. In both cases it is a viral infection on the skin or mucous membranes, resulting in clusters of vesicles with clear fluid. The distinction between the two types appears to be breaking down, as both types have been noted on the genitals. Type II can be quiescent for long periods and is contagious when it erupts.

In contrast to the "simple" herpes described above, herpes "zoster" is an acute infection of the central nervous system striking people most commonly after middle age. The virus often precipitates chills, fever, and gastric disturbances before erupting in vesicles at nerve endings on the back or the thorax. Again, the skin performs the duty of taking the brunt of the infection, but there may be neuralgic pain in addition to annoying skin problems.

If the invasion of the skin is by fungi rather than viruses, the result may be more chronic but less annoying. A common example is "athlete's foot," but this condition can occur at any part of the body where there is dead tissue, including the fingernails. On the scalp, ringworm (as the condition is technically known) can be persistent. Ringworm can also lead to other infections (dermatophytids or "ids") when the fungal infection is acute.

Parasites such as scabies and microorganisms such as lice also infect the skin, especially in areas difficult to keep clean, when there is overcrowding or insufficient hygienic conditions. Scabies is a more noticeable and debilitating condition, but the loci of lice bites and scratches are sites of organisms that cause typhus and various fevers.

The troublesome itching associated with lice and scabies, generically known as pruritis, may result from allergic reactions, insect bites, and the well-known "poisons" in the plant world: ivy and oak. But itching may also be symptom of such chronic diseases as diabetes, nephritis, cancer, and thyroid dysfunction. The latter causes should be suspected when there is no obvious exposure to an outside antagonist. Itching may also signify hormonal changes, as in pregnancy and in the change of life.

A streptococcal infection of the skin, as of the throat, usually results in swollen, red areas and accompanying fever and malaise. Known as rosacea and erysipelas, this condition occurs nowadays only in aged or chronically debilitated persons. In contrast, the loss of pigmentation, or vitiligo, has no known cause, does not signify an underlying disease, and often occurs along familial lines. It is, however, cosmetically important to blacks or when the surrounding skin is tanned.

The more common condition of dandruff, the typical manifestation of seborrheic dermatitis, affects a great portion of the population, especially those with oily skin and chronic bacterial skin infections.

Baldness, or alopecia, is a familial trait except in overt illnesses such as scarlet fever or hypothyroidism. It is usually called "premature" to distinguish it from the normal thinning and loss of hair with old age. Women rarely experience significant hair loss except for thinning, indicating that alopecia is a hormonal condition. In rare cases, acute hair loss can occur without obvious skin disorders or serious illness.

Facial rejuvenation without resort to plastic surgery has received increasing attention from females, as has hair restoration from males.

The self-esteem and social consequences of such "beauty" treatments should not be lightly dismissed. The skin and its coverings are important manifestations of good health, and maintaining the appearance of health is often conducive to the same.

WOUNDS, BURNS AND CUTS

SUGGESTED TREATMENT

Applied Nutrition **
Drink: Avoid coffee and alcohol.
Eat: Large quantities of raw fresh vegetables. Avoid white sugar, smoking, refined wheat flour, fried foods, and other junk foods.
An example of a diet for an average-weight person, thirty years old:

2100 calories	50 mg B_3
50 g protein	50 mg B_6
80 g fat	10 mg vitamin K
295 g carbohydrate	300 mcg folacin (folic acid)
Master Formula and also:	15 mg iron
25,000 IU vitamin A	500 mg calcium
1,000 IU vitamin D	200 mg magnesium
3,000 mg vitamin C	50 mg zinc
500 mg bioflavinoids	50 mcg iodine
50 mg rutin	50 mcg selenium
50 mg B_1	

Nucleoproteins:

50 mg adrenal extract	30 mg RNA extract
50 mg thymus extract	2400 mg lecithin
50 mg kidney extract	120 mg betaine hydrochloric acid
50 mg liver extract	

Aromatherapy
Use in the wounded or burned area the following formula on olive-oil base: **eucalyptus** essence 2%, **borned camphor** 0.5%, **thyme** essence 1%, **lavender** 1%. Bandage the place with this formula for two hours after cleaning the wound with alcohol 70%.

Autosuggestion
The main mental condition of this problem is self-punishment or self-hate. The affirmation should be:

I forgive and love myself unconditionally.

Color Therapy **

Use the color blue for thirty minutes followed by the ultraviolet light for another five minutes. Repeat this treatment twice per day until the wound is healed. Massage the wound with aromatherapy essence before color therapy.

Herbs

Western ****

Aloe: For burns, leaf to be opened, and its inside should be applied to cut or burn.
Marigold *(Calendula)* and **St. John's Wort** *(Hamamelis):*   As tea, capsule, or external ointment.
Acacia *(Senegal, Arabica, Vera):*   Moisture of the bark may be used externally.
Comfrey *(Symphytum officinale):*   Can aid in skin regeneration.
Hooseleek *(Sempervivum tectorum):*   Fresh leaves to be bruised and placed over burn to reduce discharge and cool inflammation.
Olive *(Olea europea):*   In form of salve or ointment for burns, scalds, and bruises.
Slippery elm *(Ulmus fulva):*   A powder mixed with water makes a good poultice for treating wounds, burns, and bruises.
Arnica montana: Compress for bruises.
Yarrow *(Achillea)* and **daisy:**   Compresses for sprains and concussions are helpful.

Chinese **

Lithospermum ointment *(Tzu-yun-kao):*   Formula of choice as a topical ointment for burns.
Coptis and Rhubarb Combination: For mild burns.
For bruises:
Cinnamon and Hoelen Formula: Formula of choice. Good for bleeding due to fluxion of wound and internal hemorrhaging.
Persica and Rhubarb Combination: For bruising, severe pain, subepidermal hemorrhage.
Coptis and Rhubarb Combination: for hemorrhage after accident.
Musk and Caechu *(Chi-li San):*   Chinese traditional contusion formula.

Homeopathy ***

For bruises:

Arnica: 3 to 30 every hour. Also **arnica** oil on unbroken skin.

Ruta: 3X for bruises of bone.

Rhus Tox: 3 to 30 for muscular bruises.

Lotion of Hamemelis (ten drops to one ounce) or **ruta** (same):   to be applied externally.

Bellis: 3X every two or three hours to female breast bruise, to be followed by **Conium 3.**

For spinal cord injuries:

Hypericum: 3X six to eight times daily.

For burns or scalds:

Urtica urens (mother tincture):   applied as lotion.

Nelson's Burn Ointment   (from Nelson's Pharmacy in London)

Cantharis Lotion   (one part to ten parts water) when there is vesication. Also take **Cantharis** 3 hourly internally.

Hepar: six to twelve four times daily for suppuration after burn.

Reflexology

In case of wounds massage the whole feet twice per day with reflexology massage device for five minutes each time as a secondary aid.

Schuessler Tissue Salts **

In case of specific injuries, bruises, or burns use the following treatment in addition to Western first aid. For immediate injuries:

Kali phosphorica 6X and **ferrum phosphorica** 6X: To mitigate shock and bleeding, take together by mouth in form of tablets (five tablets of each every ten minutes until bleeding or shock is stopped), then continue with the same remedies four times per day until condition improves.

For neglected injuries:

Silica 6X: use in the first case, then continue with **calcarea sulphorica** 6X in place of the silica. Three times per day until condition improves.

For bites and stings:

Natrum muriaticum 6X, **silica** 3X, **kali phosphorica** 12X: five tablets of each every ten minutes until condition improves.

Kali muriaticum 6X: If swelling of the part occurs, use in place of natrum muriaticum four to six times per day. This formula can be used as a lotion on the injured part.

For bleeding and cuts long after injuries:

Ferrum phosphorica: 6X five tablets every ten minutes until bleeding subsides.

Kali muriaticum 12X, **ferrum phosphorica** 6X, **kali phosphorica** 6X: In case of swelling, use every four hours until condition improves and the swelling subsides.

For nose bleed:

See Epistaxis (nosebleed).

For blood poisoning:

See Circulation Disorders.

For bruises:

Ferrum Phosphorica 6X, **kali muriaticum** 6X: For the inflammation and swelling, every ten minutes until condition improves, then continue twice per day with the same remedies until completely cured.

For bruises of the shin, ribs, and other bones:

Calcarea fluorica: 6X. Use a lotion on a gauze under a bandage every day until condition improves.

Schuessler Tissue Salts ***

For burns and scalds:

Ferrum phosphorica 3X, **kali muriaticum** 3X, **kali phosphorica** 4X: Take in tablets every ten minutes.

Kali muriaticum 6X: A solution on a piece of gauze can be used to prevent blistering. Add the lotion of kali muriaticum to the bandage for the burns.

For head injuries, falls, blows, concussions:

Ferrum phosphorica 6X, **natrum sulphorica** 6X: Take five tablets of each every ten minutes until condition improves.

Ferrum Phosphorica 30X, **natrum sulphorica** 30X, **kali phosphorica** 30X: If the concussion is serious and there is little response to treatment, take five tablets of each every fifteen minutes until condition improves.

For hernia and rupture:

Calcarea fluorica 6X, **silica** 6X: Take five tablets each every thirty minutes in the first stage. Also apply a cold compress soaked with the powder of **calcarea fluorica** 6X, **silica** 12X, and **ferrum phosphorica** 6X over the swollen area until condition improves.

For knee cap injuries from falling:

Calcarea fluorica 6X and **ferrum phosphorica** 6X: Take five tablets of each every ten minutes until pain is over. Also use the same remedies as a solution on gauze and change the solution every four hours until condition improves.

For sprains:

Ferrum phosphorica 12X, **silica** 12X, **calcarea fluorica** 12X: Take five tablets of each every fifteen minutes. Also use the same remedies as a solution on gauze over the affected area, and change the solution three times per day until condition improves.

For strains:

Ferrum phosphorica 6X, **calcarea fluorica** 6X, **kali muriaticum** 6X, **Kali Phosphorica** 6X: Take five tablets of each every thirty minutes until condition improves, then continue with the same remedies every four hours for another two weeks.

For sunstroke:

Natrum muriaticum 30X: Take five tablets every ten minutes.

Ferrum phosphorica 12X, **silica** 12X: Take five tablets of each every hour.

Natrum muriaticum 30X: Make a cold compress of water and natrum muriaticum 30X; all over the head. Change this compress every four hours until condition improves.

PSORIASIS

SYMPTOMS

Bumps and scales on the skin, from the scalp to the buttocks, with no obvious cause and with long-term effects.

SUGGESTED TREATMENT

Acupuncture and Acupressure **

GB 34, SP 10, TW 6, GV 9, LI 4, HT 7, LU 9, K7.

Applied Nutrition ****

Drink: Pure mineral water, herb tea, and fruit or vegetable juices. Avoid dairy products, coffee, tea, alcohol, cocoa.

Eat: Mainly fresh vegetables, very little fresh fruit, whole grains, seeds, cereals, sprouts, soy proteins, seafish two to three time per week, two or three organic eggs per week (from free-range chickens). Avoid all meat products, dairy products, white sugar, white flour, white rice, dried foods. Also, if condition permits, commence the diet with three days juice fasting. In many cases a naturopathic physician will recommend longer periods of pure water fasting—up to twenty-one days or more—but it must be done under supervision of a professional. And then continue with a pure vegetarian diet. Start the first day eating 25% of the daily recommended diet, then the second day eat 50% of the daily diet. The third day eat 75% of the daily diet, and in the fourth day eat the whole recommended diet, which should be low in protein. An example of a diet for an average-weight person, thirty years old:

1900 calories	50 mg vitamin B_1
40 g protein	50 mg vitamin B_2
70 g fat	50 mg vitamin B_3 (niacinamid)
278 g carbohydrate	50 mg vitamin B_6
Master Formula and also:	200 mg vitamin B_{12}
50,000 IU vitamin A	2,000 mg pantothenic acid
1,000 IU vitamin D	300 mcg folic acid
1,000 IU vitamin E	50 mcg biotin
5000 mg vitamin C	50 mg cholin
800 mg bioflavinoids	

Minerals:

800 mg calcium	40 mg zinc
500 mg magnesium	40 mg potassium
100 mg phosphorus	20 mg manganese
15 mg iron	100 mcg iodine
100 mcg chromium	50 mcg selenium
4 mg copper	40 mcg molybdenum

Enzyme Formula:

Betaine hydrochloric acid 100 mg every meal	65 mg pepsin
75 mg pancreatin	50 mg lipase
120 mg bile extract	50 mg papain

Nucleoproteins extract:

15 mg pituitary extract	40 mg RNA extract
50 mg adrenal extract	3,600 mg lecithin (very helpful
60 mg thymus extract	in psoriasis)
60 mg kidney extract	10–20 garlic capsules daily

Aromatherapy

Use externally **lavender** 2% in a distilled water base. After the water solution apply a cream containing 1,000 g **almond** oil and 250 g white **wax,** + 750 g distilled **water,** 20 g essence of **lavender,** + 5 g **aspic,** + 10 g **bergamot** + (*Hydrastis* 5 g + *Fumaria officianalis* 120 g) phytotherapy.

Autosuggestion ****
The main mental reason for this condition is emotional insecurity, being afraid to be touched. The affirmations should be:

> *I am completely secure in my feelings.*
> *I love myself unconditionally.*
> *Others love me unconditionally.*
> *I am accepted and loved in this world.*

Bach Flowers **

Pine: For those with psoriasis who suffer guilt and blame themselves for everything.
Crabapple: The cleansing remedy.

Color Therapy **
Use the color blue for thirty minutes twice per day followed by ultra-violet light for ten minutes. In this condition the treatment is long and should be given continuously, six days per week for three to six months. Before treatment it is recommended to massage the skin and lesions with vegetable oil together with aromatherapy.

Herbs

Western ***
Fumaria, calendula: For cleansing, in tea or capsules.
Hydrastis and **echinea:**   Add when inflammation is involved.
Valeriana or **Avena sativa:**   Add if person is uptight.

Chinese ***
Cinnamon and Astragalus Combination *(Kuei-chih-chia-huang-chi-tang):*   For those of weak physique and when disease has not progressed too far.
Coptin and Gelatin Combination *(Huang-lien-ah-chiao-tang):*   For weak patients with red and arid infected areas.
Siler and Platycodon *(Fang-Ofeng-tung-sheng-san):*   Add three g of rehmannia to those strong and constipated.
Tang-kuei and Gardenia *(Wen-ching-yin):*   For those with itchy, dry, and coarse skin. Their infected areas bleed.
Bupleurum and Schizonepeta: For psoriasis and tinea alba when blisters and suppurations are present.

Homeopathy ***

Psorinum 200:   A single dose acts better on chilly individuals, by physician only.
Sulphur: More for the hot type.
Arsenicum album 3X to 30X: Every four hours.
Graphites 6X: Every six hours for syphilitic psoriasis.

Hydrotherapy

For this condition sweating in a sweating sauna for a few minutes per day, increasing daily the period of time in the sauna, is very important. Start with two minutes daily and slowly increase the daily time in the sauna to ten or fifteen minutes. Drink two or three glasses of mineral water before the sauna and two or three glasses after the sauna. Many people who suffer from this condition do not sweat enough. Expose the whole skin to a warm and dry desert atmosphere for thirty minutes twice per day.

Reflexology

The reflexology treatment of this disease requires pressing the points of the liver, kidneys, lymph glands, lungs, pituitary, and nervous system.
The treatment should include the following points:
   2, 3, 24, 25, 18, 42, 16, 52.
Press each point two minutes twice per day in both hands and feet for four to eight months.

Scheussler Tissue Salts

Natrum sulphorica 6X, **natrum muriaticum** 12X, **silica** 30x, **ferrum phosphorica** 12X, **kali muriaticum** 12X: In case of psoriasis use the formula four times per day in the first month.
Natrum muriaticum 12X: Continue for another two months, twice per day, five tablets every morning and evening.

ECZEMA

SYMPTOMS

More severe reddening, sometimes crusting and ulceration of the skin of face, hands, and feet.

SUGGESTED TREATMENT

Acupuncture and Acupressure **

GV 14, LI 4, LI 1, SP 6, SP 9, K 10, UB 38, CV 12, LiV 14, CV 14, CV 4, ST 25, UB 13, UB 23.
Moxa may be applied to GB 21, UB 13, UB 22, UB 23.

Applied Nutrition ****
Before starting the diet check for food allergy with a cytotoxic blood test. And as in most skin disorders, it is recommended to start the diet with three days of juice fasting in combination with enemas of water and **lobelia** herb. Then discontinue the enemas and gradually start the diet therapy. Attention to allergens confirmed by blood test should be made; avoid all foods causing allergy.
Drink: Avoid dairy products.
Eat: Diet should be rich in fiber. Avoid dairy products, meat, white sugar, and white flour products.
An example of a diet for an average-weight person, thirty years old:

1800 calories	300 mg bioflavinoids
40 g protein	1,200 mg pantothenic acid
60 g fat	2,400 mg lecithin
275 g carbohydrate	120 mg hydrochloric acid
Master Formula and also:	50 mg zinc
1,000 mg vitamin C	

Aromatherapy
In this case use the essence of **camomile** 2% in a vegetable oil base. Massage the skin affected once per day until condition improves. This treatment is recommended in combination with color therapy.

Autosuggestion *
The main mental condition for this problem is oversensitivity that hurts the personality and inner feelings. The affirmation should be:

I am at peace, secure and safe in this world.

Color Therapy
In this case use a combination of blue, orange, and red (each one for ten minutes daily). Use these colors directly over the affected area.
If there is inflammation in addition to the eczema, use the color blue for twenty minutes daily and then continue with the orange and red for ten minutes each color.

Before treatment massage the affected area with vegetable oil containing aromatherapy.

Herbs ***

Western

Urtica
Rosemary   Use in combination
Stellaria   1:1 ratio as tea or tincture
Burdock   2–3 times daily.
Cleaver

Chinese

Bupleurum and Schizonepeta Formula: Effective for small, itchy red pimples with slight secretions.
Pueraria Combination: In initial stage of acute eczema inflammations and itching.
Persica and Rhubarb: For chronic eczema, severe itching, constipation.
Siler Combination: Good for eczema of head or face.

Homeopathy ***

Rhus-ven: 3X every six hours. This medicine shouldn't be discontinued in spite of aggravation, only changed to 30.
Oleander: For scalp eczema, 6 every six hours.
Graphites: 6 every six hours. Ointment of graphites 3X is good for palms and hands. 6X for chronic eczema behind ears.
Arsenicum: For chronic dry eczema, 3 every six hours.
Sulphur: 3X every six hours for eczema marginatum.

Reflexology

In case of eczema massage the following points as a general reinforcement of the body glands:
2, 3, 18, 19, 17, 22, 20, 21, 51, 52, 42, 43.
This treatment should be with the help of reflexologer device for hands and feet.
For hand reflexology hold the device between both hands and while pressing it with both hands open move one hand ahead so the device presses different points each time. Now move the second hand. Continue these movements with both hands so that the device reaches the whole palm of both hands. Do this treatment for seven minutes twice per day until condition improves.

Massage both whole feet with reflexology device twice per day, morning and evening, for seven minutes each time until condition improves.

Reflexology Code

2 — Pituitary
3 — Cerebrum
18 — Heart
19 — Spleen
17 — Solar Plexus
22 — Pancreas

20 — Adrenal Gland
21 — Kidney
51 — Thymus
52 — Autonomic Nervous System
42 — Upper Lymph Glands
43 — Lower Lymph Glands

Schuessler Tissue Salts

In case of eczema use twice per day (morning and evening), fifteen drops each:

Kali muriaticum 12X
Kali sulphorica 12X

Calcarea sulphorica 12X
Silica 12X

Use this remedy until condition improves.

ACNE VULGARIS

SYMPTOMS

Spontaneous and short-lived inflammation and swelling of spots on the face.

SUGGESTED TREATMENT

Acupuncture and Acupressure **

SP 10, GV 4, UB 23, UB 22, UB 20, LiV 4, K 7, CV 12, LU 1, LU 7.

Applied Nutrition ****

The diet and fasting are very important, as in many cases of skin disorders. The diet should start with three days juice fasting.
Drink: Avoid all dairy products, alcohol, coffee, tea, cocoa.
Eat: The diet should be rich in fresh raw vegetables, whole grains, cereals, seeds, and sea fish, with minimal fruit and organic eggs (two or three weekly). Avoid all dairy products, meats, poultry, fried foods,

smoking, table salt, white sugar, refined white flour. The food should be well chewed before swallowing.

An example of a diet for an average weight-person, thirty years old:

2100 calories
45 g protein
70 g fat
325 g carbohydrate
Master Formula of vitamins and minerals and also:
25,000 IU vitamin A
400 IU vitamin D
1,000 IU vitamin E
3,000 mg vitamin C
500 mg bioflavinoids
50 mg vitamin B_2
50 mg vitamin B_3

50 mg pABA
10 mg biotin
15 mg iron
50 mg zinc
50 mcg selenium
100 mg pituitary extract nucleoprotein
100 mg adrenal extract nucleoprotein
100 mg thymus extract nucleoprotein
2,400 mg lecithin

Aromatherapy

In this condition use a combination of **juniper** and **lavender.** Massage in a base of olive oil with 10% of **juniper** essence for ten minutes over the affected area on the skin, then bathe the place with **lavender** water 2%. Continue the treatment with **lavender** cream—1,000 g almond oil, 250 g white **wax,** 750 g distilled **water,** 20 g essence of **lavender**—once per day before going to sleep.

Autosuggestion

The main mental condition for this problem is not accepting, or disliking, the self, or feelings of self-hate. The affirmation should be:

I accept and love myself unconditionally.

Repeat this affirmation thirty times every four hours daily.

Bach Flowers

Crabapple 4 drops once daily.

Color Therapy

Apply the color red for fifteen minutes and continue with yellow color locally another fifteen minutes. Do this treatment daily, once per day. If there is skin inflammation with the acne, commence the treatment with the color blue for twenty minutes per day and then continue with the red and yellow.

Herbs ***

Western

Echinea, hydrastis: As anti-inflammatory herbs.
Calendula and **stellaria:** Add for cleansing.

Chinese

Use sulphur-containing cleansers.
Tang-juei and Paeonia Formula with Coix: Good for those who are anemic or pale.
Siler Combination *(Ching-shang-fang-feng-tang):* For red acne.

Homeopathy ****

Carbo vegetabilis: 6X every six hours for young people with acute stage.
Thuya: 30 3X in one day might be helpful.
Sulphur: A lotion or ointment in one teaspoonful to one ounce to be applied locally.
Kali bromium: For chronic acne, 30 every four hours.

Reflexology

In this condition massage the whole feet on a reflexology massage device three times per day for seven minutes each foot. Also massage the points for three minutes each point twice per day until condition improves:

42, 43—lymphatic system, 24—liver, 25—gall bladder, 18—heart and blood circulation, 19—spleen, 52—central nervous system.

Schuessler Tissue Salts

Silica 12X and **kali muriaticum** 12X: Use the combination (five tablets of each) every morning and evening until condition improves.

CONTACT DERMATITIS

SYMPTOMS

Appearance similar to acne, but on other parts of the body.

SUGGESTED TREATMENT

In cases of acute of chronic dermatitis that results from direct skin contact with chemicals and allergens like soaps, detergents, organic solvents, antimicrobials (especially neomycin), topical antihistamines, anesthetics, and preservatives, avoid reexposure to these irritants; use natural-source cosmetics (or better, eliminate cosmetics entirely). Use protective gloves if the occupation involves contact with allergens. Try to change the occupation or job.

Applied Nutrition **
Use the same diet therapy as in the eczema treatment.

Aromatherapy
Use the same treatment as in the case of eczema.

Autosuggestion *
Repeat the following affirmation twice per day for twenty minutes:

> From day to day I am better and healthier in every way. Every day my skin is stronger and healthier.

Bach Flowers *

Crabapple: For cleansing, 4 drops once daily.

Color Therapy
Use the same treatment as in the case of eczema.

Herbs **

Chinese

Pueraria Combination
Bupleurum and Schizone peta Combination: For allergic dermatitis.

Hydrotherapy
The use of water is very important in the first stage of contact dermatitis to remove the external cause of this problem. Use a cold jet of water directly on the affected part of the body (only if the affected part is not wounded). Then continue with hot water for a few seconds and back to cold water. In case of general skin affection the use of sauna bath every day in the first week is useful (five minutes the first day, then slowly increase the time in the sauna to ten minutes; then continue with cold bath and back to sauna for another ten minutes). Drink two glasses or more of fresh water before and after every sauna. Never take a sauna on a full stomach. The sauna should not be used by people suffering from heart problems or circulatory or tubercular diseases.

Reflexology

Use the same treatment as in the case of eczema as a secondary aid.

Schuessler Tissue Salts

Kali muriaticum 6X: five tablets every ten minutes in the first hours after the contact with chemicals.
Kali muriaticum 6X and **natrum phosphorica** 12X: Use every morning, noon, and evening after condition improves, five tablets of each for another three weeks.

BOILS, FURUNCULOSIS, and CARBUNCLES

SYMPTOMS

Serious swelling of skin infections resulting in discharge of pus and eventual scarring.

SUGGESTED TREATMENT

Acupuncture and Acupressure *

GV 12, GV 10, LI 4, UB 40 (Bloodletting) LI 11, and ST 36.
Carbuncles on back:
GB 21, ST 36, GB 41, LiV 2, LiV 3, HT 3.
For carbuncles around mouth:
Moxa LI 4.
On hands:
Moxa Li 11.
Ear Acupuncture:
Neurogate, Adrenal, subcortex, Occiput, and points associated with location of problems.
Acupuncture is supplementary to lancing.

Applied Nutrition ***

In this case, after three days juice fasting the recommended diet therapy is the same as in the treatment of eczema.

Aromatherapy

In case of boils use the following combination on the infected area twice per day until condition improves: **Lavender**—eight parts, **ca-**

momile—four parts, **myrrh**—two parts, **thyme**—two parts, in vegetable oil (preferably olive oil).

Autosuggestion

The main mental reason for boils is being angry at the self without being able to express the feeling. Repeat the following affirmation twenty times twice per day:

I am at peace and love with myself and my surroundings.

Color Therapy **

Use the color light blue over the point of infection for thirty minutes twice per day until condition improves. In case of carbuncles use also indigo and violet for ten minutes each daily before the blue light.

Herbs

Western

Clevers (Gallium)   **Aloe**
Echinea

Chinese

Take in 1:1 tincture or in capsules, three times daily. Or take 10 drops in glass of water twice daily.
For facial boils:
Bupleurum and Schizonepeta Formula: Effective only during initial stage for mild facial boils.
Astragalus and Platycodon: Alternate formula.
For carbuncles:
Angelica and Mastic Combination
Cimicifuga and Gleditsia

Homeopathy ***

GUNP: For boils, three tablets of 3X.
Arnica: 3X twice daily as preventive remedy for those with tendency to boils.
Phytolacca: 7X every four hours for boils after fever.
Antharacinum: 30 every two hours for carbuncles in general.
Silica: 6X every eight hours for carbuncles in general when there is a discharge.

Hydrotherapy

Heat boils with water as hot as you can comfortably stand a few times a day until the boils become mature and the pus is getting out. You can add to the hot water 10% of **lavender** extract, or one tablespoon of **sea salt** to a glass of hot water.

Reflexology **

Massage the following points five minutes twice per day until boils disappear:

42, 43–upper and lower lymph glands; 18–heart and blood circulation; 9–spleen; 24–liver; 25–gall bladder; 52–central nervous system.

Schuessler Tissue Salts

Ferrum phosphorica: 30X in case of furuncles or carbuncles; use in sugar tablets. Take five tablets every hour until boil is mature and continue with **ferrum phosphorica** twice per day after the boil opens and the pus is drained out, then for another two weeks.

IMPETIGO

SYMPTOMS

Contagious infection of face and hands with open sores, especially in young people.

SUGGESTED TREATMENT

Acupuncture *

LI 2, Li 5, Li 11, LI 4, TW 6, GV 14, SI 3, UB 17, UB 38, ST 38.
Ear points: Allergy, Lung, Endocrine

Applied Nutrition **

The diet should be the same as in the case of psoriasis. Also, it is recommended to use fully vegetarian diet in this condition.

Aromatherapy

Use crushed **garlic** 50% in olive oil base. Let it macerate for four days and then rub into the infected area, being careful not to rub in or near the eyes. For children use crushed **garlic** 20% in olive oil base; after ten minutes wash with cider **vinegar** 5% in cup of water. Repeat this treatment twice per day until the condition improves. If the skin (especially the face) is too sensitive to garlic aroma, use instead **lavender** 10% in olive oil base, and for children use 3% **lavender** in olive oil base.

Autosuggestion
Repeat the following affirmation twenty times twice per day:

> *From day to day I am healthier and stronger in every way.*

Bach Flowers
Crabapple 4 drops once a day.

Color Therapy
Use the color red for fifteen minutes followed by the color blue for another fifteen minutes. Repeat this treatment twice per day until condition improves. In the case of children less than ten years old five minutes of these colors should be used, also twice per day.

Homeopathy

Viola tricolor: 3X every four hours for new facial impetigo.
Cicuta Virosa 3:   3X three times daily for burning pain.
Mezereum: 30 for eruptions with discharge.
Antimonium Tartaricum: 6X to 12X twice daily for general impetigo.
Arsenicum: For marked debility.

Reflexology
In this case the treatment as a secondary aid is the same as in the case of eczema.

Schuessler Tissue Salts
Use the following remedies every hour, ten tablets of the combination:

Kali muriaticum 12X
Kali sulphorica 12 X
Calcarea sulphorica 6X
Silica 12X
Ferrum phosporica 30X

Continue until condition improves and then continue with this formula another month, twice per day.
For children give two tablets every hour until the condition improves.

HERPES SIMPLEX

SYMPTOMS

Clusters of small sores on the lips and other well-exposed areas of skin, often called "cold sores," with characteristic redness and persistence.

SUGGESTED TREATMENT

Applied Nutrition ***

Use the same diet as in the case of eczema.

Aromatherapy

Bathe with distilled water containing 2% of the **geranium** essential oil. Do this treatment before the color therapy, but only once per day. Continue the treatment until condition improves.

Autosuggestion

The affirmation in this case is the same as in the case of impetigo.

Color Therapy ***

Use the following colors ten minutes each, one after the other, all over the body: blue, red, and indigo.
Repeat the treatment twice per day until condition improves.

Reflexology *

As a secondary aid, use the same treatment as in eczema.
In the case of pain or neuralgia, massage point 55—general pain for five minutes every hour until condition improves. Then continue four times per day for another month.

Schuessler Tissue Salts **

Powder the parts affected with dry cornstarch after applying Vaseline and give **kali muriaticum** 12X and **natrum muriaticum** 12X: in alternation, five tablets of each every two hours.
Kali phosphorica 12X and **ferrum phosphorica** 6X: In case of pains, take in place of **kali muriaticum** and **natrum muriaticum** until pains disappear, and then continue with the first group of remedies.

HERPES ZOSTER (SHINGLES)

SYMPTOMS

Chills and fever associated with a virus, often gastric problems, finally sores on the back or on the thorax.

SUGGESTED TREATMENT

Acupuncture ***

GB 30, GB 31, GB 40, GB 43, or: GB 34, LI 4, ST 36, TW 5, ST 4, UB 38.
Ear points: Adrenal, Lung, Occiput, Internal Secretions

Herbs **

Chinese

Pueraria combination: For initial stage and vesicle eruptions or for prodromal stage with feverish symptoms.
Minor Bupleurum Combination: Within one or two weeks of onset and vesicle eruption.
Major Bupleurum Combination: For strong people.

ALOPECIA (BALDNESS)

SUGGESTED TREATMENT

Acupuncture and Acupressure

Moxa: GV 20, UB 10, UB 23, CV 12, CV 4, LI 4
Also massage or acupuncture:
   LU 7, GV 14, GV 12, UB 13, LI 11, LU 6, LU 9.
Ear points: Lungs, internal secretions, zero point (Nogier). Shen-men.

Herbs

1:1 ratio as tea or tincture. 3 cups of tea daily, 10 drops in glass of water three times daily.

Western

Marigold (Calendula)
Aloe and **nettles** *(Urtica urens/divica):* Excellent blood and skin cleaners.

Chinese

Bupleurum and Dragon Bone Combination: Effective for round alopecia. Good for those of strong constitution and nervousness.
Cinnamon and Dragon Bone: For round alopecia. For weak person with vertigo.
Siler and Platycodon Formula: For delicate physique and alcoholics or the constipated.

Homeopathy *

Kali carbonicum: 6X for dry, falling hair.
Phosphorum acidum: 1X every six to eight hours for alopecia stemming from depression.
Bryonia: 1X every eight hours for very greasy hair.

RINGWORM AND SUPERFICIAL FUNGUS INFECTIONS

SYMPTOMS

Commonly seen as athlete's foot or redness of the scalp, persisting as a severe itch on dead tissue.
Ringworm includes:

1. Ringworm of scalp and body (Tinea Capitis and Tinea Corpons or Tinea Circinata)
2. Tinea Cruris (Jock Itch)
3. Tinea Manum and Tinea Pedis (Dermatophytosis) Tinea of Palm and Soles—Athlete's Foot
4. Tinea Unguium and Candidal Onychomycosis (Nails Fungi)
5. Tinea Versicolor (Pityriasis Versicolor)
    (Furfur infection of the skin, usually of trunk)
6. Cutaneous Candidiasis (Moniliasis)

In order to help other therapies to overcome this problem, follow these recommendations:
Keep the skin, nails, scalp, or any affected area dry and clean. As moisture favors the growth of fungi, a cool climate is preferable. Use rubber gloves or rubber boots as appropriate when washing with water. Try to prevent excessive perspiration, to avoid moistening the skin or the affected part. After perspiration, wet parts, or bath, dry the affected part of the body very carefully, sometimes with the aid of hot air from hair dryer (dry the scalp for a short time and the nails for a longer

time, until very dry between the nails and the nail bed). Socks and other clothing should be changed often. Wear sandals or other open shoes in case of Tinea pedis. Skin secretions or wet parts should be dried as soon as possible with clean towels. In a nervous type of person it is recommended to avoid excessive perspiration by meditation and/or biofeedback.

For athlete's foot, place small wads of cotton between the toes at night.

SUGGESTED TREATMENT

Acupuncture

LI 4, SP 10, ST 36, GV 10.

Applied Nutrition
Take the same diet therapy as in the case of eczema.

Aromatherapy
Use the essence of **geranium** 5% in olive oil base and massage the affected part of the skin once per day until condition improves.

In case of nails fungi use crushed **garlic** 50% in olive oil base. After macerating the garlic with the oil for four days use this formula on a bandage around the affected nails daily for a short time each day.

In case of ringworm of the scalp use **geranium** 2% on olive oil base and rub the scalp well with the oil before bathing. Leave on for twenty minutes daily until condition improves.

Autosuggestion
Repeat the affirmation:

> *From day to day I am happier, healthier, and stronger in every way.*

Twenty affirmations three times per day.

In cases of nervous types it is important to repeat the following affirmations twenty times after the first one:

> *I love myself unconditionally.*
> *I am calm and relaxed in every way.*

Color Therapy
Use the following colors one after the other on the affected area locally: blue—fifteen minutes, indigo—ten minutes, violet—ten minutes, ultraviolet—five minutes. Repeat the treatment daily until condition

improves. In some cases, especially in nails fungi, the treatment might take between three and eighteen months.

Herbs

Western

Juniper
Elecampane   1:1 ratio in capsules
Burdock   or tincture

Chinese

Ma-Huang and Coix Combination: For thin patients with dandruff.
Forsythia Combination: For more serious lesions (dry).
Bupleurum and Schizonepeta Combination: For suppurative trichphyton accompanied by itch and pus.
Persica and Rhubarb Combination: For severe inflammation and constipation.
Lithospermum Ointment

Homeopathy ***

Tellurium: 6X every four hours for ringworm of body.
For ringworm of scalp and hairy parts,
Sepia: 1X, a paste for nightly application.
Chrysophan Acidum: John Clark recommends this ointment for night and morning. There is intense staining with this.

Hydrotherapy

Use sauna bath twice per week if any of the ringworm forms on the skin. Drink two glasses of pure water before the sauna and two glasses of pure water after the sauna. In cases of nails fungi soak the whole affected nails in hot water with **sea salt,** as hot as you can bear without suffering, once per day for five minutes, and then rinse well and dry with hot air.

Hypnotherapy

Hypnotherapy can be very useful in treating ringworm problems in any part of the body.

Reflexology

As a secondary aid, give a general massage of the whole feet, twice per day for seven minutes each foot. Use reflexology massage roller device and in the hands press or massage point 52—autonomic nervous system twice per day.

Schuessler Tissue Salts

Kali muriaticum 12X powder: Apply on the affected part of the body mixed with carbolated Vaseline, twice per day on hands or skin. In athlete's foot use the powder of **kali muriaticum** 12X mixed with dusting and drying powders between clean socks and feet. In nails fungi use **kali muriaticum** 12X mixed with Vaseline, and in the scalp use **kali muriaticum** 12X mixed with vegetable oil; rub the scalp for twenty minutes before washing, and after washing dry well and apply **kali muriaticum** 12X powder.

LICE AND SCABIES

SYMPTOMS

Noticeable as lice bites and scratches, which can lead to typhus infections and fever.

SUGGESTED TREATMENT

For scabies, the patient should be isolated; bed and clothes should be laundered to avoid contamination.

Applied Nutrition
The diet therapy in this condition is the same as in the case of eczema.

Aromatherapy
For lice, rub the whole body with the following combination in olive oil base: crushed **garlic** 10%, **lavender** essence 3%, **thyme** 2%, **rosemary** 4%. Do this treatment once per day until condition improves. For scabies, use same treatment as for ringworm.

Autosuggestion
Use the same affirmation as in the case of impetigo.

Color Therapy *
For lice, use the colors ultraviolet, blue, and violet for ten minutes each, one after the other. Repeat this treatment twice per day until condition improves.

For scabies, use blue, ultraviolet, and violet all over the body for fifteen minutes each.

Herbs

Western ****

For lice:

Aniseed: Use oils

Sassafras and **quassia** *(Picrasma excelsor):*   Use a mixture oil. 1:1 ratio.

All for *external* application.

For scabies:

Tansy *(Tanacetum vulgare):*   A strong decoction can be taken internally as well as by external application.

Homeopathy *

Sulphur: 3 to 30 four to six times daily and/or sulphur ointment nightly.

Lavender oil or **balsam of Peru:**   Choose either for painting over local itch.

Staphysagria: 3X to 30X twice daily for lice of scalp, moist discharge.

Sabadilla: Homeopathic shampoo of tincture for daily use.

Reflexology

Use the same treatment as in the case of eczema.

Schuessler Tissue Salts

For lice, use the same treatment as in the case of impetigo.

For scabies, take three times per day ten tablets of the following:

Ferrum phosporica 3X	**Natrum phosphorica** 3X
Kali muriaticum 3X	**Silica** 6X
Kali sulphorica 6X	

PRURITIS (ITCHING)

SUGGESTED TREATMENT

External irritants—rough clothing, synthetic clothing, occupational contacts—should be avoided or removed. Soaps and detergents should not be used by persons with dry or irritated skin. Nails should be trimmed and clean. To prevent scratching, unnecessary medications should be discontinued, since many medications produce pruritis. Try elimination of external factors and irritating agents. It is often successful in giving complete relief from pruritis if the pruritis is of idiopathic or allergic origin. In cases of pruritis as a symptom of another specific dermatologic disorder or as a symptom of an internal disease such as lymphoma, Hodgkin's disease, hepatic or biliary disease, diabetes mellitus, nephritis, drug intoxication or habituation, or skin dryness, treat the specific disease or disorder and then the pruritis will disappear.

Acupuncture and Acupressure **

SP 6, SP 10, LI 11, K2, GB 20, UB 25, LiV 8.

Applied Nutrition **

In case of pruritis caused by internal disease, treat the specific disease by diet therapy. But in case of idiopathic pruritis or allergic pruritis it is important to avoid any allergy food causing this problem, so check the food-allergy cytotoxin blood test. Sometimes it is not the food that is responsible for allergy or disease but chemicals added to the food, so avoid any chemicals in your diet.

If condition permits, start the diet with three days of juice fasting and continue with vegetarian or macrobiotic diet.

Drink: Dairy products. Avoid coffee, alcohol, any stimulants.

Eat: Mainly fresh raw vetegables, whole grains, cereals, seeds, sprouts, some fresh fruits, sea fish, dairy products. Avoid any stimulants, smoking, refined white flour, white sugar, and other refined or processed foods. An example of a diet for an average-weight person, thirty years old:

1900 calories	3,000 vitamin C
40 g protein	500 mg bioflavinoids
70 g fat	1,000 mg panthothenic acid
378 g carbohydrate	600 mg calcium chelated
Master formula of vitamins and	400 mg magnesium chelated
minerals and also:	20 mg zinc chelated
10,000 IU vitamin A	15 mg iron chelated
400 IU vitamin D	2,400 mg lecithin
1,000 IU vitamin E	

Aromatherapy

Use the essence of **chamomile** 2% in olive oil base and massage once per day over the affected area. Or if the pruritis involves the whole body, then wash with boiled water and **thyme** *(Thymus vulgaris)* essence 2 g and **lavender** essence 2 g, essence of **rosemary** 2 g, and 50 g of sodium bicarbonate. Repeat this washing three times per week.

Autosuggestion **

In case of pruritis caused by nervous tension, depression, etc., repeat the following affirmation twice per day:

> *From day to day I am more calm and relaxed in every way. My skin and body are clean and healthy.*

Color Therapy

Use the following colors in any case of pruritis for relieving this symptom, ten minutes per color, one after the other: blue, violet, green. Also massage the affected area with distilled water energized with green color once per day before sleep.

Herbs

Western **

Elecampane   1:1 ratio as infusion 1 teaspoonfull
Burdock   3 times daily
Thyme   or tincture 10 drops in glass of water
Wild thyme   twice daily

Chinese

Cinnamon and Ma-Huang Combination: For initial stage of pruritis.
Major Blue Dragon Combination: For young men with night pruritis.
Tang-Kuei and Tribulus Combination: For "senile" pruritis.
Gentiana Combination: For pruritis of vulva. An external compress of **Sophora Combination** *(Ku-sheng-tang)* can be applied if itching is severe.

Homeopathy

Radium bromide: 30X once a week for pruritis of anus. Same for pruritus vulva.

Hydrotherapy

In case of pruritis it is important to stimulate the skin by hot and cold showers, alternating a few seconds of hot water following a longer period of cold water. Repeat this process four to seven times once per day before the bath of aromatherapy.

Once or twice per week use a sauna bath to let the toxins in the skin get out by perspiration. The sauna's hot air stimulates the skin and is very helpful in treating pruritis symptoms if the pruritis is the result of another internal disease or disorder. Do not treat by sauna unless you have consulted and checked for the specific problem causing pruritis.

Reflexology

This treatment is mainly symptomatic unless including in the treatment the main disease treatment.

Massage the whole feet twice per day for ten minutes each foot and also by using a metal comb and combing the back of the hand from the wrist to the fingers, downward, for seven minutes each hand, twice per day until condition improves.

ROSACEA AND ERYSIPELAS

SYMPTOMS

Swollen red throat, face, and upper body resulting from strep infection.

SUGGESTED TREATMENT

Acupuncture and Acupressure *

GV 14, SP 10, K 10, PC 8, LI 4, LI 11, ST 36, SP 6.

Applied Nutrition ***

The diet should be the same as in the case of psoriasis.

Aromatherapy

The treatment should be the same as in the case of acne vulgaris.

Color Therapy *

The treatment should be the same as in the case of acne vulgaris.

Herbs ***

Western

Urtica
Calendula—Marigold 1:1 ratio as infusion 3 caps daily or as tincture
Fumaria Officinalis 10 drops in glass of water 3 times daily

Chinese **

Puraria and Carthamus Combination *(Ko-ken-hung-hua-tang):* This formula is taken for a very long time.
Coptis and Scute Combination *(Huang-lien-chieh-tu-tang):* For minor cases with only flushing.
External mixture—1 g sulphur, 1 g apricot seed, and 0.5 g calomel: Mix these components with honey; apply daily and wash in morning for eight to twelve months.

Homeopathy **

Sulphur: 200 as single dose.

Reflexology

The treatment should be as in the case of Herpes Simplex, three or four times per day as a secondary treatment.

Schuessler Tissue Salts

Take five tablets twice per day of each of the following remedies until improvement of the symptoms:

Natrum muriaticum 6X	**Kali muriaticum** 6X
Natrum sulphorica 6X	**Silica** 12X

VITILIGO AND LEUKODERMA

SYMPTOMS

Loss of pigmentation, often inherited, usually on exposed parts of the body.

SUGGESTED TREATMENT

Applied Nutrition *

The diet should be balanced, avoiding all refined foods. In case of vitiligo associated with other disorders use the diet therapy appropriate to the disease. In other cases:
Eat: A diet rich in fiber, fresh raw vegetables, white cereals, sea fish, dairy products, cereals, and a little fruit.
An example of a diet for an average-weight person, thirty years old:

2,000 calories
50 g protein
80 g fat
270 g carbohydrate
Master formula and also:
25,000 IU vitamin A
1,000 IU vitamin D
1,000 IU vitamin E
50 mg vitamin B_2

500 mg PABA
500 mg pantothenic acid
120 mg nucleoprotein desiccated liver
3 tablets glutamic acid hydrochloride
100 mg brewer's yeast in powder or in tablets
200 mg of amino acid tyrosine

Aromatherapy

In case of vitiligo use the essence of **bergamot** 2% in olive oil base. Massage this essence twice per day on the affected area. Do not use bergamot essence when exposing yourself to the sun rays, as pigmentation can occur. This oil increases the photosensitivity of the skin.

Autosuggestion *

Repeat the following affirmations twenty times each, twice per day:

> From day to day I am healthier in my body, skin, mind, and soul in every way.
> I love myself unconditionally.

Color Therapy

In case of vitiligo use the following colors one after the other for ten minutes each: green, orange, red. Apply locally on the affected area. If the vitiligo is near the eyes, the treatment should be much shorter, about one or two minutes each color.

Herbs **

Chinese

Cinnamon and Astragalus Combination: For initial state of disease.
Cinnamon and Hoelen Formula

Reflexology

In cases of vitiligo attention should be paid to the diseases or problems causing the vitiligo; then treat the associated disease.

For vitiligo associated with hyperthyroidism or hypothyroidism the treatment should be in the points:

18 – heart and blood circulation, 19 – spleen,
20 – adrenal gland, 21 – kidney, 22 – pancreas,

24 – liver, 52 – autonomic nervous system,
11 – parathyroid, 13 – thyroid.

Massage each point for three minutes daily in the first week and then twice per day, three minutes each point.
For vitiligo associated with pernicious anemia the treatment should be by massaging the following points twice per day, three minutes each point:

18 – heart and blood circulation, 19 – spleen,
24 – liver, 25 – gall bladder, 52 – autonomic nervous system.

For vitiligo associated with diabetes mellitus the treatment should be massage of the following points three minutes each, twice per day:

18 – heart and blood circulation, 19 – spleen,
20 – adrenal gland, 21 – kidney, 22 – pancreas—massage this point seven minutes twice per day—24 – liver, 25 – gall bladder, 42, 43 – upper and lower lymph glands.

For other diseases and disorders associated with vitiligo massage the following points twice per day, three minutes each:

18 – heart, 19 – spleen, 20 – adrenal glands, 21 – kidney, 22 – pancreas, 24 – liver, 25 – gall bladder, 42, 43 – upper and lower lymph glands, 52 – autonomic nervous system.

Schuessler Tissue Salts
Take the following combination in cases of vitiligo and other primary pigmentary disorders:

Kali muriaticum 12X   **Silica** 12X
Kali sulphorica 12X   **Calcarea fluorica** 12X
Calcarea sulphorica 12X

If the vitiligo is associated with other diseases or disorders, check the appropriate disease for the specific treatment and give the combination of the treatment for vitiligo as above and the other specific treatment.

NEURODERMATITIS

SUGGESTED TREATMENT

The area of skin lesions should be protected and covered. The patient should avoid stress and negative emotional situations.

Acupuncture **

PC7, GB 38, LI 2, LI 4, LI 11, SI 3, SI 5, SP 6, SP 10, UB 17, UB 40, ST 36.
Ear points: Adrenal, Lung, Occiput, Internal Secretion

Applied Nutrition ***

Avoid all food stimulants such as alcohol, beer, coffee, tea, tobacco, etc. The diet should be the same as in the case of eczema.

Aromatherapy *

Use the combination of **camomile** 2%, **hyssop** 1%, **geranium** 3% in oil base on the lesions once per day until improvement of the skin lesions occurs.
Also use one drop of **camomile** 5% on brown sugar tablets once per day, two tablets.

Autosuggestion **

Use the following affirmations three times per day:

> *I am completely relaxed and happy.*
> *Love and forgiveness, I let others be themselves and I am free.*

Color Therapy

Apply locally twice per day blue, orange, and red, five minutes each, one after the other for two to three weeks.

Herbs **

1:1 ratio of tincture 15 drops in 1 glass of water 3 times daily

Western

Cheese-rennet
Wild pansy
Plantain

Chinese

Lonicera and Forsythia Formula: To be taken for one to two months.
Silkworm Molt Combination: For head eczema, ugly pimples, and secretions.
Tang-kuei and Arctium Formula: To be taken only if previous two formulas fail.

Homeopathy **

Sulphur 6X: For simple lichen
Apis 3X: For urticatus lichen, every two to three hours.
Rumex crispus: When red itchy pimples are present, 30 every six hours.

Reflexology

Treat as a secondary treatment the following points twice per day for three minutes each on both hands and feet:

18—heart and blood circulation, 19—spleen, 20—adrenal gland, 21—kidney, 24—liver, 25—gall bladder, 42—upper lymph glands, 52—autonomic nervous system

Schuessler Tissue Salts

Take the following remedies, five tablets each, three doses per day:

Kali muriaticum 6X	**Natrum phosphorica** 3X
Kali sulphorica 6X	**Silica** 6X

SEBORRHEIC DERMATITIS AND DANDRUFF

SYMPTOMS

Flakiness of scalp tissue commonly called "dandruff," especially with oily skin.

SUGGESTED TREATMENT

Applied Nutrition ***

The diet therapy in this condition is the same as in the case of eczema.

Aromatherapy

Use the essence of **geranium** 2% in distilled water base by bathing the affected part three times per week before sleep. Continue with **sage** *(Salvia officinalis)* 10% essence in olive oil base and massage the affected parts twice per week. Allow two hours before washing out the olive oil from the scalp.

Autosuggestion **

The main mental reason for seborrheic dermatitis and dandruff is the lack of security and love. The affirmation should be:

I am in love of myself.
I am emotionally secure and safe.
I always get attention in a positive way.

Repeat one or more of these affirmations twice per day, twenty times each.

Color Therapy

Use locally the following colors for ten minutes each, one after the other, once per day: blue, orange, red.
Also use on scalp or any other affected area water energized with blue color for two hours. Then massage the scalp with this energized water. Sunlight for ten minutes daily is also important in this condition.

Reflexology

Use the same treatment as in the case of ringworm.

Schuessler Tissue Salts **

In cases of seborrheic dermatitis or dandruff take the following remedies twice per day, five tablets

Kali sulphorica 12X   **Kali phosphorica** 12X
Natrum muriaticum 6X   **Silica** 12X

Continue with this treatment until condition improves.

FACIAL REJUVENATION

SUGGESTED TREATMENT

Acupuncture and Acupressure ***

Acupuncture and acupressure can help balance facial muscular tone and improve blood circulation and nutritional supplementation to skin and muscles. These will help to revitalize the skin and by improving facial color/complexion and muscular tone decrease wrinkling and give a younger-looking skin.
ST 2, ST 3, ST 4, ST 5, ST 6, ST 7, ST 10, ST 12, LI 17, LI 18, LI 19, UB 1, UB 2, GB 1, GB 12, GB 14, TW 17, TW 23, GV 26, CV 24, Yin Tang, Tai-yang.

Applied Nutrition ****

Commence this diet with three days of our rejuvenating juice fasting. Then continue with our diet.

Drink: Pure mineral water.
Eat: Fresh green salads, raw vegetables, fresh fruits, whole cereals and beans, seeds, and a little sea fish. Avoid all stimulants, sweets, salts, and canned or conserved foods. An example of a diet for a person of average weight, thirty years old:

2,200–2,500 calories   100 g fat
50 g protein   275–310 g carbohydrate

Master formula of vitamins and minerals, and also:

1 tablet B_{50} chelated
100 mg vitamin C   1,000 IU vitamin E
2 tablets multiamino minerals

Enzymes daily:

80 mg betaine hydrochloric acid   55 mg pepsin
100 mg pancreatin   60 mg lipase
Bile extract   90 mg papain

Nucleoprotein formula of extracts:

10 mg pituitary   40 mg pancreas
50 mg adrenal   40 mg kidney
50 mg heart   Ribonucleic acid (RNA)
40 mg thymus

Autosuggestion
Repeat the following affirmation twenty times daily:

> From day to day I am stronger, healthier, happier, and more relaxed in every way.

Breathing Therapy
One of the most important things in rejuvenating the skin is oxygen. In order to have enough oxygen the breathing exercises are very important.
Breathe deeply in and out, ten to fifteen continuous breaths every morning and evening in the open air. If this exercise is done at home, use an ionization machine for better air.

Exercises ****
An old yoga system for a better appearance involves face and neck exercises. By practicing fifteen or twenty-five minutes daily your face muscles become stronger, and the whole appearance of the face becomes younger. The wrinkles diminish in most cases after a few months of regular practice.

Exercises are to be done one after the other, five to ten times each, and the skin should be clean and dry.

Frontal muscles: Put your hands on the eyebrows while exhaling. Try to raise your eyebrows as much as you can. At the same time resist this movement with your hands. Repeat this exercise five times daily.

Frontal muscles (piramidal):   Put your fingers on the space between the eyebrows and while exhaling try to close the space between the eyebrows, at the same time resisting this movement with your fingers. Repeat this exercise ten times daily.

Eyelids: Put your fingers on the upper and lower lids, and while softly resisting the closing of the eye, try to close the eyelids. Open the eyes. This exercise should be done very carefully and without much effort of the eyelids. Repeat this exercise twice per day, five times each session.

"Paranasal" Superficial Muscles (located in the side of the nose):   In this exercise, put your fingers on the sides of the nose and try to raise your mouth and nose upward while resisting the movement with your fingers. Repeat this exercise ten times daily.

Orbicular des levres (mouth muscles):   Put your fingers in the sides of the mouth—both sides—and open the mouth to the sides (like smiling). Then close your mouth as much as you can while resisting this movement with your fingers. Repeat this exercise ten times twice a day.

Masseter muscles (jaw muscles):   Put your hands on the sides of the mouth, about four or five fingers on each side from the corners of mouth. While making a gum-chewing movement, resist it with your hands, pushing downward. Repeat this exercise fifteen to twenty times twice a day.

Mentalis and triangularis muscles (chin):   This exercise is excellent for a double chin. The tongue should be raised as much as you can while sucking the tongue and raising up the chin. Then, while raising the chin, stretch the muscles of the digastricus anterior (double-chin muscles) and make them as hard as you can for a few seconds. Repeat this exercise three or four times a day.

Lower Face: Try to open and close the mouth while resisting this movement with your hands. Repeat this exercise ten times twice a day. In this exercise hold the chin with both hands.

Neck muscles: Move your head up and down while resisting movement:

- downward by placing your hands under the chin and lifting the face with your hands while lowering the head
- upward by placing your hands on the back of the head (occipitalis)

and trying to lower the head while raising the head at the same time. Repeat this exercise ten times twice a day.

Neck muscles (sides):   Move your head left and right while resisting this movement with your hands placed on the temporals. Repeat this exercise ten times twice a day.

Spine and whole-body exercises (stretching):

- while sitting on a chair try to touch the sky with your hands for a few seconds, then relax.
- while sitting on a chair try to touch the floor with your hands for a few seconds, then relax.
- repeat the same exercise with your head, trying to touch the sky and the floor for a few seconds.

Repeat these exercises twice or more per day, three or four times each.

Herbs

Western ***

Comfrey: Lotion for wrinkles due to nutritionally deficient skin. Apply twice daily morning and evening

Kelp: Has silicon to help reduce wrinkling fast. Two tablets a day

Fig *(Ficus carica):*   A good fruit to eat to soothe skin.

Alkanet *(Alkanna tinctoria):*   Powder or ointment to soothe and soften the skin. Apply nightly.

Chinese **

For freckles and black spots, **Cinnamon and Hoelen formula Pearl Cream** for nightly use.

Hydrotherapy **

For rejuvenating the head and face, it is recommended (if health conditions permit) to use the vapor bath twice per week, two to five minutes each time.

The vapor pot should be placed on a chair. The person sits in front of the pot. The upper part of the body is undressed. A sheet is thrown over the upper body and the vapor pot together, so that the steam can escape. Breathe in through the mouth and nose a few times (three to twenty times), slowly increasing the number of breaths in the vapor. Add to the water twenty-two drops of the following aromatherapy combination:

Frankincense—5 drops   Lavender—4 drops
Jasmine—2 drops   Melissa—3 drops

Myrrh—4 drops   Rose—2 drops
Patchouli—2 drops

in vegetable oil base.

Reflexology **
Press and massage the following points twice per day for two minutes each:

1—Sinus, 2—Pituitary gland, 3—Cerebrum, 6—Eye, 7—Temple, 11—Parathyroid, 13—Thyroid, 16—Lung, 18—Heart and Blood Circulation, 19—Spleen, 20—Adrenal Gland, 21—Kidney, 24—Liver, 42, 43—Lower and upper lymph gland

Schuessler Tissue Salts
For rejuvenating the skin cells take the following combination twice per day, three to five tablets or drops.

Kali muriaticum 6X   **Kali phosphorica** 6X
Kali sulphorica 6X   **Ferrum phosphorica** 6X
Calcarea sulphorica 6X   **Natrum muriaticum** 6X
Silica 6X

In one tablet or in spirit aqua.
In taking this combination the wrinkles in the face diminish slowly after a few months of regular use.

SKIN CARE

SUGGESTED TREATMENT

The skin is the mirror of your health. If you have a healthy body and mind, your skin will probably be healthy, clean, and elastic, your eyes bright, your hair shining, your smile happy, your body athletic, your nails and teeth clean.

There are many theories that treat body and mind before any cosmetic treatment. We prefer to combine health and beauty care. This chapter is intended for both men and women who want to look and feel better.

Applied Nutrition ***
The diet should be the same as for facial rejuvenation.

Aromatherapy

Use the extracts of the plants according to the skin condition.

Normal skin: Use **rosemary** 1% and **camomile** 1% in steam bath for five minutes twice a week. Use this steam bath only if there are no thread veins and if health condition permits steam bath.

Greasy skin: Use **rosemary** 3% and **sage** 2% in steam bath for five minutes twice a week.

Dry skin: Use **rosemary** 2% and **geranium** in vegetable oil base once a day as a massage three times per week.

Combination skin: Follow the treatments for both dry and greasy skin twice a week.

Autosuggestion

Repeat these affirmations twenty times daily:

> *From day to day I am better and better in every way.*
> *From day to day my skin is healthier, cleaner and stronger in every way.*

Cleaning, Toning, Moisturizing, and Special Treatments of the Face

Normal, healthy skin: Smooth, soft, fine, and elastic skin. You can see occasional spots or marks but no real problems of the skin.

Cleanse—light cleansing cream
Tone—light skin tonic
Moisturize—light liquid moisturizer
Special treatments—weekly mask or light steam facial
Greasy skin: Face quickly becomes shiny. Skin looks greasy. Prone to open pores, red spots, and marks, especially around the nose.
Cleanse—medicated cleanser twice per day
Tone—apply astringent in greasy areas twice per day
Moisturize—a light liquid moisturizer
Special treatment—twice per day use a mask or steam facial, five minutes twice a week.
Dry skin: Flaky and dull, the skin looks papery and dry.
Cleanse—massage in rich cleansing cream and wipe off with cotton wool.
Tone—very gentle toner, diluted more than usual if skin is very dry.
Moisturize—light moisturizing during the day with a rich nourishing cream at night
Special treatment—moisturize face once a week with honey, avocado, or egg yolk for twenty minutes, then wipe off and tone and moisturize the face.

Combination: A greasy panel down the center of the face with dryish areas on cheeks and around the eyes. This is the most common condition of the face.
Cleanse—use a light cream, then continue with soap on greasy areas.
Tone—light toning lotion
Moisturize—liquid moisturizer all over the face
Special treatment—once-a-week face mask and steam bath once or twice a week.

Color Therapy and Aromatherapy

If the skin is normal, expose your body for ten minutes twice a day to the sunlight, after massaging the body with **vitamin E** oil 2% mixed with wheat germ oil as a base.
In case of dry skin, start with sunlight for five minutes twice per day.
If your skin is greasy, start with fifteen minutes per day of sunbath and add **rosemary** extract 2% to vegetable oil.

Reflexology **

A general massage all over the feet and hands with reflexology roller device twice per day for five minutes each foot or hand. Also press and massage the same points as in the face-lifting treatment.

Schuessler Tissue Salts

Take twice per day the following combination:

Silica 3X	**Natrum sulphorica** 6X
Ferrum phosphorica 6X	**Magnesium phosphorica** 6X
Natrum muriaticum 6X	**Kali phosphorica** 6X

Five tablets or drops each morning and evening for the first month.

· 7 ·

THE REPRODUCTIVE
AND URINARY SYSTEMS

Up to ten percent of all hospital admissions are for the treatment of the genitourinary system. Infections frequently occur in women, but males have distinct structural problems as well. This area of medicine demands careful diagnosis and often specialized techniques.

Problems in dysuria—which is difficulty or painful discharge of urine—are common. Such problems may indicate food poisoning, low-grade infections, or a variety of dietary changes. Most people are aware of their own history of such problems. When the problems become intense or prolonged, care should be taken to get more specific diagnoses. Inflammation in the bladder commonly causes prostatitis in males and cystitis in females. Persistent pain in voiding may be the result of other diseases: syphilis, multiple sclerosis, or diabetes.

With incontinence, infections or major disease states may be the underlying cause. Incontinence may also be a congenital trait. Males over seventy or under five years of age may be considered normal candidates for incontinence (or bedwetting, in the latter case). After five, bedwetting (eneuresis) not due to obvious emotional problems should be considered a functional problem.

Various chronic conditions, such as forms of diabetes, kidney disorders, and even potassium depletion, may cause an abnormal, diluted flow of urine, or polyuria. In hematuria, blood in the urine also points to serious problems. Tumors account for about one in five cases. Other conditions are hemorrhage in the bladder or severe problems in the urethra or kidneys. For women, blood in the urine is difficult to identify as from the urinary tract, the vagina, or the rectum.

When there is inflammation of the kidney, or nephritis, the symptoms may be so varied as to defy accurate diagnosis. Various parts of the kidney may be affected, in either acute or chronic ways. Problems in voiding may also be accompanied by fever, flank pains, nausea, and vomiting.

Urinary tract infections are the common currency of this field. They occur so frequently, in varying degrees, that few patients can distinguish them from ordinary problems associated with poor dietary habits and stress. Bacteria exist to some degree in all urinary tracts; the seriousness of the problem is always a matter of degree. Thus cystitis may easily be a matter of definition. The only overt sign of such disorders is a burning sensation during urination.

The kidneys are subject to an acute disorder popularly known as "kidney stones." (The Latin root for the English "kidneys" is "renus," while the Greek is "nephros." Thus diseases of the kidneys are sometimes referred to as "renitis" and sometimes as "nephritis," while the glands that rest on top the kidneys are named with the appropriate Latin or Greek preposition—hence, the adrenals and the epinephrines secreted by them.) Renal colic, or an attack of kidney stones, typically is a severe cramp in one side of the back, radiating to the abdomen and lower thigh. Small stones may be passed for years with no such complications, but large stones usually require surgery for removal. Chronic infection as well as family history may predispose one to kidney stones.

Inflammation of testes and prostate problems are common in postpubescent males, the latter resulting in a common operation at middle age. Extreme tenderness in the prostate gland may result from infections, which are not chronic. Massage and hot baths may be helpful or harmful, depending on the exact condition of the prostate.

The reproductive system in both men and women holds out many challenges to medicine. Surgery may be helpful in many cases, but alternative medical approaches have a great part to play.

The reproductive cycle in females begins with the first menses and continues through to menopause and the cessation of reproductive possibility. Delay in beginning menstruation or subsequent missing of periods may be tolerably normal or may indicate a problem. Uterine abnormalities account for most cases of dysmenorrhea—discomfort in menstruation—or primary or secondary amenorrhea.

In recent years, premenstrual tension, or premenstrual syndrome (PMS), has received great attention in the media as a distinct medical problem. Casually dismissed as "in the mind" in former days, PMS is now believed to affect the majority of women of childbearing age at the specific time of five to eight days prior to menstruation. Bloating, breast tenderness, edema leading to weight gain, and various psychological disorders are common. The well-known fluctuations in female sex-hormone levels during the reproductive period would indicate a wide variety in biochemical reactions and mood changes. Bleeding during this period typically signifies pregnancy but may also point to disease conditions in the uterus or ovaries.

The other major reproductive problems of women are mastitis (infection of the breast) and insufficient lactation (for a newborn). Frigidity, the inability to experience sexual satisfaction, and infertility affect more women than men. Men, however, should be thoroughly tested first in cases of inability to conceive—to rule out the possibility of insufficient sperm due to functional problems or infections. Of the ten percent of couples in the United States unable to conceive, four percent suffer from male gonadal insufficiency.

Male insufficiency may be due to a low sperm count (oligospermia), complete absence of sperm in the semen (azoospermia), or no ejaculate at all (aspermia). These in turn may be the result of testicular atrophy (from infection, alcoholism, etc.), drug toxicity, prolonged fever (resulting in increased testicular heat), hypothyroidism, adrenal problems, testicular abnormalities such as undescended testes, or various obstructions of the seminal tract. Sufficient levels of sperm count and motility are well established.

Investigation of causes of female infertility is more time-consuming and expensive. Regular ovulation is the first requisite. It is more difficult to evaluate the functioning of the reproductive tract for the ability to unite the sperm and ovum in the oviduct.

The distinctly male problem of premature ejaculation may require psychological counseling as well as medical attention to the possibility of such inflammations as protatitis and urethritis. The typical progressive frustration felt by the female partner may aggravate already severe psychological problems of the male, resulting in discouragement and feelings of inferiority, leading to impotence or at least impaired sexual performance. In rare cases, desensitization of the penis through mechanical means may be helpful.

The condition of menopause, or change of life, is biologically a female phenomenon, although there are psychological components of the syndrome that may appear in some males in middle to late-middle age. Natural menopause is a normal result of declining ovarian function between ages forty-five and fifty. So-called artificial menopause may follow surgical removal or irradiation of the ovaries. Premature attrition of the follicles in the ovaries may cause symptoms of menopause before the age of forty. The intensity of symptoms varies substantially from woman to woman, as does their duration. The most common and annoying symptom is the abrupt rise in temperature, with sweating, known as hot flashes. Headaches, insomnia, palpitation, numbness, and even vertigo occur frequently. Fatigue and irritability often alternate with nervousness and excitability, crying spells, and general depression. The possibility of organic disease as the cause of one or more of these symptoms should not be dismissed. It is always possible that menopausal symptoms may never appear or may last for as short a time as a few months.

DYSURIA

SYMPTOMS

Difficult or painful discharge of urine.

SUGGESTED TREATMENT

Acupuncture and Acupressure **

1. CV 2, CV3, CV 4, CV 5, CV 9, UB 31, UB 32, UB 33, UB 34, UB 38, UB 47, HT 8, K 4, K 5, ST 36.
2. UB 28, UB 31–34, K 1, K 4, K 5, K 11, Liv 8, CV 5, CV 9, UB 20.

Ear points—Shen-men, Zero, Kidney.

Herbs ***

capsuels 1 X3 daily, infusion 1 X3 daily or 1:1 ratio of all 3 herbs in tincture 10 drops in glass of water X3 daily

Western

Berberry *(Uva ursi)*, **dandelion** *(Taraxacum)*, and **Yarrow** *(Achillea)* may be effective.

Chinese ****

Rehmannia 8 Formula: When there is kidney atrophy and for dysuria in last trimester of pregnancy.
Polyporus Combination: For painful and dripping urination.

Homeopathy

Cantharis: 3X every three hours for painful, drop-by-drop urination.

Camphor: 3X every one to three hours for acute strangury.
Copaiba: 3 every half hour for women with strangury.

SUGGESTED TREATMENT

Applied Nutrition

Drink: Mineral or boiled fresh water. Avoid any stimulating beverage such as alcohol, beer, coffee, or tea.
Eat: A lot of fresh vegetables, fruits, whole cereals with beans (well-cooked). Avoid sugar and reduce animal protein. Also avoid salt in the food.

An example of a diet for an average-weight person, thirty years old:

2,000 calories	400 IU vitamin E
40 g protein	50 mg B_6
80 g fat	15 mg zinc
280 g carbohydrate	Nucleoproteins
Master formula of vitamins and	60 mg adrenal
minerals and:	40 mg thymus
3,000 mg vitamin C	40 mg kidney

Aromatherapy

Use the aromatherapy extract of:
Black pepper—if the dysuria is accompanied by vertigo and fever.
Cedarwood—if the dysuria is accompanied by cancer, gonorrhea, or cystitis.
Juniper—if the dysuria is accompanied by nervous disorders, urinary tract infections, kidney stones.

Autosuggestion

Repeat the following affirmations twice per day:

> *I release the old ideas and welcome the new life.*
> *From day to day I'm healthier and better in every way.*

Color Therapy

Use the following color radiation locally for twenty minutes each color, one after the other each day: yellow, blue, violet.

Reflexology ***

To relieve this symptomatic condition, massage and press the following points in the hands and feet every hour for two minutes each point until condition improves:

20—Adrenal, 21—Kidney, 32—Urinary Tract, 33—Bladder, 43—
Lower Lymph Gland, 44—Uterine Tube—Spermatic Duct, 26—

Uterus—Prostate, 49—Sex Hormones, 52—Autonomic Nervous System, 55—General Pain

Schuessler Tissue Salts
Use the following combination to relieve this symptom, twice per day, ten tablets each time until condition improves.

Natrum sulphorica 3X   **Kali muriaticum** 6X
Natrum muriaticum 6X   **Ferrum phosphorica** 6X

INCONTINENCE

SUGGESTED TREATMENT

Acupuncture **

1. UB 32, UB 53, UB 23, LI 3
2. UB 23, SP 6, UB 33

Can use these two groups in rotation.
Moxa—UB 22, UB 27, LI 3, UB 67
Also add LI 4, LiV 3
Ear points—Bladder, Urethra, External Genitalia,
Sympathetic
Additional points - Kidney, Spleen, Triple Warmer
Acupuncture is effective for this condition. Must find underlying cause.

Herbs *

Western
Combine **horsetail** *(Equisetum arvense),* **agrimony,** and   1:1 ratio
sweet sumac *(Rhus aromatica).* Drink as tea three to four
times a day or take three capsules a day.

Chinese ***
Rehmannia 8 Formula and Cervus (deer antler; add three g):   Good
for incontinence, nocturia, cold extremities.
Rehmannia 6 Formula: For cloudy urine, dry throat.

Homeopathy **

Belladonna: 3 every four to six hours for nocturnal incontinence.
Benzoic acid: 3X every four to six hours when urine is very smelly
and hot.

Kreosotum: 3 every eight hours for children when they are not easily awakened.
Verbascum thapsus: 3 every four hours for constant dribbling.
Gelsemium: 6X when prostate is enlarged and/or bladder stone is present.
Causticum: 3 to 6 for involuntary loss while coughing or laughing.

INCONTINENCE AND ENURESIS (BEDWETTING)

SUGGESTED TREATMENT

Acupuncture and Acupressure

For children only acupressure is recommended.
For chills and bedwetting - Massage and Moxa:
CV 3, CV 4, and LiV 1, GV 20.
Add also: UB 23, UB 47, UB 28, ST 36, SP 6, K 3.
LI 4 and GV 20 are important in acupuncture treatment.
SP 9, LU 7, LI 6 too.
Ear points: Bladder, Brain, Sympathetic, Urethra, Occiput.

Applied Nutrition

The diet should be as in the case of dysuria. The beverages should be given in less quantity, and for children avoid or reduce drinks before sleep.

Aromatherapy

Use two drops each of **cypress** and **pine** in a vegetable oil base, and massage the lower area.

Autosuggestion

Use the same affirmation as in the case of dysuria.

Bach Flowers

Rock rose: For hysterical children.
Aspen: For those with fears of unknown origin.
Walnut: For those seeking protection.

Color Therapy

Use the following colors daily, one after the other, fifteen minutes each, applied locally: blue, green.

Herbs ***

Western

Bearberry 1:1 ratio five drops of mother tincture in glass of water
Horsetail twice daily for two months only. *

Passiflora or oats: Because of psychological factors like fear, etc.,
add for relaxation.

Chinese

Minor Cinnamon and Paeony Formula
Pueraria Combination

Reflexology **

Use the same treatment as in the case of dysuria, but three times per
day in place of every hour.

Homeopathy ****

Sabadilla: 6X to 30X when urine is thick and clay-colored.
Ferrum phosphorica: 6X for weak sphincter muscle.
Gelsemium: Choice for hyperactive, nervous children.
Belladonna: 3C every eight hours for children with bedwetting in
early night hours.

Schuessler Tissue Salts

Take twice per day the following remedies in combination, ten tablets
each time:

Calcarea phosphorica 12X
Natrum muriaticum 12X
Ferrum phosphorica 12X

LEUKORRHEA

SUGGESTED TREATMENT

Acupuncture and Acupressure **

GB 26, SP 6, CV 6
If there is yellow smelly discharge, add:
LiV 2 and SP 9.
If patient is tired, add:

CV 4 and ST 36.
Electro Acupuncture:
Moderate frequency for ten to fifteen minutes after connecting one point of trunk to one on lower limb.
Moxa is useful on: GV 4, CV 3, CV 8.
Ear points: Uterus, Bladder, Shen-men.

Applied Nutrition **

The diet therapy should be the same as in the case of premenstrual tension.

Aromatherapy

Make a bath with the following extracts daily with ten drops as follows: **bergamot**—four drops, **eucalyptus**—four drops, Lavender—two drops.

Bach Flowers **

Crabapple   four drops once daily.

Color Therapy

Use blue and green colors daily for twenty minutes each.

Herbs ***

Western

Beth root (*Trillium pendulum erectum*):   Checks secretions. Infusion over dried powder of the root of this herb.
Billberry (*Vaccinium myrtillus*):   For washing the vagina.
American bittersweet (*Cleastrus scadens*):   Both root and bark in decoction are reported to be effective.
Buchu: in infusion or ten to twenty tincture drops.
Ergot (*Claviceps purpurea*):   Widely used for this condition, fifteen to thirty drops of extract daily.
Witch hazel (*Hamamelis*):   In infusion or ointment.

Chinese ***

Gentiana Combination: For yellow discharge due to endometriosis, vaginitis, and vaginal trichomoniasis.
Cinnamon and Hoelen Formula: For acute and chronic leukorrhea with lower abdominal pain.
Tang-kuei and Eight Herb Formula (*Pa-wei-tai-hsia-fang*):   for

chronic leukorrhea with yellow or white discharge with mild anemia, or when caused by gonoccoccus or trichomoniasis.

Tang-kuei and Evodia Combination: For water leukorrhea.

Homeopathy **

Pulsatilla: 3X every four to six hours for simple white mucus discharge (mostly in blond females).

Fagopyrum: 3X to 12X for yellow discharge and pruritus vulvae.

Sepia: 6X four times daily for greenish, offensive discharge.

Alumina: 6–30 for irritating, burning white discharge before or after period.

Borax: 3–30 for clear white discharge in midcycle.

Magnet Therapy

In evening north pole on CV 4 and morning strong magnets on soles of feet.

Reflexology

Press and massage the same points as in the case of amenorrhea.

Schuessler Tissue Salts

Kali muriaticum: 12X three times per day in case of discharge of non-irritating mucus of milky-white color.

Kali phosphorica: 6X to 12X three times per day in case of yellowish, acrid, and scalding discharge.

Kali sulphorica: 6X to 12X three times per day in case of yellowgreenish discharge.

Natrum muriaticum: 6X to 12X three times per day in the case of watery, irritating discharge.

Natrum phosphorica: 6X to 12X three times per day in case of creamy or honey-colored or acrid and sour-smelling discharge.

Calcorea phosphorica: 6X to 12X three times per day in case of albuminous mucus, worse after menses.

HEMATURIA (BLEEDING INT HE URINARY TRACT)

SUGGESTED TREATMENT

Acupuncture ***

1. LI 4, PC 7, CV 4, CV 6, UB 23, K 7, ST 36.
2. K3, SP 10, UB 23, UB 27, UB 28, LiV3, ST 36, LI 4, PC 7.

Ear points: Adrenal, Liver, Kidney, Bladder.

Applied Nutrition *

Commence the diet with three days juice fasting, then continue with the rejuvenating diet. An example of a diet for an average-weight person, thirty years old:

1,800 calories	50 mg vitamin B_1
40 g protein	50 mg vitamin B_2
70 g fat	50 mg vitamin B_6
252 g carbohydrate	100 mcg vitamin B_{12}
Master formula and:	100 mg vitamin B_{15}
25,000 IU vitamin A	*Nucleoprotein*
1,000 IU vitamin D	60 mg kidney
1,000 IU vitamin E	40 mg adrenal
3,000 mg vitamin C	40 mg ribonucleic acid extract
300 mg bioflavinoids	

Aromatherapy

1. Use the following combination and massage the lower part of the body. In vegetable oil base: **nettle** 1%, **pine** 2%, **horsetail** 1%, **wild thyme** 3%.
2. Take one drop of the following on brown sugar tablet daily, every morning and evening, for three weeks: **milk thistle, potentilla, cinnamon.**

Autosuggestion

As for most of the urinary system, use the general affirmation:

From day to day I am healthier and better in every way.

Repeat this affirmation twenty times twice per day.

Color Therapy

Use the following combination of colors one after the other for twenty minutes, three or four times per day until blood is stopped and condition improves: blue, violet, ultraviolet.

Herbs

Chinese

Polyporus Formula

Homeopathy

Terrebinthina   3 every two hours.
Hamamelia: 1 every two hours when painful.

Reflexology

Press and massage the following points twice per day, five minutes each point:

20—Adrenal Glands, 21—Kidneys, 24—Liver, 32—Urinary Tract, 33—Bladder, 43—Lower Lymph Glands, 52—Autonomic Nervous System

Schuessler Tissue Salts

Take the following combination three times per day:

Kali phosphorica 12X   **Calcarea phosphorica** 6X
Kali muriaticum 12X

POLYURIA

SYMPTOMS

Often seen as light-colored urine, irregular flow of urine, or obstructions in urinating.

SUGGESTED TREATMENT

Acupuncture *

SI 1, ST 36, UB 21.

Applied Nutrition

The diet should be given according to the specific disease or disorder.

Autosuggestion

Repeat this affirmation twice per day:

> *From day to day I am better and better in every way.*

Color Therapy

Should be applied according to the specific disorder that causes the polyuria. But to relieve the stress feelings, use the following rays for fifteen minutes each one, once per day: blue, violet.

Herbs

Chinese ***

Rehmannia 8 Formula: For profuse urination with cold extremities. Also for diabetic polyuria.
Ginseng and Gypsum Combination: For polyuria accompanied by fever, sweating, and thirst.

Homeopathy ***

Causticum: 3X for night urge in older people.
Carlsbad: 6 every eight hours for urge after water consumption.
Ignatia: 3 every eight hours for after-coffee urge.
Scilla: 1 every three to four hours for polyuria in diabetes, or
Murex: 6 four to six times daily if mostly night frequency.
Syzygium: 1X (gtt. v.) every eight hours for diabetes mellitus.

Reflexology

Use the same treatment as in the case of dysuria.

Schuessler Tissue Salts

To cure this problem the primal cause should be diagnosed and treated accordingly. But to relieve the symptoms, take the following remedies three times per day, ten tablets each time:

Natrum muriaticum 12X
Kali phosphorica 6X

NEPHRITIS (KIDNEY STONES)

SYMPTOMS

Severe cramps in one side of the back, radiating to the abdomen and thigh.

SUGGESTED TREATMENT

Acupuncture **

UB 23, K 7, SP 6, K 9, ST 41, UB 26, ST 28, CV 9
Ear points: Shen-men, Kidney, Triple Warmer, Occiput

Applied Nutrition ****

This diet should be rich in carbohydrate and fat with little protein and sodium.

An example of a diet for an average-weight person, thirty years old:

1,800 calories	Nucleoprotein extracts
25 g protein	60 mg kidney (twice per day)
80 g fat	40 mg ribonucleic acid
245 g carbohydrate	40 mg adrenal
Master formula of vitamins and	10 mg pituitary
minerals and:	

Aromatherapy

Use the following combination in vegetable oil base as a massage oil: **eucalyptus**—2%, **juniper**—2%, **geranium**—1%, **thyme**—2%. Massage the back area of the body once per day.

Autosuggestion

Repeat the general affirmation used in the case of hematuria.

Color Therapy

Use the following colors locally, fifteen minutes each color, twice per day: blue locally, blue and green generally, violet locally and generally.

Herbs ***

Chinese

Hoelen Five-Herb Formula: For oliguria after drinking. No edema present.

Major Blue Dragon Combination: For acute nephritis with severe edema, headache, anxiety.

Minor Blue Dragon Combination: Effective for fever, oliguria, and edema in acute nephritis.

Bupleurum and Dragon Bone Combination: For cases with no edema but with hypertension, palpitation, and constipation.

Minor Bupleurum Combination with Hoelen and Coptis: For chronic nephritis with albinuria.

Stephanie and Ginseng Combination: For chronic and degenerative nephritis.

Homeopathy **

Arsenicum: 3 every two to four hours for tubular nephritis, 9 after scarlatina.

Mercurius: 3 every two hours.

Reflexology

Press each point for ten minutes three times per day in case of chronic nephritis:

20—Adrenal gland, 21—Kidneys, 18—Heart and Circulation, 24—Liver, 32—Urinary Tract, 33—Bladder, 52—Autonomic Nervous System.

Schuessler Tissue Salts

Take the following remedies twice per day, ten tablets each, until condition improves:

Kali muriaticum 6X   **Ferrum phosphorica** 12X

ENDOMETRITIS

SUGGESTED TREATMENT

Acupuncture **

GB 26, CV 3 joined to CV 2, SP 6, SP 8, UB 23, GB 27, ST 29, ST 36. Ear points: Adrenal, Internal secretion, Ovary, Uterus, External Genitals.

Applied Nutrition

Use the same diet therapy as in the case of premenstrual tension.

Aromatherapy
Use a bath with the following extracts once per day, ten drops in total:
bergamot—four drops, **camomile**—four drops, **juniper**—two drops.

Color Therapy
Use the following colors locally, one after the other, once per day until condition improves: blue—twenty minutes, indigo—ten minutes, violet—ten minutes.

Herbs ***
Garlic to eat on a daily basis; Kyolic capsules 1 x 3 daily; Echinea as decoction 1 x 3 daily or tincture 10 drops daily x 3 in glass of water.

Western

Garlic and **echinea:** Antimicrobials in tincture 10 drops in glass of water x 3 daily.
Cleavers *(Galium):* Should be used in lymphatic drainage.

Chinese ***

Gentiana Combination: For acute or chronic endometritis due to bacterial infection.
Cinnamon and Hoelen Formula: When due to retained placenta, myoma of uterus with leukorrhea, and difficult or excessive menstruation.
Persica and Rhubarb Combination: For severe endometritis.
Rhubarb and Moutan Combination: For the most serious cases of endometritis.

Homeopathy **

Arsenicum album: 3X four times daily.

Magnet Therapy
Strong magnets applied in morning on palms. In the evening apply magnets to SP 6 acupuncture point, north pole right side and south pole left side.

Reflexology **
Press the same points as in the case of amenorrhea.

Schuessler Tissue Salts
Take the following three times per day until condition improves, five tablets each:

Ferrum phosphorica 12X   **Kali phosphorica** 12X
Natrum muriaticum 12X

URINARY TRACT INFECTION, URETHRITIS, AND CYSTITIS

SYMPTOMS

Burning sensation during urination is the most common sign. Frequency and urgency are also common symptoms.

SUGGESTED TREATMENT

Acupuncture and Acupressure **

1. UB 23, UB 28, LI 3, SP 6, UB 32, Liv 8.
2. UB 23, K9, ST 29, UB 58, LI 3.
    Ear points - Kidney, Bladder, Urethra
    Also add: Subcortex, Neurogate, Sympathetic

Applied Nutrition **

The food should be low in salt and protein, rich in carbohydrate and fat. The diet is the same as in the case of nephritis.

Aromatherapy

Use the following combination on brown sugar tablet base, two tablets daily: **eucalyptus**—3%, **juniper**—2%, **thyme**—2%.

Autosuggestion

Repeat the following affirmations twice per day:

> *I love myself unconditionally.*
> *From day to day I am healthier and healthier in every way.*

Color Therapy

Use the following colors locally, ten minutes each, one after the other: blue, green, violet, ultraviolet.

Herbs **

Western

Bearberry, couchgrass, and **yarrow:**   Separately or as a combination. As capsules 1 x 3 daily 1:1 ratio

Chinese

Polyporus Combination: For acute and chronic cystitis, strangury, and tendency to dribble after urination with pain and occasional hematuria.

Gentiana Combination: For severe inflammation with painful urination.

Lotus Seed Combination: For turbid and residual urine, loss of appetite, and general fatigue.

Hoelen Five-Herb Formula: For turbid urine, thirst.

Homeopathy

Cantharis: For acute inflammation use 3 every two hours.

Cantaris: When chronic use 3 to 6 every six hours.

Benzinum Acidum: If urine has a very strong horselike smell, take 3X every six hours.

Borax: For pungent smell, 6X every eight hours.

Reflexology

Press the same points as in the case of nephritis twice per day.

Shuessler Tissue Salts

Use the following combination, ten tablets twice per day. Continue this treatment until condition improves.

Kali muriaticum 12X	**Kali phosphorica** 12X
Ferrum phosphorica 12X	**Magnesium phosphorica** 12X

NEPHROLITHIASIS

SUGGESTED TREATMENT

Applied Nutrition ***

In case of alkali stones:

Eat: Mainly foods containing acid, such as whole rice, whole bread, eggs, cheese, sea fish, beans, seeds, whole green salad.

In case of acid stone:

Eat: Mainly food containing alkali, such as almonds, fruits, fresh salads, baking powders.

An example of a diet for an average-weight person, thirty years old:

2,000 calories	285 g carbohydrate
60 g protein	Master Formula of vitamins and
100 g fat	minerals and:

25,000 IU vitamin A   50 mg vitamin B₃
50 mg vitamin B₁   1,000 mg vitamin C
50 mg vitamin B₂

Aromatherapy
Use the following on brown sugar tablets, one drop of each extract:
fennel, geranium, hyssop.

Color Therapy
Use the following colors twice per day for ten minutes each time locally all over the lower body: violet, blue, ultraviolet.

Herbs ****
As capsules, 1 three times daily as separate herbs or 1:1 as combination 1 three times daily.

Western
Pellitory of the Wall *(Parietaria diffus):*   Also effective for kidney stones and gravel.
Buchu: An infusion may prove helpful.

Homeopathy ***

Odimum canum: 30 every fifteen minutes when passing renal calculus with agonizing pain.
Berberis: 6 every fifteen minutes for violent pains from kidneys to urethra.

Reflexology **
Press the following points four to six times per day for one to two minutes each:

   20—Adrenal Gland, 21—Kidneys, 32—Urinary Tract, 33—Bladder.

Schuessler Tissue Salts
Take the following remedy, five tablets every hour, until the stones dissolve:

Calcarea phosphorica 12X   **Natrum sulphorica** 12X

AMENORRHEA AND DYSMENORRHEA (MENSTRUAL PERIOD DISORDERS)

SYMPTOMS

Late or missed menstrual periods and discomfort in menstruation are relative problems that may indicate a range of underlying causes, from insufficient dietary fat to pregnancy.

SUGGESTED TREATMENT—AMENORRHEA

Acupuncture and Acupressure ****

Shiatsu-Acupressure:

Massage first GV 4 and UB 23. Then UB 22, UB 31–34, UB 47, CV 6, CV 4, SP 10, GV 20, GB 20, ST 27. Massage on K3, K7 when chills of lower limbs are present.

Acupuncture:

UB 23, LI 7, SP 6, UB 17, SO 10, ST 30, SP 8, LiV 8.

For cessation of periods:

1. Moxa GV 2, K 6
2. LI 11, ST 36, TW 6

Ear points: Endocrine, Kidney, Liver, Spleen, Neurogate, Subcortex

Applied Nutrition ****

The diet therapy should be the same as in the case of orchitis.

Aromatherapy

For amenorrhea take the following extracts in vegetable oil base: **camomile**—2%, **clary**—1%, **fennel**—1%, **pennyroyal**—2%. Massage the pubis, sacrum, and external vagina with these extracts before the color therapy.

Color Therapy

To treat this problem use ten minutes of the following light over the pubis, the sacrum, and into vagina with the aid of a vaginal speculum after massaging with aromatherapy: blue—ten minutes each place, violet—ten minutes each place.

Herbs

Western ***

Pennyroyal and **tansy:**   Infuse (capsules are good, too) and drink daily (three to five times) until period begins.

Blue cohosh *(Caulophyllum thalicroided)* with **false unicorn root** *(Chamamelirium luteum):*   Effective in regulating periods and toning uterus.

Rue *(Ruta gravelones):*   An infusion may be added or drunk separately.

Chinese

Tang-Kuei Four Combination: Formula of choice for amenorrhea and anemia, general fatigue.

Homeopathy

Pulsatilla: If period doesn't arrive until puberty, 3X three times daily.

Cyclamen: For blondes who are depressed and have headache, 30 three times daily.

Reflexology ***

Press the following points twice per day for three minutes each:

> 44—Uterine Tube, 46—Ovary, 47—Uterus, 48—Vagina, 49—Sex Hormones, 52—Autonomic Nervous System.

Schuessler Tissue Salts

Take the following combination twice per day, five tablets each, morning and evening:

Magnesium phosphorica 12X   **Kali phosphorica** 6X
Calcarea phosphorica 12X

SUGGESTED TREATMENT—DYSMENORRHEA

Acupressure ****

For menstrual pains begin massage or acupressure on:
> UB 2, UB 23, UB 31, UB 32, UB 33, UB 34, UB 48. Follow to CV 3, CV 4, CV 6, ST 27, LI 4, K 3, SP 6.

Acupuncture

LI 4, SP 6, ST 29, LI 7, ST 36, UB 23, LI 6. Also UB 18, UB 24.
Begin treatment one week before menses.
Use Moxa on LI 4, LI 2 and M-CA-18 (Zigong).
Ear points—Neurogate, Ovaries, Endocrine, Shen-men.

Aromatherapy

For dysmenorrhea, massage with the following extracts:
camomile—3%, clary—1%, jasmine—1%, marjoram—2%.
Massage the same way as in the case of amenorrhea.

Herbs

Western ***

Cramp bark *(Viburnum opulus):*   The herb of choice in decoction (two teaspoons). This herb combines well with **Black haw Bark** *(Viburnum prunifolium).*
Pasque flower *(Pulsatilla),* infused, and **valeriana:**   May be considered in case of tension.

Chinese ****

According to Chinese herbology, dysmenorrhea (with lower abdominal and lumbar pain) is categorized into pre-, mid-, and postmenstrual pain.
The causes might be organic, inflammatory, or emotional. Chinese herbal formulas are for use in those with anemia and depleted vitality.
Tang-kuei and Paeonia Formula: For dysmenorrhea caused by narrow opening of cervix or anemia.
Cinnamon and Hoelen Formula: Helps in case of anteflexion or uterine retroflexion, myoma of uterus.
Persica and Rhubarb Combination: For dysmenorrhea due to inflammation, postmenstrual pain. Effective for lower abdominal pain.
Cinnamon and Persica Combination: For dysmenorrhea caused by endometritis, oviduct inflammation, and pelvic peritonitis.
Tang-Kuei, Cinnamon, and Paeonia Formula: For severe abdominal pain, lumbar pain, and pain after or at end of menstruation.

Homeopathy ***

Lachesis: 200 one dose.
Borax: For pain in groin area, six 4 to 6 times daily.
Viburnum opulus: For cramps, 3 every hour.

Aconitum: 30 hourly for severe pain.
Caulophyllum: 3X to 6X hourly for abdominal pain.

PREMENSTRUAL TENSION

SYMPTOMS

Bloating, tenderness in the breasts, water retention, and often manic-depressive reactions during five to eight days before menstruation. Bleeding may indicate pregnancy or sometimes a disease condition.

SUGGESTED TREATMENT

Applied Nutrition **

Drink: Avoid all stimulants such as coffee, alcohol, etc.
Eat: Fresh vegetables and fruits. Reduce protein intake. Avoid salt and all stimulants in your food.
An example of a diet for an average-weight woman, 140 pounds, twenty-five years old:

1,700 calories	50 mg vitamin B_1
35 g protein	50 mg vitamin B_2
60 g fat	50 mg vitamin B_3
255 g carbohydrate	100 mg vitamin B_6
Master formula of vitamins and minerals and:	500 mcg folacin
	1,000 mg pantothenic acid
25,000 IU vitamin A	*Nucleoprotein formula*
1,000 IU vitamin D	60 mg adrenal
1,000 IU vitamin E	60 mg thymus
3,000 mg vitamin C	40 mg ribonucleic acid
500 mg. bioflavinoids	120 mg betaine hydrochloric acid

Aromatherapy
Put into the bath ten drops of the following extracts daily at the beginning of stress feelings related to menstruation:
camomile—2 drops, **lemon**—4 drops, **rosemary**—2 drops, **lavender**—2 drops.

Autosuggestion **
Repeat the following affirmations twice per day, twenty times each:

I accept myself as a beautiful woman.
I accept myself as a feminine woman.
I am healthy, and all is well in my body.

Bach Flowers ***

Impatiens: For stress and tension. 4 drops once daily.

Breathing Therapy
If the pain, tension, or stress is too strong, you can relieve those feelings by breathing in and out deeply and continuously, ten breaths each hour until condition improves.

Herbs ***
Four drops 3 times daily for three to six weeks

Western

Skullcap *(Scutellaria)* and **valeriana:**   Can help ease premenstrual tension. Both in infusion.

Chinese ***

Tang-Kuei Four Formula: Formula of choice.

Hydrotherapy
Hot baths in the lower body can relieve the pain and tension.

Hypnotherapy **
Hypnosis can be very helpful in relieving fear and mental stress before menstruation. Also, it can be very helpful to use self-hypnosis to control the stress, fear, and pain.

Reflexology **
Press during the month, daily, the following points, three minutes each point in the feet and hands:

> 44—Uterine Tube, 45—Groin, 46—Ovary, 47—Uterus, 46—Vagina, 49—Sex Hormones

Schuessler Tissue Salts
Take the following combination twice per day, ten tablets in sugar tablets:

Magnesium phosphorica 12X   **Natrum muriaticum** 6X
Ferrum phosphorica 12X   **Silica** 6X
Kali phosphorica 12X

MENORRHAGIA AND METRORRHAGIA
(ABNORMAL UTERINE BLEEDING)

SUGGESTED TREATMENT

Acupuncture ★★★
 LI 7, SP 6, UB 20, UB 18, SP 1.
Also add:
 GV 4, LI 4, SP 10, LiV 1, GV 20.
Special menorrhagia formula:
 LiV 2, LiV 5, SP 5, SP 6, CV 3, CV 4.
Metrorrhagia formula:
 CV 2, CV 6, LiV 3, SP 6, SP 10, HT 5, K 8, K 10, UB 58.
General ear points: Uterus, Subcortex, Endocrine, Ovaries.

Applied Nutrition ★★
Take the same diet therapy as in the case of premenstrual tension.

Aromatherapy
Use the following extracts in a base of vegetable oil and massage all
the lower area of the body before the color therapy: **cinnamon** 2%,
cypress 5%, **juniper** 2%, **pine** 2%, **geranium** 2%. Use the formula
in combination with the color therapy.

Color Therapy
Use the following colors fifteen minutes each every hour until condition improves: blue, violet, indigo.

Herbs

Western ★★★

For menorrhagia:
American cranesbill *(Geranium maculatum):*   In decoction.
Beth root *(Trillium erectum):*   In decoction.
Periwinkle *(Vinca major):*   In infusion.
For metrorrhagia: use the same, but you may add **Chasteberry** *(Vitex
agnus-castus)* in infusion.

Chinese

Cinnamon and Hoelen Formula: For scarce menses.
Tang-kuei and Paeony formula: For both meno- and metrorrhagia.

Homeopathy **

Ficus religiosa: 7X every four to six hours for metrorrhagia with light-colored reddish blood.
Camomile: 6X every two to four hours when metrorrhagia is with dark flow accompanied by pain.
Vinca major: For bleeding long after menses stops.

Reflexology

To stop the bleeding symptomatically press the following points three minutes each hour until the bleeding is stopped:

46—Ovary, 47—Uterus, 48—Vagina, 18—Heart, 52—Autonomic nervous system.

Schuessler Tissue Salts

Use the following remedies in sugar tablets every hour until condition improves, ten tablets each time.

Ferrum phosphorica 30X   **Kali phosphorica** 30X
Calcarea phosphorica 30X

MASTITIS

SUGGESTED TREATMENT

Acupuncture **

LI 17, SI 1, ST 18, PC 6, TW 10
Use Moxa in early stages, using crushed paste of garlic or onion on the affected tissue. Afterwards apply Moxa stick for ten to fifteen minutes.
Ear points: Mammary Glands, Adrenal, Neurogate, Subcortex

Herbs ***

Chinese

Pueraria Combination with Gypsum: At early stage when accompanied by fever, swelling, and pain.
Minor Bupleurum Combination: For women with fever and no appetite after taking formula No. 1.
Astragalus and Platycodon Formula: When there is suppurative swelling.
Lithospermum and Oyster Shell Formula: For chronic mastitis when cancer is *not* suspected.

Homeopathy ****

Calcarea fluorica: 30 twice weekly for severe nodular mastitis.
Aconite: 3 to 6 every four hours at very acute stage.
Byronia: 6 when breast is hard and painful.
Hepar Sulphurus Calcareum: 3X to 30X is the choice when abscess developed.
Silica: 3X to 30X every eight hours when there is chronic mastitis with discharge.
China: 3X every two hours for overflow of milk.

MASTITIS AND INSUFFICIENT LACTATION

Applied Nutrition **

Eat: Fresh green salads, fresh fruits, cereals, beans, seeds, and sea fish.
An example of a diet for an average-weight woman, twenty-five years old:

2,400 calories	10,000 IU vitamin A
70 g protein	100 IU vitamin D
100 g fat	1,000 IU vitamin E
305 g carbohydrate	50 mg vitamin B complex
Master formula of minerals and	3,000 mg vitamin C
vitamins and:	300 mg bioflavinoids

Aromatherapy

Take the following extracts in vegetable oil base and massage the breast and chest daily before the color therapy: **camomile** 5%, **eucalyptus** 2%.

Color Therapy

Radiate over the chest locally the following colors after massaging the breast with aromatic extracts in vegetable oil base. Once per day with each color until condition improves. Blue—thirty minutes, indigo—ten minutes.

Reflexology ****

Press the following points three minutes each twice per day until condition improves:

20—Adrenal Gland, 21—Kidney, 24—Liver, 25—Gall Bladder, 42—Upper Lymph Glands, 16—Lung Breast Chest.

Schuessler Tissue Salts
Take the following remedies in combination, ten tablets three times per day until condition improves.

Ferrum phosphorica 12X   **Kali phosphorica** 12X
Calcarea phosphorica 12X

INSUFFICIENT LACTATION

SUGGESTED TREATMENT

Acupuncture ***

LI 17, ST 18, SI 1, UB 18, UB 20, ST 36
Also:
Moxa on SI 1, LI 17, LI 18

Herbs **

Western

Caraway *(Carum carvil):*   Infusion
Fennel *(Foeniculum):*   Infusion
Aniseed *(Pimpinella anisum):*   Infusion
Can combine above.
Also **Fenugreek** *(Foenum greckum):* Effective.

Chinese ***

Pueraria Combination: An old-time lactogogue. For women who have enough milk but can't feed due to obstruction and back pain.
Cnidium and Tang-kuei Combination: Increases vitality and milk production.
Dandelion Combination *(Pu-kung-ying-tang):*   For underdeveloped breasts.

PREGNANCY AND LACTATION

SUGGESTED TREATMENT

Applied Nutrition ****

This diet should be well-balanced, rich with protein, vitamins, and minerals.
Drink: Dairy products. Avoid alcoholic beverages, coffee.
Eat: Fresh green vegetables, fresh fruits, whole cereals, beans, seeds,

sea fish, low-fat meat, dairy products, eggs. Avoid white sugar, candies, white wheat flour, saturated lipids, salty foods, refined carbohydrates.

An example of a diet for an average-weight woman, twenty-five years old (in the last six months of pregnancy the weight should be increased about three to four pounds per month):

2,600 calories	400 IU vitamin D
105 g protein	400 IU vitamin E
75 g fat	2,000 mg vitamin C
375 g carbohydrate	300 mg bioflavinoids
10,000 IU vitamin A	B_{50} complex—one tablet daily.

Chelated Minerals

2,000 mg calcium	50 mg zinc
1,000 mg magnesium	90 mg potassium
20 mg iron	30 mg manganese
200 mg phosphorous	100 mcg iodine
200 mcg chromium	100 mcg selenium
3 mg copper	40 mcg molybdenum

Enzyme formula

120 hydrochloric acid	60 mg pepsin
100 mg pancreatin	80 mg lipase
100 mg bile extract	80 mg papain

Nucleoprotein formula

20 mg pituitary extract	50 mg thymus extract
50 mg adrenal extract	50 mg pancreas extract
50 mg heart extract	50 mg kidney extract
50 mg ovarian extract	50 mg RNA extract

Autosuggestion

Repeat the following affirmations twice per day during pregnancy, ten times each:

I love myself and my child unconditionally.
Peace, joy, and relaxation to me and my baby.
Health, strength, and love I send to my baby and myself.

During lactation repeat the following affirmations three times per day loudly and softly so your baby can hear you, too:

I give you all my love and happiness.
I am at peace, with joy and happiness while feeding you.

Schuessler Tissue Salts

Kali phosphorica: 3X to 12X for nervous tension during pregnancy. Take five tablets twice per day.
For morning sickness and vomiting of undigested food during pregnancy take:

Ferrum phosphorica: 6X to 12X, five tablets twice per day
Natrum muriaticum: 6X to 12X, five tablets twice per day

Natrum phosphorica: 6X to 12X, five tablets twice per day
Natrum sulphorica: 6X to 12X, five tablets twice per day

Calcarea phosphorica: 12X, five tablets twice per day for weakness, weariness, poor assimilation of foods.
In the period of pregnancy and lactation take daily the following remedies to aid the normal development of the child and mother—five tablets each once per day:

Kali phosphorica: 12X
Calcarea phosphorica: 12X

Ferrum phosphorica: 12X

INFERTILITY

SUGGESTED TREATMENT

Acupuncture ★★★

LiV 3, LiV 8, St 36, SP 6, GV 4, GV 3, CV 3, CV 4, CV 6, UB 20, UB 23.
Ear points: Kidney, Subcortex, Internal Secretion, Shen-men.

Herbs ★★★★

Chinese

No help in case of aspermia or blocked oviduct. Women who aren't pregnant due to endometritis, pilviperitonitis, and uterine dislocation can *hope* for pregnancy.
Tang-kuei and Paeonia: For defects in uterine development, and for anemia.
Cinnamon and Hoelen Formula: For infertility due to ovaritis, endometritis, and malposition of the uterus.

Homeopathy ★★★★

Borax: 6 when there is leukorrhea.
Silica: As a constitutional remedy.
Aurum: For tired people with lack of sexual desire and depression.

INFERTILITY, NONORGANIC

SUGGESTED TREATMENT

Applied Nutrition **
The diet should be rich in protein, fat, vitamins, and minerals. Avoid stimulants and smoking. Sample diets for men and women follow.
For a man:

2,500 calories	110 g fat
80 g protein	300 g carbohydrate

For a woman:

1,900 calories	90 g fat
60 g protein	210 g carbohydrate

For both:

Master formula of vitamins and minerals	50 mg magnesium
	50 mg phosphorus
B$_{50}$ complex—one tablet daily	10 mg iron
1,000 IU vitamin E	100 mcg chromium
25,000 IU vitamin A	90 mg potassium
1,000 IU vitamin D	30 mg manganese
2,000 mg vitamin C	100 mcg iodine
20 mg zinc	100 mcg selenium

Enzyme Formula

100 mg hydrochloric acid	50 mg pepsin
100 mg pancreatin	50 mg lipase
50 mg bile extract	50 mg papain

Nucleoprotein Formula

20 mg pituitary extract	50 mg thymus extract
50 mg adrenal extract	50 mg pancreas extract
50 mg heart extract	50 mg kidney extract
30 mg ovaria/testis extract	60 mg ribonucleic acid extract

Aromatherapy
Use the following combination in a vegetable oil base once per day before the color therapy and to massage the lower part of the body: **cinnamon** 5%, **clove** 5%, **onion** 2%, **garlic** 2%.

Breathing Therapy
As a secondary aid, breathe twice per day for ten times each exercise, in and out continuously and deeply, with full inhalation of air and full exhalation of the air.

Color Therapy
Use the following colors fifteen minutes each, one after the other daily: red—fifteen minutes, yellow—fifteen minutes, green—fifteen minutes. Use this color therapy after the aromatherapy.

Reflexology *
Press the following points three times per day, five minutes each point:

44—Spermatic Duct—Uterine Tube, 46—Groin, 46—Testicle-Ovary, 47—Uterus-Prostrate, 48—Vagina-Penis, 49—Sex Hormones, 2—Pituitary.

Schuessler Tissue Salts
Take the following remedies per day, ten tablets each time:

Silica: 30X   **Silica:** 12X
Calcarea sulphorica: 12X

MENOPAUSE

SYMPTOMS

Abrupt changes in temperature ("hot flashes"), often accompanied by sweating, headaches, palpitation, and insomnia, in women as ovarian function declines at age forty-five to fifty. In severe cases there can be numbness, vertigo, depression, and irritability manifested in crying spells and manic behavior. Duration of symptoms varies from a few months to several years, with daily or weekly episodes.

SUGGESTED TREATMENT

Acupuncture and Acupressure
For hot flashes use: **
UB 10, GV 20, GB 20, LI 17, ST 11, CV 17, CV 12, CV 4, ST 27, CV 3, GB 21, UB 15, UB 23, UB 47, UB 33, UB 29, LI 4, ST 36, UB 60, SP 6, K3, K 9
Ear points: Shen-men, Neurogate, Internal Secretion, Adrenal

Applied Nutrition ***
The diet should be rich in minerals and vitamins.
Drink: Avoid stimulants like coffee, alcohol, etc.

Eat: Green vegetables, fruits, whole cereals, and beans. Avoid any stimulant food.

An example of a diet for an average-weight woman at age fifty:

1,900 calories	*Nucleoprotein Formula*
55 g protein	50 mg adrenal extract
80 g fat	50 mg ovary extract
240 g carbohydrate	50 mg thymus extract
Master formula of vitamins and	50 mg RNA extract
minerals and	

Aromatherapy

Take internally on a base of brown sugar tablets one drop of the following remedies:

For hot flashes: **camomile**—two drops per day.

For cold flashes, nervousness, mental depression, etc.: **cypress**—one drop daily and **fennel**—one drop daily.

Autosuggestion ***

Repeat the following affirmations twice per day, twenty times each:

> *I am perfect in all changes of cycle.*
> *I love my body unconditionally.*
> *I accept my age with love.*

Breathing Therapy

In cases of hot and cold flashes, breathe continuously for ten breaths, connecting the inhalation to the exhalation.

Color Therapy

For hot flashes use blue for fifteen minutes twice per day.

For cold flashes, anemia, or debility use red for fifteen minutes twice per day and green for ten minutes twice per day.

For depression, anxiety, or worry use blue for fifteen minutes twice per day and green for ten minutes twice per day.

Herbs

Western ***

Passion flower *(Passiflora):*   The herb of choice. Take ten to twenty drops of the extract a day or in infusion three times daily.

A mixture (tea or capsules) can be made of the following herbs and taken for a few months:

Wild yam *(Dioscorea)*   Oats *(Avena sativa)*
Chasteberry *(Vitex agnus castus)*   Liferoot *(Senecio aureur)*
Black cohosh *(Cimicifuga)*

Valeriana, passiflora or **skullcap** *(Scutellaria)* can be added when there is nervousness.

Chinese ***

Bupleurum and Paeonia Formula *(Chia-wei-hsiao-yao-san):* Very effective for menopausal disturbances with emotional instability, fatigue, headache.
Persica and Rhubarb Combination: When constipation is also present.

Homeopathy ***

Ignatia: 3X to 6X every six to eight hours for hot flushes and constipation.
Lachesis: 6X four times daily for flushes that are worse in morning and for mental irritation.
Sulphuricum Acidum: 3X to 5X four to six times daily for evening flushes.
Fabiana imbricata: 6 every two to four hours for sudden sweating.
Valeriana: 3X four times daily for insomnia and irritability.
Pulsatilla: 3X to 30X for changing temperament.
Veratum viride: Recommended for controlling flashes.

Hypnotherapy

To reduce the tension and the bad feelings at the menopause period hypnotherapy can be very helpful.

Reflexology **

In cases of hot flashes, cold flashes, weakness, and mental depression due to menopause press the following points every hour, two minutes each point until condition improves. Then continue with the same points twice per day. For hot and cold flashes:

2—Pituitary, 11—Parathyroid, 13—Thyroid, 20—Adrenal Gland, 44—Uterine Tube, 46—Ovary, 47—Uterus, 49—Sex Hormones

For weakness and mental problems:

2—Pituitary, 20—Adrenal Gland, 44—Uterine Tube, 46—Ovary, 47—Uterus, 49—Sex Hormones, 51—Thymus, 52—Autonomic nervous system

Schuessler Tissue Salts

For hot and cold flashes take five tablets of each remedy every hour until condition improves, then continue with the same remedies twice per day:

Kali sulphorica 12X   **Ferrum phosporica** 6X
Kali phosphorica 12X

For nervousness and mental depression or irritability, anxiety, and fainting take five tablets of each remedy every hour until condition improves, then continue with the same remedies twice per day:

Kali phosphorica 12X   **Natrum muriaticum** 12X

For weakness, anemia, or loss of weight, take five tablets of each remedy every hour until condition improves. Then continue with the same remedies twice per day.

PROSTATITIS

SUGGESTED TREATMENT

Acupuncture and Acupressure

1. UB 23, UB 28, LI 4, SP 6
2. In acute cases: LI 6, SP 10, SP 9, K3, K6
For chronic: GV 2, LI 3, GV 20, K 12, SP 6
Can use warm-needle technique.
Ear points: Kidney, Bladder, Urethra, Pelvic Cavity

Applied Nutrition ***
Take the same diet therapy as in the case of orchitis.

Aromatherapy
Onion—put three drops of essence of onion into a spoonful of gourd oil and take daily upon awakening.
Massage daily the lower region before the color therapy with **pine** 2% in vegetable oil base.

Color Therapy **
Radiate the lower part of the body once per day, ten minutes each color: blue, green, violet.

Herbs

Western ****

Saw Palmetto Berries *(Serenoa serrulata* or *Sabal serrulata):* Excellent tonics for gonads. A decoction tea of a half teaspoon of berries three or four times daily.
Echinea: The condition also calls for an anti-inflammatory herb like this.
Hydrangea, horsetail, echinea, couchgrass: A mixture two to three times daily is good for prostatomegaly.

Chinese ***

Persica and Rhubarb: With enlarged or hypertrophic prostate.
Rhubarb and Moutan Combination: For prostatitis and constipation with tendency to bleed.

Homeopathy ****

Thuya: 3X every two hours for acute inflammation
Pulsatilla: 3X every two hours.
Sabal serrulata: 3X every three to four hours for acute or chronic prostatomegaly and burning sensation when urinating.

Reflexology **

Press the same points as in the case of orchitis.

Schuessler Tissue Salts

Take the following remedies three times per day, five tablets each:

Ferrum phosphorica 6X   **Natrum sulphorica** 12X
Calcarea fluorica 12X

EPIDIDYMITIS AND ORCHITIS

SUGGESTED TREATMENT

Acupuncture *

1. LiV 3, LiV 5, LiV 8, GB 27, SP 12, ST 36, UB 38
2. For orchitis: CV 4, CV 6, LI 4, LiV 1, LiV 8, SP 6
3. CV 4, GB 27, GB 28, GB 29, GV 1, SP 10, SP 12

Ear points—Adrenal Gland, Internal Secretion, Testicle, Shen-men, External Genitalia

Herbs ***

Western

Anti-inflammatory herbs are useful.
Echinea, in decoction or capsules, three times daily, and **yarrow** in infusion, one to three times daily are choice herbs.

Chinese

Gentiana Combination: For inflammation, swelling, and pain in abdomen and genitalia. Specific for gonococcal orchitis.
Cinnamon and Hoelen Formula: Add six g **coix** for prolonged testicle swelling.
Minor Bupleurum Combination: For orchitis caused by mumps or tuberculosis.
Moutan and Persica: For severe inflammation in patients with strong physique.

Homeopathy ****

Pulsatilla: 3X every hour for acute orchitis.
Aconitum: 3X every hour when there is fever.
Songia tosta: 3X every two to four hours when there is pain and swelling of testicles.

IMPOTENCE

SUGGESTED TREATMENT

Acupressure and Acupuncture ***

Moxa is very effective on:
UB 22, UB 23, GV 4, UB 31–34
Acupressure/puncture and moxa should be applied to:
K 16, CV 3, CV 4, LiV 11, LiV 9, SP 6, ST 36, K3
An acupuncture formula that aims at strengthening and relaxing:
LI 4, SP 6, LiV 5, HT 7, GV 4.
Ear points: External Genitalia, Testicles, Endocrine, Subcortex, Neu-rogate

Herbs

Western **

Damiana Sarsaparilla and **gotukola:** Tonics. 10 drops of tincture 1:1 x 3 daily

Passiflora: Add if due to nervousness as infusion three times daily.

Chinese ****

Bupleurum and Dragon Bone: For impotence, heart problems, vertigo

Rehmannia Eight Formula: For weak, tired people.

Rehmannia Six: For milder cases.

Lycium Formula *(Huan-shao-tan):* Increases vigor and sexual desire.

Ginseng Panax

Homeopathy ***

Nux vomica: 3X to 6X every four to six hours when due to nervousness and digestive troubles.

Lycopodium: 30X three times daily for long-term impotence.

Arnica: 3X six times daily if caused by traumatic injury.

Agnus castus: For early stages of problem.

Sabal serrulata: For the elederly.

IMPOTENCE AND FRIGIDITY

SUGGESTED TREATMENT

Applied Nutrition *

Use the same diet therapy as in the case of infertility.

Aromatherapy

Massage the whole body with the extracts of **clary** 5%, **jasmine** 3%, **rose** 5% in vegetable oil base, once per day before the color therapy.

Autosuggestion

Repeat the following affirmations twice per day, twenty times each:

> *I let the strength of my sexuality operate with easy joy.*
> *I enjoy and love sex.*

Sex makes me feel great.
From day to day my sexual powers become stronger and stronger.

Color Therapy

Radiate the following colors, twenty minutes each, one after the other all over the body: red, orange, green.

Hypnotherapy

Hypnotherapy can be very useful in treating problems in which emotional factors are important.

Schuessler Tissue Salts **

For frigidity use the following combination twice per day, five tablets each time:

Natrum muriaticum 6X   **Silica** 6X
Ferrum phosphorica 6X

PREMATURE EJACULATION

SYMPTOMS

Rapid sexual arousal and orgasm in the male.

SUGGESTED TREATMENT

Acupuncture and Acupressure **

Massage point CV 1 while male is on his back during lovemaking.
In general, massage/press/puncture:
   UB 23, SP 6, LiV 8, ST 36, UB 20, K 3, HT 7, CV 3, CV 4, CV 6, UB 24, UB 17, GV 4, UB 31–34.

Applied Nutrition

Use the same diet as in the case of infertility.

Aromatherapy

Use the same as in the case of impotence.

Autosuggestion ***

Repeat the following affirmations twice per day, twenty times each:

I am in full control of my feelings.
From day to day I am better and better in all my sex activities.

Bach Flowers

Agrimony: For fear of bad sexual performance.

Herbs

Chinese
Tonic decoction: To stabilize emotions.

Homeopathy **

Conium, selenium 200, and **zinc metalicum:**   The choice remedies.
Sepia: 3-30 when there is aversion to sex.

Hypnotherapy

In this condition the treatment of choice should be hypnotherapy.

Reflexology

Use the same treatment as in the case of impotence.

Schuessler Tissue Salts

Use the same treatment as in the case of impotence.

· 8 ·

THE IMMUNE SYSTEM AND SYSTEMIC DISEASES

The immune system has become, in the eighties, what vaccines and antibiotics were in the forty years prior: a new perspective on defenses against disease in the mind of the public. We should resist the temptation to find immune reactions behind every ailment. Yet it is becoming increasingly clear that immunology has helped explain a large number of previously unrelated conditions. The most promising advances against such systemic disease as cancer have, in fact, come from this relatively new branch of medicine.

The immune system may be considered to include every defense mechanism in the body, beginning with the skin. It is more precise to limit this system to two general types of biochemical reactions that result in response to "attacks" from foreign substances, or what we commonly call *infections*. There are two types of biochemical reactions because there are two types of "delivery" systems in the body: the blood and the lymphatic networks. Immune reactions are accordingly classified as either of the antibody type (immunoglobulins) carried in the blood system (humoral), or of the cellular type (lymphocytes) carried in the lymph system. When antibodies are not produced in sufficient quantities, or when lymphocytes are not adequate, distinct types of disease, or infections, may overcome the body. There are five types of immunoglobulins thus far identified (Ig—for Immunoglobulin—G, M, A, E, and D). Deficiencies in these may result from inherited conditions or may be transient—the latter most often in the fourth to twelfth week of life. Lymphocytes may be inadequate because of deficiencies in the thymus, where lymphocytes are produced. Finally, deficiencies in either antibodies or lymphocytes may be acquired, as in the acquired immune deficiency syndrome, or AIDs.

Allergies are the most commonly known types of immune reactions, although many so-called allergies are really sensitivities. A food sensitivity, such as to shellfish, may indicate simply a problem in food metabolism. Although wheat and milk sensitivities are quite common, one must again resist the temptation to ascribe vitually every condition, from overweight problems to alcoholism, to such sensitivities. The mechanism involved in a true allergy results in *tissue injury* by virtue of a number of interactions between antibodies or lymphoid cells and the invading agents, or *antigens*. It is an unusual interaction: First there is exposure to the antigen, then an alteration in sensitivity to that antigen, and finally, on a second or third exposure to the antigen, a harmful reaction to the change in sensitivity that causes tissue damage. For example, in a type I reaction, the first contact between antigen (or allergen) and antibody may change the body's sensitivity by producing extra histamine. Then, on a second contact, the antigen releases the histamine—with the well-known "hay fever" results. (This highly simplified description cannot do justice to the complexity of the mechanisms involved, nor does it attempt to explain why this sort of defense reaction has evolved.) In other interactions between antigen and antibody, the cells to which the antigen is affixed are destroyed, or the resulting complexes become toxic.

A streptoccocal infection that commonly affects children (with resulting reactions by the immune system), known as rheumatic fever, has now been identified as part of a quite distinct syndrome *in which the defense mechanism attacks the body*. The immune system fails to recognize itself as friend and treats itself as foe. (Further examples of such "autoimmune" disease will be mentioned later.) In rheumatic fever, malnutrition and genetics may well be contributing factors. The resulting inflammation often affects the large joints, the brain, and especially the heart, causing valve damage.

Inflammation of the joints is a specific symptom of rheumatoid arthritis—also an example of autoimmunity. Here the tenderness and observable thickening of the joints appears to be the direct result of "colonization" of the synovial membrane in the joints by lymphocytes and plasma cells—our normal loyal defenders. A virtually universal symptom is stiffness in joints after inactivity, but fatigue and depression are also frequent. As the colonization proceeds, usually in both sides of the body, the joints readily lose their range of motion, and disabling deformities may develop rapidly.

The mechanism of diabetes mellitus is clearly an insufficient production of insulin, or at least an insufficiency in the blood. Yet autoimmunity may also play a crucial role in the adult-onset version of this disease. In children diabetes usually occurs abruptly, but in adults there is no clear line that identifies the condition, and it is often tolerated with simple dietary changes. Insulin regulates carbohydrates in the bloodstream and is in turn produced in the pancreas and removed from the bloodstream by receptors along its course. The autoimmune system may affect the functioning of this entire regulatory system. For all these reasons, various therapies for diabetes often seem unrelated or contradictory. Any condition that increases insulin demand may predispose to diabetes: obesity, hyperthyroidism, infection, pregnancy. Typical symptoms of adult-onset diabetes are constant hunger and weakness with subsequent weight loss, thirst, and frequent urination.

Many of these symptoms also characterize malfunctions of the thyroid gland. An overactive or enlarged thyroid (hyperthyroidism) typically results in hyperactivity, nervousness, and sensitivity to heat, while the opposite occurs in hypothyroidism. Some types of low-thyroid functioning have been identified as autoimmune responses, but in many cases surgery or radiation therapy are responsible.

When the immune system breaks down, either for genetic reasons or because of a viral attack (acquired, or AIDS), the body is literally defenseless against any number of diseases. It appears that cancer is the first disease to strike in such cases. Accordingly, a strong immune system may well be the necessary, though not always sufficient, protection against cancer.

Cancer, or neoplasm, is the proliferation of cellular growth not normal to the body. These "wayward cells" may spread rapidly to many sites in the body—metastasis—a process that precludes any treatment by removal of the tumors through drugs (chemotherapy), surgery, or irradiation. Although this is the final, morbid progression of the disease, it is not clear whether the ultimate causes of all neoplasms are the same at the molecular level. Hence cancer is commonly thought to be many diseases. The proximate causes we now are aware of are sometimes genetic, as in multiple polypsis of the colon or breast; or viral, as in leukemia; or nutritional, as in gastric cancer and breast cancer in societies with high-fat diets; or chemical, as a result of carcinogens such as coal tar and cigarette smoke; or physical, as a result of overexposure to X rays. The response of the host immune system can be a specific as well as a general factor; certain tumors create new antigens when under attack. Increasingly it is believed that cancers precipitated by any of the factors mentioned above can be kept under control by the "immunological surveillance" of a strong host system—

in short, that we all have some sort of cancer some of the time, just as we all have viruses, yet our immune systems are one step ahead of them for most of our lives.

Chinese Herbology for immuno deficiency and Autoimmune

1. *ASRTRA 8 Formula*—an energy tonic. Has been used by Immune Enhancement Project and the Quan Yin clinic in San Francisco for treatment of ARC patients. It improves sleep, digestion and appetite according to reports from users and practitioners. *Dosage:* 3 tablets twice daily.

Formula: Astrogalus
Atractylodes
Schizardra
Ligustrum
Ganoderma
Eluthero
Ginseng
Codonopsis
Licorice

2. *Power mushroom*—enhances immune system and promotes digestion—mild diuretic.

Dosage: three tablets two times daily.

Formula: Ganoderma (Reishi)
Lentinus (Shiitake)
Silver fungus (white ear)
Polyporus
Hoelen (poria).

3. *Astragalus Ten plus*—There are reports that patients with *Chronic Epstein Barr Virus* (CEBV) Syndrome responded well to this product by Cascade mushroom products at ITM, Portland, Oregon).

Dosage: In powder: one tablespoon two times daily
In tablets: four to five tablets three times daily.

Formula: Ginseng
Astragalus
Cistanche
Ganoderma
Morus fruit
Lycium fruit
Ophiopogan
Ligustrum
Licorice
Eluthero
Ginseng

Schizandra
Ho-shou-wu
Atractylodes

4. *Bioherb*—A special extract of high-quality Ganoderma Lucidum used as modulator for immune system in Japan. Given to patients with *cancer* to enhance immune functions and to help regulate autoimmune processes for patients with Myasthenia Gravis.

Dosage: one to three tablets at a time, twice daily.

Formula: Ganoderma concentrated extra (13:1)

ALLERGIES

SYMPTOMS

Persistent sneezing or coughing, with difficulty breathing, in the presence of a food or substance in the air to which a person is sensitive. Severe reactions, such as to shellfish, can result in choking and even paralysis.

SUGGESTED TREATMENT

Homeopathic Preventative Medicine

Preventative Remedies:

for whooping cough: Pertussin 30
for measles: Morbillinum 30
for mumps: Parotidinum 30
for influenza: Influenzinum Co. 30
for chicken pox: Varicella 30
for common cold: Oscillococcinum 200

This should be perscribed by an experienced practitioner only.

FOOD ALLERGIES

SUGGESTED TREATMENT

See General Immune and Systematic Disorders.

Applied Nutrition ****

See General Immune and Systematic Disorders. If the food allergy is too large, consisting of many kinds of food, then "food rotation" should be applied, changing the types of food every seven days to avoid dependence and allergy.

The diet for seven days' rotation should be as follows:

Day 1

Food Family	*Foods*
Apple	apple, pear, quince
Mulberry	mulberry, fig, breadfruit
Honeysuckle	elderberry
Olive	olives (black and green)
Gooseberry	currant, gooseberry
Potato	potato, tomato, eggplant, peppers (red and green), chili pepper, paprika, cayenne
Lily	garlic, onion, asparagus, chive, leek
Grass	wheat, corn, rice, oats, barley, rye, wild rice, cane, millet, sorghum, bamboo shoot
Buckwheat	buckwheat, rhubarb
Bovidae	milk products—butter, cheese, yogurt, beef, lamb
Mint	basil, savory, sage, oregano, horehound, catnip, spearmint, peppermint, thyme, marjoram, lemon balm
Oils	olive, corn, butter
Tea	elder, mint, catnip
Juice	from the above-listed fruits and vegetables

Day 2

Citrus	lemon, orange, kumquat, citron, grapefruit, lime, tangerine
Parsley	carrot, celeriac, parsley, anise, parsnip, celery, dill, cumin, coriander, caraway, fennel
Pepper	white pepper
Nutmeg	mace
Walnut	walnuts, black walnut, pecans, hickory nuts, butternuts
Birds	chicken, goose, quail, and their eggs
Oils	fats from birds, as little as possible; oils from any walnuts listed above
Sweeteners	orange honey

| Tea | comfrey, fennel |
| Juices | from the above-listed fruits and vegetables |

Day 3

Grape	all varieties of grapes and raisins
Rose	strawberry, raspberry, blackberry, dewberry, loganberry, youngberry, boysenberry, rose hip
Legume	pea, black-eyed pea, dry bean, string bean, carob, soybean, lentil, licorice, peanuts, alfalfa
Flaxseed	flaxseed
Suidae	pork
Arrowroot	arrowroot
Oil	peanut, soy
Sweetener	carob syrup, clover honey
Tea	alfalfa, rose hip
Juices	from above-listed fruits and vegetables

Day 4

Heath	blueberry, huckleberry, cranberry, wintergreen
May Apple	may apple
Papau	papaw, papaya, papain
Composites	lettuce, chicory, escarole, artichoke, dandelion, sunflower, tarragon, oyster plant (salsify)
Morning Glory	sweet potato
Laurel	avocado, cinnamon, bay leaf, sassafras, cassia
Protea	macadamia nut
Beech	chestnut
Orchid	vanilla
Fungus	mushrooms, yeasts, brewer's yeast
Spurage	tapioca
Oil	avocado
Tea	sassafras, papaya
Juice	from the above-listed fruits and vegetables

Day 5

Pineapple	pineapple
Gourd	watermelon, cucumber, cantaloupe, pumpkin, squash, melons, zucchini
Purslane	purslane, spinach
Mallow	okra, cottonseed

Cashew	cashew, pistachio, mango
Pedalium	sesame
Mollusca	abalone, snail, squid, clam, mussel, oyster, scallop
Crustacea	crab, crayfish, lobster, prawn, shrimp
Oils	cottonseed, sesame
Tea	fenugreek
Juices	from the above-listed fruits and vegetables

Day 6

Banana	banana, plantain, arrowroot
Pomegranate	pomegranate
Ebony	persimmon
Palm	coconut, date, date sugar, sago, palm cabbage
Pepper	black pepper, peppercorn
Nutmeg	nutmeg
Beet	beet, chard, spinach, lamb's quarters
Birch	filbert, hazelnut
Bird	turkey, duck, pigeon, pheasant, and their eggs
Oils	coconuts
Sweeteners	date sugar, beet sugar
Juice	from the above-listed fruits and vegetables

Day 7

Plum	plum, cherry, peach, apricot, nectarine, almond, wild cherry, fresh or dried in small amount
Mustard	mustard, turnip, radish, horseradish, watercress, cabbage, kraut, Chinese cabbage, broccoli, cauliflower, Brussels sprout, collard, kale, kohlrabi, rutabaga
Yam	yam, Chinese potato
Brazil Nut	Brazil nut
Conifer	pine nut
Bovidae	lamb
Sweetener	buckwheat, safflower, sage honey
Tea	safflower tea, maté
Juice	from the above-listed fruits and vegetables

HYPOGLYCEMIA

SYMPTOMS

Lightheadedness, fast heartbeat, often following a high-carbohydrate meal.

SUGGESTED TREATMENT

General: According to some theories, low blood sugar is one step before diabetes, so the treatment should be as in the case of diabetes. In the treatment by alternative methods we mainly balance the many activities of the body. The treatment should include aromatherapy, autosuggestion, color therapy, hydrotherapy, reflexology, and Schuessler tissue salts as given under General Immune and Systemic Disorders.

Applied Nutrition
The diet should be well balanced, as in diabetes diet therapy.

Acupuncture *
Same points as for dizziness, fatigue:
    ST 36, SP 6, ST 25, K 3, UB 20, UB 23, CV 12, CV 6

Herbs

Chinese ***

"Decoction of Three Shells to Recover the Pulse" *(San-chia-fu-mai-tang):* For hypoglycemia, anemia, dizziness.

RHEUMATISM, ARTHRITIS, AND GOUT

SYMPTOMS

Rheumatoid arthritis: inflammation of joints, usually in the elderly, with observable thickening of the area and tenderness. Stiffness is an early signal, with eventual fatigue, deformity, and often depression.

SUGGESTED TREATMENT

General: Keep body dry and warm. Use the ionizator while sleeping. The patient should be calm and relaxed, free from worries, frights, and stress. Usually a psychological treatment is very helpful.

Acupuncture/Acupressure ****

In acupressure try to improve blood circulation for rheumatic conditions. First press/massage in regions of pain. Then:
For elbow and wrist pain:
  LU 5, PC 3, HT 7, PC 7, LU 9, TW 10, LI 11, LI 5, TW 4
For ankle pain:
  SP 5, KI 3, ST 41, UB 60

Acupuncture

For arthritis of jaw:
  ST 7, SI 19, TW 17, LI 4
For arthritis of vertebrae:
  M-BW-35 (yiayi) corresponding to area of pain, UB 51, UB 40, GV 26
For arthritis of shoulder:
  LI 15, TW 14, M-VE-48 (yianneiling), SI 11, TW 3, GB 34
For arthritis of elbow:
  LI 11, TW 10, LI 4
For arthritis of wrist and metacarpal fingers:
  TW 5, LI 10, LI 5, TW 4
For arthritis of lumbosacral:
  GV 3, M-BW-25 (Shigizhuixia), UB 30, UB 26, UB 40, UB 60
For arthritis of sacroiliac:
  UB 27, UB 28, local sore points
For arthritis of hip:
  GB 29, GB 30, GB 34, GB 39
For arthritis of knee:
  M-LE-27 (heding), M-LE-15 (xixia), ST 35, ST 34, ST 36, GB 34, SP 9.
For arthritis of ankle:
  ST 41, GB 40, GB 41, K 3, UB 60, GB 35, K 8.
For arthritis of metatarsophalangeal:
  M-LE-41 (shangbafeng), SP 4, UB 65, GB 38, SP 5
Ear points: Sympathetic Neurogate
         Points of tenderness corresponding to region of pain in body.
For Gout:
  UB 35, UB 28, CV 4, ST 36, points of tenderness in affected regions.
For swelling around big toe and ankle:
  LiV 4, K 2, LiV 2, L 3, K 7.
Also add:
  ST 36, LV 4, UB 28.
Sciatic Pain

For lateral pain:
  GB 29, GB 30, GB 34, GB 39, UB 58, LI 4.
For pain along quadriceps muscles:
  ST 30, ST 34, ST 36, LI 4, ST 37, ST 39.
For pain along back of leg:
  UB 51, UB 40, UB 60, UB 63.
Ear points: Sciatic, lower back, points of tenderness.

Applied Nutrition **

Use the diet in General Immune and Systemic Disorders.

Aromatherapy **

Massage the whole body with the following extracts in vegetable oil base, once daily before color therapy: **camomile** 8%, **cypress** 4%, **hyssop** 4%, **pine** 4%, **eucalyptus** 4%.

Autosuggestion

Use the tape cassette in General Immune and Systemic Disorders.

Color Therapy **

Radiate the following colors twice per day, one after the other, all over the body: blue—thirty minutes, green—fifteen minutes, yellow—ten minutes (locally).

Herbs

Western ***

Bogbean, black cohosh, celery seed, meadowsweet, yarrow: A complex capsule or infusion.
Wild yam or **guaiacum:**   Add or use separately when there is severe inflammation.
St. John wort: Oil or ointment can be rubbed into pain areas.
Lavender, marjoram, rosemary, peppermint: A mixture of essential oils for passage.
Buchu and **sarsaparilla:**   For chronic rheumatism.
Paraguay tea *(Ilex paraguayenesis):*   Infusion.
Fireweed *(Erechtites hieracifolia):*   Oil to be applied to painful area.
Burdock root, celery seed, yarrow, thuya: A mixture (infusion/capsules/tincture) for gout.
Balm of Gilead *(Populus candicans):*   Ointment for pain.
Couchgrass *(Agropyrum repens):*   Use root in decoction.

Chinese **

Coix Combination: For acute or subacute chronic rheumatic pain, difficulty moving the hands and feet, Arthralgia, muscle pain, paralysis.

Pueraria Combination: For initial stage of neuralgia, chronic rheumatic pain, sore shoulders, facial neuralgia.

Ma-Huang and Coix Combination: For chronic rheumatic pain, neuralgia, muscle pain.

Cinnamon and Atractylodes Combination: For people of little physical strength with no serious muscular distension, a tendency to perspire, oliguria or frequent urination, painful swelling of the limbs, joints.

Rehmannia Eight Formula: For cold arms and legs in the elderly; especially for pain in the lower limbs and lower back.

Clematis and Stephania Combination: For chronic disease with occluded blood, pain in the arms and legs, joint pain, neuralgia, lower-back pain, muscle pain; especially for sciatica and pain in the legs.

Tang-kuei and Anemarrhena Combination: For reddening, swelling, and pain of the muscles around the joints.

Persica and Rhubarb Combination: For people whose normal complexion is dark and reddish, with headaches, constipation, menoxenia, and sciatica.

Tu Huo and Vaeicum Combination: For pain in the loins and knees, chills, numbness, weakness, neuralgia.

Clematis and Carthamus Formula: For chronic multiple joint pain, pain in the arm and leg joints, neuralgia.

Homeopathy

Guaiacum   3X, every four hours in gout.

Benzinum acidum: 3X every four hours in gouty subjects with high-smelling urine.

Arctium: 6X, every four hours for pain in joints, colalgia, neuralgia.

Aconitum: 3, every hour in rheumatic subjects with fever, restlessness, anxiety.

Bryonia alba: 3 for pain worse with movement, part sensitive to touch.

Pulsatilla nigricans: 3, every hour in women and children with pain worse by heat, better by cold.

Apis mellifica: 3X for much swelling, little pain.

Hepar sulphuris calcareum: 6, four d when suppuration has taken place.

Mercurius sulphuricus: 6, every four hours for rheumatic synovitis.

Berberis vulgaris: 1X, every four hours for chronic synovitis of the knee.

Mercurius: 12, every two hours for pain and swelling of joints, worse at night, profuse sweat, pericardial complications.

Sulphuricum: 1–30, every two hours when the pains are worse at night, by warmth.

Rhus toxicodendron: 1–3, every hour for restlessness and pain improving with movement.

Dulcamarta: 3, hourly for subacute rheumatism due to cold and wetness.

Kalmia latifolia: 3 T 3h for acute nonfebrile rheumatism with migratory pains.

For gout:

Belladona: 3X, every half-hour.

Mother Tincture of Colchicine: a hot compress with several drops.

Colchicine: 3X, every two to four hours for great weariness, nausea, shoutings and tearings in muscles and joints worse with movement, better at night. Tearings in legs, feet, and toes with swelling.

Pulsatilla nigricans: 3, every two hours when gout flies about from joint to joint.

Sabina: 3, every two hours when connected with uterine disorder

Reflexology ***

Massage and press the same as in rheumatic fever, three or four times a day. If in pain, press points 52–55 every hour as in rheumatic fever.

Schuessler Tissue Salts

Take the following remedies three or four times per day, ten tablets each:

Ferrum phosphorica: 6X to 30X. In the first stages of the disease in case of pains, fever, heat, redness, quickened pulse in every part of the body.

Kali muriaticum: 6X to 30X in the second stage of the disease together with **ferrum phosphorica** with swelling of the joints when movement increases the pains.

Natrum phosphorica: 6X to 30X. Take with the **ferrum** and **kali muriaticum.**

Calcarea fluorica: 6X. When enlargement of the joints appears from one of these diseases.

Silica: 6X. To reduce accumulation of urates lodgings around the joints and muscles, especially in gout.

RHEUMATIC FEVER

SYMPTOMS

Inflammation of the large joints, often with damage to the brain or heart, resulting from autoimmune reaction, usually in children.

SUGGESTED TREATMENT

General: Stay in bed until all signs of active rheumatic fever have disappeared. Also keep the body warm and dry until improvement.

Applied Nutrition **

The diet therapy should be the same as in General Immune and Systemic Disorders.

Aromatherapy

Massage the painful parts of the body with the following extracts in vegetable oil base: **origans** 8%, **pine** 4%.

Color Therapy ***

Radiate the following colors one after the other all over the body until condition improves: blue—thirty minutes, yellow—fifteen minutes, green—fifteen minutes.

Reflexology **

Press and massage the points given in General Immune and Systemic Disorders three times per day. To alleviate pain, press every hour, three minutes each point in each hand until pain is over:
55—General pain, 52—Autonomic nervous system

Schuessler Tissue Salts

Take five tablets three times per day of each remedy until condition improves:

Ferrum phosphorica 30X   **Natrum sulphorica** 30X
Natrum phosphorica 30X

DIABETES MELLITUS

SYMPTOMS

In adult-onset diabetes, constant hunger or thirst with frequent urination; sometimes weakness and subsequent weight loss, but often unexplained weight gain.

SUGGESTED TREATMENT

General: Hygienic care is very important, with particular attention to the feet and toes. The skin must be kept scrupulously clean and dry. Tight shoes should be avoided. Do not apply local heat to legs and feet because it may lead to gangrene. Care for the mouth and teeth by brushing well at least three or four times per day; a mouthwash should be used before and after eating. Regular bowel movements are important. The mental side is also very important; the patient should be free from stress and fears. Many cases of diabetes start after some past trauma. To solve these conflicts it is important to use psychotherapy; see Personality Disorders.

Acupuncture ***

M-BW-12 (Yishu), UB 13, UB 20, UB 23, ST 36, K3
For excessive thirst add:
LU 11, LU 10, UB 17
For increased appetite accompanied by emaciation of muscles add:
M-BW-10, UB 21, CV 12
For frequent urination add:
CV 4, K7, K 5.
Ear points:
For thirst: Endocrine, Lung, Thirst
For hunger: Endocrine, Stomach, Hunger
For frequent urination: Endocrine, Kidney, Bladder

Applied Nutrition ****

Reduce the weight in obesity cases.
Drink: Vegetable juices, unsweetened dairy products. Avoid juices, sweetened fruit juices, coffee, alcohol, beer.
Eat: Fresh vegetables, whole rice, beans, soy protein, poultry, sea fish, potato, unsweetened dairy products, seeds. Avoid any refined sugar, candies, dried fruits, honey, cakes, biscuits, white wheat bread.
The diet should be 50% whole rice, 30% fresh vegetables, 10% beans, 5% seeds, 10% sea fish.
The calories should be calculated according to the weight, age, and type of physical work.
An example for an average-weight person, thirty years old:

1,800 calories	80 g fat
60 g protein	210 g carbohydrate

Master formula of vitamins and minerals and all the supplements given in General Immune and Systemic Disorders.

Take every meal a handful of *Trigonella foenum graecum*, known also as "Chilve" in Arabic, as seeds or sprouts.

Aromatherapy

Massage the whole body with the extract of **eucalyptus** 4%, **geranium** 4%, **juniper** 4% in vegetable oil base. Repeat this massage daily before hydrotherapy.

Autosuggestion

Repeat the same tape recorder cassette twice per day as in General Immune and Systemic Disorders.

Color Therapy

Radiate the following colors twice per day, one after the other all over the body: green—thirty minutes, yellow—fifteen minutes.

Herbs

Western ****

Use plants with hypoglycemic activity, such as allspice, artichoke, banana, barley, bugleweed, burdock, cabbage, carrot, ginseng, lettuce, lily of the valley, nettles, oats, olive, onion, papaya, pea, spinach, sunflower, sweet potato, turnip, wormwood (this list was compiled by Fransworth et al., in *The Holistic Herbal* by David Hoffman, published by Findhorn Press).

Goat's rue *(Galega officinalis):* Infusion/tincture has hypoglycemic activity.

Garlic: Good.

Fenugreek and **corn silk** *(Zea mays):* Helpful in tea/capsules.

Buchu: May be taken in early stages of problem.

Dandelion *(Taraxacum):* Stimulates pancreatic activity.

Chinese ****

Rehmannia Six Formula: Formula of choice for fatigue, polyuria, thirst, vertigo, tinnitus, weakness of kness, edema.

Rehmannia Eight Formula: For weaker people, cold arms and legs, presdyopia, edema, difficult urination.

Ginseng and Gypsum Combination: For dry mouth, thirst, initial stage of diabetes mellitus.

Siler and Platycodon Formula: For strong people. Prevents diabetes mellitus.

Homeopathy ***

Codeinum: 3X four to six times daily for depression and skin irritation.
Syzygium: 1X every eight hours as a general remedy.

Hydrotherapy **
A daily warm bath is very important in order to keep the patient clean and warm.

Reflexology
Massage the whole feet softly twice per day for five minutes. Press the following points twice per day, three minutes each point:

2—Pituitary, 3—0 Cerebrum, 4—Cerebellum, 20—Adrenal Gland, 21—Kidney, 22—Pancreas (five minutes this point), 24—Liver

Schuessler Tissue Salts
Take ten tablets of each twice per day:

Kali phosphorica 3X first week
                      6X second week
                      12X third week, and continue with this potency
Natrum muriatirum 12X
Ferrum phosphorica 6X

Sport
In this condition physical exercise is a must. At least one hour a day or running, swimming, or general athletics is very important.

HYPERTHYROIDISM AND HYPOTHYROIDISM

SYMPTOMS

Hyperactivity generally results from an enlarged or overstimulated thyroid gland, and the opposite in the case of low thyroid functioning. This sort of hyperactivity is often manifested in nervousness and sensitivity to temperature changes.

SUGGESTED TREATMENT

General: Avoid any stress and allow freedom from worry in both hyper- and hypothyroidism. The main purpose is to balance the thyroid gland's activity by various methods.

Applied Nutrition **

Take the same diet therapy for hypothryroidism and hyperthyroidism. If overweight in the hypo, then reduce the calorie intake accordingly. The quantity of iodine mineral intake as a supplement should be reduced in hyperthyroidism to 10 mcg daily.

The diet therapy otherwise is the same as in General Immune and Systemic Disorders.

Aromatherapy

For hypothyroidism, massage the neck before the color therapy with massage oil base for the following extracts: **basil** 4%, **bergamot** 2%, **lavender** 2%.

For hyperthyroidism, massage the neck before the color therapy with massage oil base for the following extracts: **juniper** 4%, **cedarwood** 4%, **neroli rose** 4%.

Autosuggestion

Repeat the same tape recorder cassette as in the case of General Immune and Systemic Disorders.

Color Therapy ***

For hypothyroidism, radiate the following colors one after the other twice per day until condition improves: green—fifteen minutes locally, yellow—ten minutes locally, red—twenty-five minutes locally.

For hyperthyroidism, radiate the following colors one after the other twice per day until condition improves: green—fifteen minutes locally, blue—twenty-five minutes locally, indigo—ten minutes locally.

Reflexology **

In both cases press the following points twice per day, three minutes each point, except Nos. 11 and 13, six minutes each point twice per day:

2—Pituitary, 2—Cerebrum, 4—Cerebellum, 8—Neck, 10—Throat, 11—Parathyroid (six minutes twice per day), 13—Thyroid (six minutes twice per day), 20—Adrenal gland, 21—Kidney, 24—Liver

Schuessler Tissue Salts

Take twice per day the following remedies, ten tablets each:

Calcarea fluroica 3X first week
6X second week 12X third week

Kali muriaticum 12X
Silica 12X

HYPERTHYROIDISM

SUGGESTED TREATMENT

Acupuncture and Acupressure **

PC 5, SP 6, N-HN-43 (Qiying), M-BW-35 (yiayi)
From 3rd to 5th cervical vertebra.
For too much sweat add HT 6 and K7.
For palpitation or insomnia add HT 7 and N-HN-54 (Anmnian)
For sexual problems and restlessness add LiV 3 and GB 20
For tachycardia add PC 6.
Ear points—Neurogate, Subcortex, Endocrine, Thyroid, Heart, Lung
Moxa—50 cones—indirectly on LU 3.

Herbs

Western

Bugleweed *(Lycopus europaeus):*   Major herb for this problem. Ten
drops in water three times daily.
Nettles *(Urtica):*   Infusion three times daily.
Valerian: Tincture ten days—or three capsules daily.
Yarrow *(Achillea):*   Infusion or ten drops three times daily.
Kelp: is also recommended. Tablets, one three times daily.

Chinese ***

Baked Licorice Combination *(Chich-kan-tsao-tang):*   Formula of
choice for lack of vitality, palpitations, gasping, irregular pulse.
Bupleurum and Dragon Bone Combination: For insomnia, pal-
ipitations, mental instability.
Bupleurum and Peony Formula *(Chia-wei-hsiao-yao-san):*   For
menoxenia, heavy head, vertigo, insomnia, palpitations, cold feet.

HYPOTHYROIDISM

SUGGESTED TREATMENT

Acupuncture **

Ear points: Thyroid, Internal Secretion, Brain, Shen-men

Herbs

Western

Bladderwrack
Damiana
Kola vera
Nettles   1:1 ratio ten drops daily three times
Oats
Wormwood

A combination is good.

Chinese ***

Rehmannia Eight Formula
Vitality Combination: For edema, hypothyroidism, nephritis.

CANCER AND MALIGNANT GROWTH

SUGGESTED TREATMENT

General: In all kinds of cancer and malignant growth the mental component is very important. The patient should help fight this disease by staying calm and relaxed. Do meditation to reduce stress, fears, hate, and anger as much as possible. Also visualizing yourself healthy, running, swimming, or doing other activities. Meditate three times per day, fifteen to thirty minutes each time.

Acupuncture and Acupressure

For pain due to cancer: ****
   Ear points: Heart, Subcortex, Sympathetic, Liver, Shen-men, points corresponding to regions of disease.
For stomach cancer: **
   UB 18, UB 20, UB 21, UB 23, UB 22, UB 25, PC 6, ST 26, CV 12, CV 15, LiV 2.

Applied Nutrition **

The diet should be macrobiotic.
Drink: Pure water and herb tea. Make deep colonic enemas twice in the first week, then one deep colonic per month.
Eat: Whole cereals, 70%; 20% cooked vegetables; and 10% fresh vegetables and sprouts.
An example of a diet for an average-weight person, thirty years old:

2,000 calories
40 g protein
80 g fat
280 g carbohydrate

Master formula of vitamins and
minerals and all the supplements
given in General Immune and
Systemic Disorders

Autosuggestion ****

Repeat the tape recorder cassette three times per day as in General
Immune and Systemic Disorders.

Color Therapy ***

Repeat the following colors twice per day, one after the other all over
the body and locally: green—twenty minutes, yellow—ten minutes,
violet—twenty minutes, blue—ten minutes.

Herbs

Western

Fifteen drops in glass of water four to six times daily, six days a week,
under physician's guidance.

Madagascan periwinkle: The source of the drugs Vinblastine and
Vincristine, used for leukemia. There are detoxifying herbs—alternatives that might aid the body via cleansing to get rid of certain cancer-
ous growths.

Burdock, blue flag, and **yellow dock** are specific to aid elimination
by the kidneys.

Cleavers and **dandelion**

Echinacea and **poke root:**   Lymphatic and anti-inflammatory herbs

Guaiacum (decoction) and **sweet violet:**   Antineoplastics, but there
is no certainty as far as their efficacy.

In the book *The Treatment of Cancer with Herbs* by John Heinerman
(Orem, Utah: Biworld Publishers, 1984) there are the following recommendations to minimize chemotherapeutic side effects:

Siberian ginseng
Sarsaparilla
Wild Oregon grape

Chinese

For breast cancer:

Lithospermum and Oyster Shell *(Tzu-ken-mu-li-tang):*   For lym-
phadenoma, anemia, weak malignant skin disorders.

Tang-kuei Sixteen-Herb Combination: For cervical lympha-
denopathy, goiter, fibrocystic disease.

W.T.T.C. *(Lo-shih-sho):*   To prevent postsurgical metasteses.

For stomach cancer:

W.T.T.C.:   Formula of choice. It is used in Japan in initial stage of gastric cancer and also to prevent relapse after surgery.

Six Major Herb Combination: Given in conjunction to improve appetite.

For leukemia, the objective of treatment is remission.

Ginseng, bupleurum and Longan Combination *(Chia-wei-kuei-pi-tang):*   Effective for bleeding, anemia, fatigue, splenomegaly, hepatomegaly.

Lithospermum: Ten grams is added to the above formula to treat malignant ulcer. In his book *The Medical Service of Modern Chinese Herb Medicine* the author Chen-chu-lin outlines the following for leukemia:

Ginseng and Succinum Formula: For patients with splenomegaly.

Ginseng and Longan Combination: For hemmorrhage.

Chin-chiu and Bupleurum Combination *(Chin-chiu-fu-lei-tang):*   For patients with fever.

Tortoise Shell and Phaselous Combination *(Pieh-chia-chih-hsiao-tou-tang):*   For patients with edema, ascites, oliguria, shortness of breath.

The journal of the American College of Traditional Chinese Medicine (2, 1982) reports on a combination of Chinese herbal medicine and radiotherapy in the treatment of nasopharyngeal carcinoma in 2220 cases.

The Chinese *Prescription of Destagnation* consisted of ten herbal drugs:

Radix salviae miltiorrhizae	15–24 g
Radix paeoniae rubra	10 g
Radis angelica sinesis	10–12 g
Radix astragali	15–30 g
Rhizoma ligustici wallichii	10–12 g
Flor carthami	10 g
Pueraria lobata ohwi	10 g
Semen prisae	10 g
Pericarpium citri raticulatae	10 g

Herbals were boiled and decanted and taken orally twice daily during whole radiation course.

The combined use of Chinese herbs and radiation gave a higher five-year survival (53%–21%) than that of radiation alone (24%–12%).

Authors of article recommend further study—clinical and laboratory.

For treatment of toxic side effects resulting from radiation and chemotherapy, in their book, *Treatment of Toxic Side Effects Resulting from*

Radiation and Chemotherapy, authors C. S. Cheung M.D., U Aik Kaw, and Howard Harrison recommend the following for fullness in chest and abdomen, frequent belching and hiccuping, nausea and vomiting. If there is incessant hiccuping, use the folk medication as a last resort.
Fried Semen Allii Tuberosi: Thirty to sixty g. Fry over low fire until yellow and pulverize. Dosage: 1.5 g per time. Use two or three times daily orally.
Decoction Radix Saussurea, Fructus Seu Semen Anomi in Six Gentlemen Composite: For distension and stuffiness in chest and abdomen, lack of taste, appetite loss, thin, loose, or dry stool. 1.5 g two times daily.
Normalizing Powder of Hera Pogostemi Composite: For stuffy chest, frequent vomiting, detestation of food, fatigue, and somnolence.
Pill of Fifth and Sixth Heavenly Stems: For abdominal pain associated with radiation and certain chemotherapy (Vincristine, VCR, Leucocristine), paroxysmal intense pain around navel region, and constipation as in acute abdominal emergency. One pill three times daily.

Chinese herbal formulas to combat side effects of radiation and chemotherapy resulting from inhibition of the hemopietic function of the marrow by the toxicity:
Decoction for Returning to Spleen: For weakness, laziness in moving about, dimness of head, dizziness of eyes, palpitation, restlessness, facial pallor, falling of hair.
Pill of Spotted Dragon: For dimness of head, weakness of body, soreness of back and extremities, edema of face and extremities, decreased food intake, loose stool, loss of hair.
For inflammation of skin due to radiation:
Golden Yellow Powder
Powder for Regeneration of Tissue: When there is delayed healing of ulcers.
For inflammation of oral cavity and throat:
Pills of Six Immortals
Pill of Inflammation of Throat
For inflammation of rectum:
Decoction Radix Pulsatillae Composite
Pill of Rhizoma Coptidis and Radix Saussureae Composite: Three to six g two to three times daily.
For bladder and urethral inflammation:
Powder of Eight Normalities: Use with **Powder for Leading Out the Red.**
For inflammation of lungs and mediastinum:

Decoction Herba Ephederae, Semen Armenialae Amarae, Gypsum Fibrosum and Radix Glycyrrhizae Composite.
For herpes zoster:
Single Realgar Powder: Add thirty to sixty g Realgar Powder to 100–200 ml of 75% alcohol. Stir into thin paste and apply on lesion three or four times daily.

Homeopathy

By physician only: 30X to 200X according to condition
Carcimosin: 30–200 nosode of cancer occasionally
Schirrhinum: 30–200 nosode for undoubted breast cancer, in conjunction with
Hydrastis canadensis: 1X three to four times daily.
Oleum Animal: 30 every eight hours for strong pain in nipples.
Phosphoricum: 6–30 every six hours for bone cancer.
Euphorbium: 6–30 every two hours for cancer pains.

Hypnotherapy
Very useful to reduce the pains and suffering of the patient in the last stages. Also can be very useful to implant a positive outlook.

Reflexology
Only to reduce pains. Press the points:
52—Autonomic Nervous System, 55—General Pains three to eight times per day or every hour until pain is over, for three to five minutes each point.

Schuessler Tissue Salts
Take the following remedies three times per day, ten tablets each, in all forms of tumors:

Calcarea fluorica: 3X first week 6X second week 12X third week

Silica: 12X
Calcarea phosphorica: 12X
Kali sulphorica: 12X
Kali phosphorica: 12X—for the pains of cancer and for offensive discharges.

AUTOIMMUNE DISEASES

SUGGESTED TREATMENT

Herbs

Chinese

For myasthenia gravis, according to Dr. Cheung M.D. and Brian Laforgia in the Journal of ACTCM, 1, 1982:
Decoction for Tonifying the Center and Benefiting Chi: large dosages.
Decoction of Cortex Cinnamoni and Radix Aconiti Carmichaeli
Praeparata for Regulating the Center
Fortified Pill of Buddha's Warrior Attendant
For myositis:
Decoction for Moistening the Kidney and Vitalizing Blood
For scleroderma:
Decoction for Warming the Kidney and Vitalizing Blood

- The herbs used for "Supporting the Righteousness and Eliminating Evil" seem to benefit the immune mechanism.
- **Ginseng and Radis Astragalus** seems to upgrade the immune function and at the same time inhibit growth of cancer cells.
- Decoction for Generating the Meridians has regulating action on immune mechanism.
- Chinese herbs to inhibit cancer growth and increase immune function:

Rhizoma zedoariae   *Rhizoma coptidis*
Herba oldelandia diffusa   *Grifolia*
Ramulus mori

GENERAL IMMUNE AND SYSTEMIC DISORDERS

SUGGESTED TREATMENT

General: Various disorders, mental and physical, may be associated with the immune system or systemic problems directly or indirectly. So in any case of undiagnosed disorders or allergy reactions reinforce the immune system by combining a few methods of the alternative therapy.

Applied Nutrition ***

Commence the rejuvenating diet therapy with the three-day juice fast. The food-cytotoxic test is very important in any immune system problem to avoid allergy to food and chemicals.

Drink: Avoid dairy products, alcohol, coffee, or any stimulating food.

Eat: Fresh vegetables, whole cereals, beans, seeds, fresh fruits, and a little sea fish. Avoid any processed foods, dairy products, red meats, freshwater fish, fried foods, or any stimulating food. Also avoid any food to which you found allergy.

An example of a diet for an average-weight person, thirty years old:

2,100 calories
45 g protein
100 g fat
255 g carbohydrate
Master formula of vitamins and minerals and:
Vitamins and minerals (chelated).
As in all mega-vitamin therapy, take the supplements under physician's supervision only.
75,000 IU vitamin A
400 IU vitamin D
1,000 IU vitamin E
6,000 mg vitamin C—in acute cases, up to 12,000 mg
3,000 mg bioflavinoids
100 mg Vitamin B_1
100 mg Vitamin B_2
100 mg Vitamin B_3
300 mcg folic acid
1,600 mg pantothenic acid
100 mcg vitamin B_{12}
200 mcg biotin
1,000 mg PABA
100 mg choline
100 mg inositol
50 mg vitamin B_{15}
1,200 mg calcium—in acute cases, up to 3,000 mg
600 mg magnesium—in acute cases, up to 1,500 mg
12 mg manganese

50 mg phosphorous
15 mg iron
100 mcg chromium
3 mg copper
100 mg zinc
200 mcg iodine
100 mcg selenium
Enzyme Formula
120 mg hydrochloric acid
160 mg pancreatin
150 mg bile extract
75 mg pepsin
120 mg lipase
120 mg papain
Nucleoprotein Formula
20 mg pituitary extract
100 mg adrenal extract
50 mg heart extract
150 mg thymus extract
75 mg pancreas extract
75 mg kidney extract
150 mg RNA extract
Amino Acids Formula
300 mg L-tryptophan
150 mg lystine
100 mg methionine
100 mg histidine
General Supplements
2,400 mg lecithin
200 mg night primrose oil
100 mg alfalfa
1,000 mg brewer's yeast

Aromatherapy

Massage the following extracts in vegetable oil base: **bryony** 4%, **eucalyptus** 3%, **lavender** 3%, **rosemary** 3%.

Autosuggestion ***

Repeat the following affirmations into a tape recorder cassette, twenty times each phrase, and listen to this cassette twice per day, each morning and evening:

> *From day to day all my body and mind and spirit is stronger and healthier in every way.*
> *I love myself unconditionally.*
> *I accept myself as I am.*
> *I am relaxed, strong, and healthy.*
> *From day to day I am more relaxed, healthier, stronger, and happier.*
> *I have a good, healthy defense system in my body.*
> *All the systems in my body are working perfectly.*
> *My immune system is perfectly balanced.*
> *From day to day my immune system, circulatory system, and endocrine system are healthier and better in every way.*
> *From day to day each part of my body is stronger and healthier.*
> *All of my body, mind, and spirit is balanced and healthy.*
> *I release all negatives from my life and accept only the positive, healthy, and good into myself.*
> *I am at peace. The world is good, safe, and friendly to me. I am free. I love and forgive all of my past and present life. I let others be themselves. My world is filled with joy and happiness—I am healthy and happy.*

Color Therapy **

Radiate the following colors daily, one after the other, until condition improves: orange—fifteen minutes, green—fifteen minutes, yellow—fifteen minutes.

Hydrotherapy

Take a cold bath or shower daily for a few seconds to improve the circulation and immune system.

Psychotherapy

For reducing stress, fears, phobias, and neuroses, see Personality Disorders. This can strengthen the immune system and cure or improve many allergic symptoms and disorders.

Reflexology

Massage the whole hands and feet with a massage roller twice per day, seven minutes each foot and hand.

Press the following points twice per day for three to five minutes each point. Continue daily until three months after all symptoms disappear:

2—Pituitary, 11—Parathyroid, 13—Thyroid, 17—Solar Plexus, 20—Adrenal Gland, 21—Kidney, 24—Liver, 51—Thymus, 52—Autonomic Nervous System

Schuessler Tissue Salts

Take the following remedies for any problem that may be connected with the immune system. Take three tablets of each twice per day:

Kali phosphorica 3X to 6X two to three times daily

Kali sulphorica 3X to 6X two to three times daily

Natrum muriaticum 3X to 6X two to three times daily

Natrum sulphorica 3X to 6X two to three times daily

Ferrum phosphorica 3X to 6X two to three times daily

· 9 ·

THE EYE SYSTEM

The eyes have a certain primacy in our bodily organs, not merely for their complexity in themselves but for their overwhelming importance in our understanding and enjoyment of the world. Eyes are often critical in work, significant in beauty, and essential in that unique human activity, communication.

Abnormalities in the eyes should therefore be considered in the framework of a complete physical examination. Even the psychological factors involved in impairment of sight at an early age or diminishment of reading ability in middle age should be carefully taken into account in any therapy. What is normal deterioration for a given age group should be of great interest to the patient.

Eye problems fall into five general categories: subnormal visual acuity, pain or discomfort, increased discharge of fluids, dizziness, and change of appearance. Any or all of these may affect the rest of the body, and they may affect each other.

The inflammation of the eye, or conjunctivitis, is the most common eye disorder. If it is bacterial in origin, it can be alleviated by treatment; viral conjunctivitis is self-limiting, usually lasting fron one to three weeks.

Allergies frequently cause the tearing associated with conjunctivitis. If redness persists, an inflammation of the uveal tract in the iris should be considered. Early diagnosis of uveitis is important.

Perhaps the most serious condition of the eye to be watched in diagnosis is glaucoma, which ultimately leads to blindness. It is estimated that 50,000 people in the United States are blind as a result of this disease. Glaucoma is a complex of problems causing an increase in pressure in the eye sufficient to atrophy the retina. It can be a congenital condition, the result of trauma, surgery, and the like, or of no known etiology.

Cataracts are an equally diverse set of conditions, with the common result of increasing lens opacity. They are common with aging, usually occurring in both eyes at approximately the same time.

Lifelong eye conditions are often fixed in early childhood. The common condition of myopia, or nearsightedness, for example, usually increases in teenage years and levels off before age twenty-five, regardless of factors like eyestrain or endocrine balance that are often blamed for the problem. In myopia, rays of light are focused in front of the retina, limiting the effective "far point" of the eye to about twenty feet. The size of the eyeball or the strength of the refractive power of the cornea or lens often causes the condition. In contrast, hypermetropia is the condition in which light is focused behind the retina, because of conditions the opposite of those in the case of myopia. The result is indistinct vision at all distances, but the disease is not common.

Strabismus, or "crossed eyes," results from the failure of one eye to center the image. It is a condition in about one of twenty children and should be diagnosed early for best treatment. Normal binocular vision and proper cosmetic adjustment are easily possible with early attention to the problem.

Color blindness affects a surprising proportion of the population—eight percent of males (and only one twentieth that number of females). Despite this fact, it is one of the least of eye problems. Yet it does lend support to the theory that three basic colors are necessary for color vision, since the two common types of color blindness are two-color and single-color vision. Although objects refract light in a whole range of wavelengths, certain eyes are apparently insensitive to distinct segments of the spectrum. The common types of color blindness are inherited on male–female lines.

When the optic nerve atrophies there is a directly correlated loss of vision. Many diseases, in and outside the eye itself, can be responsible, and only quite early treatment can be helpful. Systemic degenerative disease, such as diabetes or atherosclerosis, should be considered.

Eyelid infections by staphyloccocus can be internal or superficial—a sty. This abscess or boil should be treated by frequent washing. In general, tired or weak eyes require the same care, as they may be infected. Any sort of irritant to the eyes—improper prescriptions for contact lenses or glasses, work under toxic conditions, or dust, sun, and subsequent rubbing—should be taken care of before any more specific treatment is considered.

MYOPIA (NEARSIGHTEDNESS), WEAK EYESIGHT, HYPERMETROPIA (FARSIGHTEDNESS), ASTIGMATISM, DIPLOPIA, AND COLOR BLINDNESS

SUGGESTED TREATMENT

Applied Nutrition

Use whole food and avoid all the refined foods. The diet therapy should be the same as in the case of conjuntivitis.

Aromatherapy

Use the essence of rose as a compress over the closed eyes once per day for four weeks.

Autosuggestion

The main mental reason for weak eyesight is not liking or being afraid of what is happening in your own life. The affirmation for this condition should be:

> I see myself with loving eyes.
> I see clearly and with love.
> From day to day I see better and better in every way.

Color Therapy **

For any condition of weak eyesight, use the colors blue and white for twenty minutes each once per day for one to six months. Also receive sunlight in the morning and evening about one hour after sunrise and one hour before sunset with closed eyes for fifteen minutes each time for one to six months.

Exercises to Improve Eyesight (Bates Method) ****

In any case of poor/weak eyesight we can correct the situation simply by using (in addition to the previous therapies) eye exercises that will balance the optic nerves, muscles, and other parts of the eye.

The first thing to do is to avoid mental strain of any kind. Just relax and try to receive all the impressions you get from your eyes as they are, because by trying to "see perfect" you cause inner stress, which should be avoided. On the other side, continue with physical activity and work so your body is functioning properly. But in a combination of relaxation and activity any hard work should be done in a relaxed atmosphere, never under tension. The exercises are:

1. Palming—Sit down comfortably, close your eyes, and cover your eyes with your hands. Do not press the eyeballs themselves but close your eyes with your hands so that no light will be seen. While doing this exercise repeat mentally the affirmations and relax your whole body and muscles.

   Do this exercise a minimum of twice per day (better four to six times per day), five minutes each time, until condition improves. And then continue this exercise once per day for the rest of your life.

2. Swinging—Stand up with your feet apart. Keep yourself relaxed, mentally repeat the affirmations, and gently sway the whole body from side to side very slowly and gently, first clockwise and then counterclockwise. Do this exercise while your eyes are open and relaxed. Do not try to "see" anything while doing this exercise. Repeat this swinging ten times in every direction twice per day.

3. Focus—Stand up and keep yourself still without moving the head. Now look up as far as you can without straining your vision. Then look down as far as you can without straining your vision. Repeat this exercise twice per day. While doing this blink continuously several times.

4. While sitting or standing without moving the head move the eyes from left to right ten times. While doing this exercise relax your vision and blink continuously.

5. While sitting or standing look down at your right side, then up toward the left eyebrow. Repeat this exercise but start now to look down at your left side, then up toward your right eyebrow. Repeat this exercise ten times twice per day.

6. Now move your eyes around in a clockwise circle very slowly and gently, and repeat counterclockwise. Do this ten times in each direction twice per day.

7. This exercise should be helped with your finger. Hold up the first finger of the left hand about twelve to eighteen inches in front of your eyes. Now look at your finger without strain for a few seconds and then continue to look at some distant object about 30 feet from you. Repeat this exercise ten times twice per day.

8. Rotate your hand in a clockwise circle while sitting still. Then continue the same in a counterclockwise direction. Repeat this exercise ten times in each direction twice per day.

9. Lower your head toward the chest as much as you can. Then raise your head and let it fall backward as far as possible. Repeat this exercise ten times continuously, twice per day.

10. Now lower your head to your right shoulder while sitting still.

Do the same toward the left shoulder, and repeat this exercise ten times twice per day.

Notes:

1. If while doing these exercises you feel uncomfortable, with pains in your muscles or nerves in and around your eyes, stop your exercises and relax, because the most important thing in these exercises is the complete relaxation of muscles, tendons, and nerves mainly of the eyes.
2. While doing all these exercises repeat the affirmations in the autosuggestion therapy.
3. Blink as much as you can without strain or effort while doing these exercises and during the day.

Reflexology **

In all cases of weak eyesight reflexology is very helpful to restore the eyesight by balancing the nerves and muscles of the eyes.
The treatment is by pressing the following points daily, four times per day, seven minutes each point. The points are:
6, 52. In both hands.
This treatment must be continued daily for three to six months. After the eyesight is balanced, continue this treatment another year, once per day for five minutes each point.

Schuessler Tissue Salts

Natrum muriaticum: 12X in any case of poor/weak eyesight. Use five tablets twice per day for fifty days.

MYOPIA

SUGGESTED TREATMENT

Acupuncture and Acupressure ***
1. GB 20, LI 4, BL 1, ST 1
2. ST 1, N-HN-2 (xianyingming—new head and neck point) ST 36, ST 2, LI 4 [Source: Bensky A. C. Text]
3. BL 23, LI 6, GV 19, BL 2, BL 60, add K 5 for myopia in women [Source: Bensky, A. C. Text]

Homeopathy *

Phsostigma: 3X every four hours.
For hemiopia:
Lithium carbonicum: 6X if right side of objects has vanished.
Lycopodium: 6X for left side vanishing.
Muriaticum acidum: 6X for vanishing of either vertical half.
Aurum: 6X for vanishing of upper half.

ASTIGMATISM

SUGGESTED TREATMENT *

Acupuncture and Acupressure ***
   GB 1, GB 20, TW 23, ST 1, BL 1, BL 2.
For senile astigmatism:
   GB 18, LiV 4, BL 10, BL 17, K 15, LU 6
   Ear points: Eye, vision #1, Vision #2, Kidney, Liver, Occiput

Homeopathy *

Lilium tigrinum: 30 every eight hours.

WEAK EYES AND TIRED EYES

SUGGESTED TREATMENT

Acupressure and Acupuncture **
Acupressure and Shiatsu Tsubo therapy helps calm and relieve eye complaints that are a result of optical nerve tiredness.
It *cannot* and does not claim to *cure* faulty refractions in the lenses of the eyes.
There is also no claim to cure or help distant blurred vision.
Acupressure for tired eyes:
In the horizontal position (on the back) close eyes lightly and with four fingers of each hand begin to rub eye rims from inside (medial) out (lateral). The light pressure of thumbs or fingers should be directed toward the bone around eye socket. One should press gently and in a slanting direction. A continuation of the massage should be applied to points:

GB 7, GB 20, BL 10, SI 15, TW 23, Tai-yuan, Yin-tang, GB 14 (Bilateral), ST 8.
Acupuncture: Most active points and first treatment for all eye problems:
GB 4, GB 20, GB 37, and ST 36 and BC 38.
Acupuncture for tired eyes:

1. GB 3, GB 14, GB 20, GB 37, LiV 8, ST 1, ST 8, ST 36, BL 1, BL 2, BL 38, HT 2, GV 19, GV 24, SI 6, TW 23
2. PC 2, SI 6, SI 15, BL 2, BL 4, BL 21, BL 38, GB 1, GB 4, GB 16, ST 8, ST 36

Ear points: Liver, Vision I, Subcortex

Herbs

Western *

A mixed drink to help vision in general is:

½ cup orange juice
½ cup grapefruit juice
¼ cup apple juice
1½ tablespoons apple cider vinegar

2 tablespoons wheat germ oil
1½ tablespoons raw honey

This mixture (blender drink) should be sipped three to five times daily, preferably before meals (½–1 hour).
Parsley: An infusion can be drunk three or four times daily as a general eye-tonifying tea.
Rosemary *(Rosemarinus officinalis):* Infusion (one teaspoon to a cup of water as tea) three times daily, and use one drop in each eye morning and before sleep.
Red sage *(Salvia officinalis):* To clear eyes and keep them bright, use in infusion form, three cups daily.
For dimness of eyesight:
Angelica *(Angelica archangelica):* In tea, powder, or tincture.
Maple red *(Acer rubrum):* For sore eyes. Was widely used by American Indians. This herb tends to strengthen tissues and eliminate fluid discharges. Two to three ml in tincture or powder recommended.

Chinese **

For eye fatigue the formula of choice is **Atractylodes and Hoelen Combination** *(Ling-kuei-chu-kan-tang).* This formula is indicated for those with dizziness, flushing, and dry lips. Other eye indications include dacryocystitis, conjunctivitis, ocular eczema, and cataract. It is

also recommended for what is known as "pseudo-nearsightedness."
Composition:

Hoelen 6g

Cinnamon twigs 4g

Licorice root 2g

Paichu (white atractylode rhizome) 3g

Bupleurum and Dragon Bone Combination *(chai-hu-chia-lung-ku-mu-li-tang):* Very helpful for eye ache and dimness of eyesight because of neural fatigue.
Compsoition:

Bupleurum 5g

Pinellia rhizome 4g

Scute 2.5 g

Ginger rhizome 2.5 g

Jujube fruit 2.5 g

Ginseng root 2.5 g

Cinnamon twigs 3g

Oyster shell 2.5 g

Hoelen 3g

Rhubarb rhizome 1 g

Dragon bone 2.5 g

For eye fatigue due to female problems, use **Bupleurum and Peony Formula** *(chia-wei-hsiao-yao-san).*
Composition:

Tang-kuei 3g

Paeony 3g

Atractylodes 3g

Hoelen 3g

Bupleurum 3g

Licorice 2g

Moutan 2g

Gardenia 2g

Ginger 1g

Mentha 1g

Homeopathy **

In homeopathic treatment for weak eyesight it is important that the correct spectacles should be provided for adults if the reasons for the condition stem from refraction or accommodation errors. On the other hand, it is highly advised to follow up constitutional treatment for children *before* using spectacles, because the latter will fix the problem.

Baptisia: For sore eyes and difficulty in distinguishing fine things and writing at night, use 3X every six hours.

Phosphorous: If from nervous weakness or oversexual strain, 3X every four hours.

Natrum muriaticum: 6X every four to six hours is the choice for weak sight due to overstrain and use.

BLURRED VISION AND SPOTS IN FRONT OF THE EYE

SUGGESTED TREATMENT

Acupuncture and Acupressure **
1. SI 6, LI 4, BL 4, GB 20, BL 5
2. Blurred, spotty vision:
   a. LI 3, LI 4, ST 6, ST 36, SP 2, BL 1, BL 2, BL 3, TW 3, TW 18, PC1, PC 2.
   b. BL 18, BL 23, K 1, SP 2, GB 1, GB 3, GB 6, GB 14, GB 37.

Herbs

Western

For blurred vision and dimness of sight:

Angelica: May be used in tea or eye drops.

Eyebright (Euphrasia officinalis): The herb for general irritating disorders of the eye. Seven and a half teaspoonfuls of **eyebright** extract combined with same amount of **golden seal** (Hydrastis) extract may help.

Chinese

Ginseng (Panax): Has a reputation of helping when there are gray spots in front of eyes, as well as for difficulty in opening eyelids and when objects appear double.

Homeopathy ***

Lilium tigrinum: For blurred vision, appearance of veil before eyes, 30X every three hours is the choice.

Gelsemium: For blurred vision, 3X every eight to ten hours.

INFLAMMATION OF THE EYE
(NONSPECIFIC EYE DISEASE CAUSING SYMPTOMS OF REDNESS, DRYNESS, PAIN, CONJUNCTIVAL DISCHARGE, AND SPOTS IN FRONT OF THE EYE)

SUGGESTED TREATMENT

Applied Nutrition *
If the physical condition of the patient permits, it is better to commence the diet with juice fasting for three days. Then gradually commence a low-protein diet.

Drink: Avoid dairy products, coffee, tea, cocoa, alcohol.

Eat: Avoid all spicy foods, dairy products, fried foods, white sugar, white wheat flour (refined), tobacco, cigarettes, etc.

An example of a diet for an average-weight person, thirty years old:

1,700 calories	100 mg inositol
35 g protein	200 mg vitamin B_{15}
70 g fat	1,000 mg calcium chelated
193 g carbohydrate	600 mg magnesium chelated
Master formula and the following	100 mg phosphorous chelated
vitamins and minerals: **	15 mg iron chelated
4,000 mg vitamin C	100 mcg chromium chelated
100 mg bioflavinoids	5 mg copper chelated
50,000 IU vitamin A	50 mg zinc chelated
1,000 IU vitamin D	100 mg potassium chelated
1,000 IU vitamin E	30 mg manganese chelated
200 mg vitamin B_2	100 mcg selenium chelated
100 mg vitamin B_3	50 mcg molybdenum chelated
100 mg vitamin B_6	Ribonucleic acid extract
100 mg folacin folic acid	Pituitary extract nucleoprotein
500 mcg vitamin B_{12}	Adrenal extract nucleoprotein
1,500 mg pantothenic acid	Thymus extract nucleoprotein

Aromatherapy

Use the essence of **bergamot** (eight parts), **eucalyptus** (four parts), **juniper** (two parts). Take this formula by inhalation twice per day for one week in any case of inflammation of the eye, optic nerves, retina, or any other part of the eyes.

Autosuggestion

Repeat the following affirmation twenty times every morning and evening:

From day to day and from second to second my eyes become stronger and healthier in every way.

Color Therapy

In case of inflammation use blue color twenty minutes twice per day for three weeks on the eyes directly. The light should be given in thirty-second bursts sixteen to twenty times per day.

Warning: Do not expose the open eyes to a direct, powerful source of light or directly to the sunlight for any period of time. Directing the open eyes to the sun may cause ultraviolet keratitis (actinic keratitis).

Reflexology **

The treatment of reflexology as a secondary reinforcement is very important. Use the following points in both hands:
1-6-52, 54, 55.
Press each point for five minutes every two hours, especially Nos. 6 and 52.

Schuessler Tissue Salts

Natrum phosphorica: 30X in case of eye inflammation if the discharge from the eye is yellow.
Kali muriaticum: 30X if the discharge of the eye in case of inflammation is thick white mucus.
Kali sulphorica: 30X if the discharge of the eye in case of inflammation is greenish.

Take the remedies every hour until improvement of the inflammation occurs. Then continue three times per day for another three weeks with the same remedy.

CONJUCTIVITIS, UVEITIS, IRITIS, DACROCYSTITIS, AND BELPHARITIS

SYMPTOMS

Redness, often persistent, and frequent tearing.

SUGGESTED TREATMENT

Acupuncture and Acupressure **

1.   GB 20, Tai-yang, LI 4, BL 1, GB 8
2.   GB 20, BL 2, Tai-yang, LI 4, GB 37
3.   TW 23, GB 1, GB 14, BL 1, ST 2, PC 7, LI 4, LI 20, LI 5, GB 42, GB 4, GV 14, GV 12, BL 18, BL 20

Ear points: 1.   Liver, eye, vision #2
            2.   Temple, Ear Apex, Lower-blood pressure Groove
For red eyes:
    BL 60, K 3, LI 15, PC 7, BL 1, SI 3, GB 1, GB 16
    If painful, add BL 2, TW 2

For red, swollen, and painful eyes:
  BL 62, LI 15, LiV 3, LiV 8
For red, swollen, painful eyes with diminishing vision:
  apply Moxa on LI 4, LI 2, BL 18, ST 36.

Herbs

Western

Quince *(Cydonium,* or *Cydonia obconga):*   Used as a soothing lotion in conjunctivitis and eye and lid inflammations. When ripe, the quince fruit is edible.

Chinese **

Ginseng *(Panax):*   Excellent for eye inflammations in tincture, powder, tea, and tablet form.
Pueraria Combination *(Ko-ten-tang):*   The formula of choice for all eye inflammations and mostly in initial stage of any eye disease.

Homeopathy ***

Euphrasia: For acute inflammation of the margin use 1X to 3X every two to three hours.
Euphrasia lotion may be applied at three- to four-hour intervals.
Hepar sulphuris: For chronic eye inflammation, 6X every six to eight hours.
Pulsatilla: For inflammation of lacrimal sac, 3X every three hours, followed by
Clematis: 3X every two to three hours.
Aconitum: For acute conjunctivitis, 3X hourly. A local compress of **euphrasia** lotion is useful.
Mercurius corrosivus: If there is pustular inflammation or gonorrheal inflammation, use 3X hourly.
Calcarea carbonica: For granular opthlamia, 6X three times daily.
Aconitum: In keratitis, iritis, and sclerotitis, 1X to 3X every two to three hours.

GLAUCOMA

SYMPTOMS

Increasing problems of vision; accurate diagnosis difficult without laboratory diagnosis.

SUGGESTED TREATMENT

Applied Nutrition

Use the same diet therapy as in the case of inflammation of the eye. In this condition the amino minerals chelates are very important.

Aromatherapy

Use the same aromatherapy treatment as in the case of conjunctivitis.

Autosuggestion

Use the same affirmation as in the case of conjunctivitis, but at least four times per day.

Color Therapy **

Use blue light over the eyes for thirty minutes locally and daily. Also use yellow light for another ten minutes daily.

Use this technique once per day for one month. It is recommended to get the sunlight with closed eyes for a period of ten minutes after the sunrise and again before sunset.

Reflexology **

In case of glaucoma, open-angle glaucoma, and infantile glaucoma, press the following points in the hands and feet for three minutes each four to five times per day for the first two weeks, and then continue three times per day for another two months or more:

1, 2, 3, 6, 52, 54, 55.

Point number 52 only in the hands.

Schuessler Tissue Salts

As a secondary reinforcement of the eye, use the following formula three times per day:

Ferrum phosphorica 30X   **Kali phosphorica** 12X
Natrum phosphorica 12X   **Magnesium phosphorica** 6X
Natrum muriaticum 12X   **Silica** 12X

In spirit aqua (drops).
Take ten drops from this formula every morning, noon, and evening, at least thirty minutes after a meal. Use for one month.

CATARACT

SUGGESTED TREATMENT

Applied Nutrition

In many cases the best results can be achieved by a longer juice fast of six days. Then continue the same diet therapy as in the case of conjunctivitis.

Aromatherapy

Use the same treatment as in the case of conjunctivitis—externally only.

Autosuggestion

The main mental reason for this condition is mental confusion about the future, usually a very pessimistic outlook on life, not being able to see any good opportunities ahead in the future.
The affirmation for this condition should be:

> I am free to see my future in a positive way.
> My life now and in the future is filled with joy and happiness.

Color Therapy

Use blue light over the eyes for thirty minutes with closed eyes, but open the eyes and gaze into the light for a few seconds every minute. Repeat this treatment once per day for a period of one month. The color blue can be reinforced with green for fifteen minutes.
If the condition is very severe, do this treatment twice per day for the first two weeks and then continue for another month once per day.

Reflexology **

Reflexology is helpful in the early stages of cataract caused by congenital, infantile, traumatic, diabetic, or senile problems.
The treatment is the same as in the case of glaucoma but may require a longer period of therapy—between two and six months of daily pressing points.

Schuessler Tissue Salts

Use the same technique as in the treatment of glaucoma.

· 10 ·
PSYCHIATRIC DISORDERS

The focus of modern medicine since the discovery of vaccines, the development of antibiotics, and the study of vitamin and mineral deficiencies has been on "magic bullets": single therapies for single disease states. In the last few decades this emphasis has shifted to the *multifactorial* causes of illness and the *synergistic* effect of multiple therapies. The organic, the psychological, the social, the environmental, and the behavioral aspects of an illness are now routinely taken into account in the best practice. There is now general agreement in principle, if not in emphasis, that:

1. Any illness has both somatic (bodily) and psychological components—or, to put the matter another way, these are distinctions only in theory, not in practice.
2. Diagnosis should take the patient's life situation into account.
3. All illnesses are experienced with anxiety, depression, and grieving.
4. Psychiatry should always suspect organic problems; biochemical therapy should always suspect personality problems.

The "disordered personality" presents a problem in diagnosis as well as in treatment that underscores how difficult it is to put the above prescriptions into practice. Typically this person has maladaptive behavior problems that are "only" exaggerations of patterns exhibited at times by most people. He or she is not aware of any symptoms of anxiety or depression because he or she feels normal and right. He or she is "ego syntonic," feeling no need for help unless referred by family or friends with whom he or she is unable to live in harmony. Problems arise from fixed, repetitive, often self-defeating patterns of behavior. The person therefore cannot respond to stress appropriately, but rather becomes psychotic, inflexible, anxious, and unresponsive.

In contrast, the neurotic person presents childlike characteristics, often sensitive and suggestible, indulging in fantasy and introspection. In contrast with the psychotic, the psychoneurotic feels discomfort in the form of insecurity and inferiority. But the reaction is in the form of defenses, which may create the opposite impression to the casual observer. He or she craves the attention of people, including a family he or she may have difficulty living with. The defenses employed to alleviate anxiety or depression are again only exaggerations of normal behavior, but carried to extremes: (1) denial, suppression, repression; (2) rationalization and intellectualization; (3) displacement and projection (attributing to others the feelings he or she has for them); (4) reversal of effect; (5) introjection; (6) sublimation; (7) obsessive and compulsive mechanisms; (8) regression. These reactions become increasingly fixed as ways of counteracting the stresses of anxiety and depression.

Depression is common to everyone at one time or another, in varying degrees. When it persists in sustained feelings of hopelessness, lack of self-esteem, and utter reliance on others, it may be classified as a disorder. Common symptoms are changes in the person's eating and sleeping patterns, decrease in libido, and withdrawal from social contacts over time. Minor problems or setbacks reduce the sufferer to inactivity and a feeling of dependency. When he or she fails to achieve symbiotic support from others, he or she may seek relief in drugs and alcohol.

Anxiety is a more palpable psychological state than depression, although many people may experience it for a lifetime without attaching that word to their behavior. In the clinical sense, anxiety has quite specific symptoms: a sense of panic, often accompanied by sweating and palpitations, even vomiting and diarrhea. The wave of fear may pass in a few minutes or may persist in the middle of the night as a feeling of impending doom, such as death or insanity. Such attacks may also exacerbate organic disorders of bronchial asthma, peptic ulcer, chronic colitis, or enteritis. Anxiety is a frequent concomitant of psychoneuroses as well as many toxic or disease states.

Far more specific symptoms occur in a schizophrenic state than in anxiety, neurosis, or depression. The latter disorders may accompany a variety of conditions. Schizophrenia, in contrast, is a common disorder that is often exhibited in isolation from other problems. There is no apparent organic cause and no brain dysfunction. But the disassociation from reality is clear-cut: poor logical associations, limited emotional responses, ambivalence in a pronounced degree, delusions, and occasionally hallucinations. There is a continuous misperception of the world and one's place in it. Schizophrenia commonly occurs from teenage years to midlife, affecting, by some estimates, nearly one percent of the population.

Many schizophrenics also show signs of the manic-depressive syndrome, common in the more manic stages between the ages of fifteen and twenty-five, and in depressive stages from twenty-five to thirty-five. Manic-depressive behavior is the second most common of the psychotic disorders, affecting women twice as often as men and higher social or professional groups. It is characterized by wild fluctuations between these apparently contradictory states. Depression, as described above, may last for a few minutes or for days. Manic behavior is often short-lived: frenzied activity, wordiness, preoccupation with the sounds rather than with the meanings of words, flightiness, mischievousness, delusions of great achievement, and elation punctuated by irritability and anger when proposed flights of fancy are not immediately accepted. As in all the conditions described in this book, occasional outbursts of such behavior should not be interpreted too technically.

Dementia is a severe term for a class of organic brain damage with no obvious cause. In dementia, cerebral tissue is impaired, causing recent memory loss, lack of attention, poor orientation, diminished comprehension, abstraction, weakened judgment or emotional response. A deficiency of acetylcholine, a neurotransmitter, has recently been suspected as a cause of dementia. In the presenile period (up to sixty years), dementia is known as Alzheimer's disease; in addition to the above symptoms, general confusion is common in the much-publicized Alzheimer's.

Drug addiction has some elements in common with the above psychiatric disorders, primarily the need to deny an unpleasant state. Some forms of alcoholism may be classified here. As in alcoholism, genetic and other organic factors may be predominant in the dependency, if not in the initiation of the addiction. The variety of drugs has intensified in recent years with demand for greater satisfaction and the easy availability of synthetic sources. A common theme of drug dependence is the escalation of doses as the individual becomes tolerant of the initial effect of the drug. The moral, legal, and practical aspects of drug use in our society are beyond the scope of this book.

Finally, a garden-variety type of psychological disorder should be considered: insomnia. In many cases, of course, the inability to get a good night's sleep may be due to injury or illness. Chronic insomnia is another matter entirely, affecting a large percentage of the population, at least at income-tax time, in marital stress, and in old age. It is well-known that the usual over-the-counter medications are counterproductive in the long run. It is on this theme that this discussion comes to a logical conclusion, since the inability to sleep is an everyday example of how social, environmental, organic, behavioral, and psychological difficulties can contribute to a very manifest problem.

PERSONALITY DISORDERS (ANTISOCIAL PERSONALITY, IMMATURE PERSONALITY, BORDERLINE PERSONALITY, NARCISSIST PERSONALITY, AVOIDANT PERSONALITY, DEPENDENT PERSONALITY, AND PASSIVE-AGGRESSIVE PERSONALITY)

SYMPTOMS

Personality Disorders, Psychosis: Exaggerated patterns of behavior, leading to inflexibility, anxiousness, and unresponsiveness.
Neurosis: Sensitivity, childlike fantasies and suggestibility, feelings of inferiority, insecurity, leading eventually to repression and regression.

SUGGESTED TREATMENT

General: Psychological treatment is useful in most personality disorders, either in group therapy or individual treatment in various techniques such as:

1. Adlerian psychotherapy
2. Adlerian group psychotherapy
3. Art therapy
4. Assertive behavior therapy
5. Dance therapy
6. Drama therapy
7. Behavioral family therapy
8. Gestalt therapy
9. Hypnotherapy
10. Jungian group therapy
11. Modern psychoanalysis
12. Music therapy—play therapy
13. Primal therapy
14. Existential–humanistic psychotherapy

and in many more therapies, which should be done by a well-trained therapist. The social environment, such as self-help communities in a group therapy that utilize peer pressure and relationship to modify the self-destructive behavior, can be very helpful in addition to the psychological therapy.

Applied Nutrition ***

Complete blood test. Thyroid Function Test—T(3)–T(4) TSH, urine analysis, and the cytotoxic blood test, hair and nail analysis are very important to find out if there is an allergic reaction of the body or a mineral imbalance that can cause or aggravate the mental symptoms or any other physical problems that may cause these mental symptoms.

Drink: Avoid coffee, alcohol, dairy products.

Eat: Fresh green vegetables, some fresh fruits, whole cereals and beans well cooked, seeds unroasted, sprouts, and soy protein, to supply whole protein to the body. Avoid any processed food, artificial colors, stimulant food, canned foods, smoking, dairy products, meats, eggs, and fish. Poultry should also be avoided in the beginning of the therapy. Special attention should be paid to avoid foods that may cause allergic reaction, tiredness, heaviness, or any other bad feelings. The amount of protein should be calculated according to the behavior of the patient. In hyperactivity, aggression, violence—yang conditions—about 0.5 gram of protein per kilogram of body weight. In hypoactivity, passive reactions, brain fatigue, depression—yin conditions—about 1.0 gram protein per kilogram of body weight. An example of a diet for an average-weight person, thirty years old:

Yang condition	*Yin condition*
2,500 calories	1,900 calories
20 g protein	70 g protein
120 g fat	80 g fat
325 g carbohydrate	225 g carbohydrate

For both conditions of yin and yang:
Vitamins

25,000 IU vitamin A	2,000 mg folic acid
1,000 IU vitamin D	200 mcg vitamin B_{12}
1,000 IU vitamin E	1,500 mg pantothenic acid
7,000 mg vitamin C	100 mcg biotin
400 mg bioflavinoids	100 mg cholin
100 mg vitamin B_1	200 mg inositol
100 mg vitamin B_2	30 mg Paba
500 mg vitamin B_3	50 mg B_{15}
200 mg vitamin B_6	

Chelated amino mineral

500–2,000 mg calcium, according to the parathyroid function test
300–1,200 mg magnesium
100 mg phosphorous
15 mg iron
200 mcg chromium

50 mg zinc
100 mg potassium
50–200 mcg iodine, according to the thyroid function test T(3)–T(4)
100 mcg selenium
50 mcg molybdenum

Enzymes

180 mg hydrochloric acid
150 mg pancreatin
120 mg bile extract

65 mg pepsin
65 mg lipase
120 mg papain

Nucleoprotein extracts

60 mg pituitary extract
40 mg adrenal extract
60 mg thymus extract

60 mg pancreas extract
60 mg kidney extract
60 mg RNA extract

General

2,400 mg lecithin
2,000 mg brown yeast

2,000 mg alfalfa

Autosuggestion ***

In all cases of personality disorders, as in most psychological and psychiatric problems, the patient can be helped by the use of affirmations. If the patient is too depressed or is unwilling to repeat the affirmations by himself or herself, they can be recorded on a tape recorder cassette. Then listen to this cassette twice per day, twenty minutes each morning and evening. The affirmations are:

From day to day I am better and healtheir in every way.
I love myself unconditionally—for myself.
I am in full control of my body, mind, and spirit.
From day to day I am stronger and happier in every way.
I release the past. I am living peaceful and secure.
I can express myself freely and peacefully.
I relax into the flow of life and let life flow through me with ease.
I feel tolerance and compassion and love for all people and myself.
From day to day I fulfill myself in every way.
From day to day all my personal problems dissolve until they disappear.

Color Therapy

If the general reaction and behavior of the patient is yin in nature, use the colors red and yellow, twenty minutes each. If yang in nature, use the colors blue and indigo in addition to the specific colors given below.

Antisocial personality: Radiate the color pink thirty minutes twice per day. Then continue with green twenty-five minutes twice per day. Then continue with blue fifteen minutes once per day.

Immature personality and borderline personality: Radiate the colors violet for twenty minutes and chrome yellow for fifteen minutes twice per day.

Narcissist: Radiate the colors for thirty minutes and blue for fifteen minutes twice per day.

Avoidant personality and dependent personality: Radiate the colors red for thirty minutes and yellow for fifteen minutes twice per day.

Passive–aggressive personality: Radiate the colors green for twenty minutes and dark green for twenty minutes.

Homeopathy ***

Agaricus muscrius: For antisocial personality.
Sepia: 200 once only for antisocial personality.
Anacaroium: 200 for immature personality.
Sepia: 200 D for paranoid personality.
Agarius muscarius: 200 D for antisocial personality.
Anacardium: 200 D for immature personality.
Belladonna: 200 D for borderline personality.
Hyoscyamus: 200 D for narcissist personality.
Phosphorous: 200 D for dependent personality.
Nux vomica: 200 D for passive–aggressive personality.

Reflexology
Press the same as in depression, p. 298.

Schuessler Tissue Salts
In addition to the general treatment, take the following remedies in every case as follows:
Antisocial personality:
Take five tablets of each remedy twice per day, one after the other:

Calcarea phosphorica 6X   **Kali phosphorica** 6X

Immature personality:

Kali phosphorica: 12X, ten
tablets twice per day.

Borderline personality:
Take ten tablets of each remedy, one after the other, twice per day:

Natrum phosphorica 12X   **Calcarea phosphorica** 12X

Narcissist personality:
Take ten tablets of each remedy, one after the other, twice per day:

Natrum muriaticum 12X   **Natrum phosphorica** 12X

Avoidant personality:

Natrum phosphorica: 6X, take
ten tablets twice per day.

Dependent personality:

Calcarea fluorica: 12X, take ten
tablets twice per day.

Passive–aggressive personality:
Take ten tablets of each remedy, one after the other, twice per day:

Calcarea sulphorica 12X   **Natrum muriaticum** 12X

PARANOIA

SUGGESTED TREATMENT

Acupuncture
PC 5, PC 6, HT 7, K 3, LI 4, LiV 3, TW 5, TW 18
Ear—Shen-men, Endocrine, Occiput

Homeopathy

Arnica: 3X to 30X

HYSTERIA

SUGGESTED TREATMENT

*Acupuncture and Acupressure ***
PC 6, HT 7, GV 26, SI 3
If epileptic add:
LI 11, LU 11, GB 34, GB 30, LI 4, LiV 3
For insomnia and stiffness add:
LiV 1, K 1, GV 20

For constricted throat add:
  K6, CV 22.
For obstructed vision add:
  UB 1, TW 23
For hysterical aphasia add:
  CV 22
For sudden laugh-cry add:
  PC 7, LU 11, K4, SP 6
Ear points: Heart, Kidney, Subcortex, Brain Stem, Neurogate, Sympathetic.
Acupuncture is effective but should be used with Western and Chinese remedies.
For hysterical seizures:
  UB 60, SI 3
Or: GV 26, LI 4, PC 8
Or: GV 20, PC 6, TW 5

Herbs

Western **

Arrach *(Chenopodium olidum):* Use one ounce of powdered herb in one pint of water (boiling), two or three cups daily.
Asafetida *(Ferula assa-foetida linne):* The exudate of the gum resin was found helpful to relieve spasms.
Gentiana: A small amount of the powdered root or stem.

Chinese

Pinellia and Magnolia Combination: For hysteria and mental instability. May be accompanied by weak digestion or distressed throat and chest.
Ginseng and Astagalus Combination: With insomnia and weak digestion.
Licorice and Jujube Combination: For hysteria, insomnia, restlessness.

Homeopathy ***

Moschus: 3 every fifteen to twenty minutes while in attack.
Ignatia: 3 to 6, four to six times daily when there is a feeling of "lump" in throat and changes of moods.
Platinum: 6 four to six times daily when depressed.
Senecio Aureus: For females with amenorrhea and hysteria.

PSYCHONEUROTIC DISORDERS
(OBSESSIVE–COMPULSIVENESS, PARANOIA, HYSTERICAL NEUROSIS, IMPULSIVENESS, PHOBIC NEUROSIS, AND HYPOCHONDRIAL NEUROSIS)

SUGGESTED TREATMENT

General: Psychological treatment as in personality disorders, mainly in individual treatments.

Applied Nutrition **

The same as in the Personality Disorders diet.

Aromatherapy

In all cases of impulsiveness, hysteria, fears, phobias, paranoia, and obsessive–compulsive behavior, take the following extracts twice per day: **lavender** 4% **rosemary** 4% **valerian** 12% on brown sugar tablets until condition improves and the patient is relaxed.

Autosuggestion ***

The same affirmations as for personality disorders on a tape recorder cassette, twenty minutes each morning and evening. Also a personal affirmation according to the specific disorder, twenty times each affirmation. For obsessive–compulsiveness:

> I have all I need.
> My needs are secured, and all I need is secured.

For paranoia:

> I love every person in this planet, and everybody loves me.
> I have compassion for others and for myself.

For hysterical neurosis:

> I am relaxed, free, and calm.
> I am secure and protected.

For impulsiveness:

> Calm, no rush into my life.
> I take a deep breath before any action.

For phobic neurosis:

> I am secure and protected.
> I accept joy and fun as a basis of my life.

For hypochondrial neurosis:

> *I am healthy and secure in every way and part of my body, mind, and spirit.*

Color Therapy **

For obsessive–compulsiveness, radiate the following colors one after the other, twice per day: blue for thirty minutes, green for ten minutes, yellow for ten minutes.

For paranoia, hysterical neurosis, and phobic neuroses, radiate the following colors, one after the other, twice per day: blue for thirty minutes, indigo for fifteen minutes, green for fifteen minutes.

For impulsiveness, radiate the following colors one after the other, twice per day: green for twenty minutes, dark green for ten minutes, light blue for ten minutes.

For hypochondrial neurosis, in yin condition, radiate twice per day: red for twenty minutes, pink for twenty minutes, yellow for ten minutes. In yang condition of this state radiate twice per day: green for twenty minutes, blue for fifteen minutes, indigo for ten minutes.

Reflexology

Press the same points as in depression.

Schuessler Tissue Salts

For obsessive–compulsiveness, take twice daily, ten tablets each:

Ferrum phosphorica 30X   **Kali phosphorica** 200X

For hysterical neurosis: take twice per day, ten tablets each:

Kali phosphorica 200X   **Kali sulphorica** 30X
Silica 30X

For impulsiveness, take twice per day, ten tablets each:

Calcarea sulphorica 30X   **Natrum muriaticum** 200X
Natrum sulphorica 30X

For phobic neurosis, take twice per day, ten tablets each:

Kali phosphorica 200X   **Ferrum phosphorica** 30X
Kali sulphorica 30X

For hypchondrial neurosis, take twice per day, ten tablets each:

Kali phosphorica 200X   **Calcarea phosphorica** 30X
Natrum muriaticum 30X   **Natrum sulphorica** 30X

SENILE AND PRESENILE DEMENTIA (INCLUDING CONCENTRATION, LEARNING, AND MEMORY)

SYMPTOMS

Dementia–Alzheimer's Disease; recent memory loss, lack of concentration, weakened judgment, emotional disorder.

SUGGESTED TREATMENT

Acupuncture ***

1. Sedate: GV 26, LU 11, HT 8, CV 14
2. LI 4, LiV 3, TW 2, TW 10, TW 23, K 1, K 9, ST 45.

Applied Nutrition

Use the same diet therapy as in Personality Disorders. The quantity of protein should be as in yin condition, rich in protein.

Aromatherapy

Use the following extracts on a base of brown sugar tablets: **rosemary** 8%, **peppermint** 4%, **cardamom** 4%, **basil** 2%,

Autosuggestion

Use the tape recorder cassette twice per day as in Personality Disorders.

Breathing Therapy

Using the breathing exercises three or four times per day improves the mental abilities by enriching the brain with oxygen. The exercises are: Breathe in (inhale) to the count of four. Breathe out (exhale) to the count of eight. Stop breathing to the count of forty-five. Then repeat this cycle ten times.

Color Therapy *

Radiate the following colors twice per day, one after the other: yellow for twenty minutes, red for ten minutes, green for ten minutes.

Herbs

Chinese
Rehmannia Eight Combination **

Hypnotherapy

Can be very useful to improve all mental activities in presenile dementia.

Reflexology

Massage the whole feet with foot reflexology device, twice per day for seven minutes each time.

Press and massage the following points twice per day, two or three minutes each point:

1—Sinus, 2—Pituitary, 3—Cerebrum, 4—Cerebellum, 11—Parathyroid, 13—Thyroid, 17—Solar Plexus, 18—Heart, 20—Adrenal Gland, 21—Kidney, 24—Liver, 51—Thymus, 52—Autonomic Nervous System, 54—Cranial Nerves, 56—Energy

Schuessler Tissue Salts

Take the following remedies twice per day, ten tablets each:

Kali phosphorica 200X   **Natrum muriaticum** 30X
Silica 30X   **Ferrum phosphorica** 30X
Calcarea phosphorica 30X

These remedies can be taken at any age to improve poor concentration, learning abilities, and memory

DEPRESSION

SYMPTOMS

Extended feelings of hopelessness and lack of self-esteem, manifested in basic behavioral changes in eating, sleeping, social patterns, usually with loss of libido.

SUGGESTED TREATMENT

General: As in Personality Disorders, psychological treatment is recommended.

Acupuncture and Acupressure **

LI 4, UB 38, K 4, HT 3, HT 6, LiV 3, SP 6, GV 13, GV 14.
For nervous depression:
PC 8, PC 9, GB 22, GV 13, SP 6, UB 38, HT 3, HT 9, ST 36, K 27.
Ear points: Shen-men, subcortex, adrenal

Applied Nutrition ***
The same diet therapy as in Personality Disorders.

Aromatherapy
Take the following essences once per day on a brown sugar tablet:
camomile 6%, **jasmine** 4% **bergamot** 4%.

Autosuggestion ****
Repeat the same as in Personality Disorders, and also the following affirmations ten times:

I am more and more happy in every cycle of my life.
I enjoy living on this planet.

Breathing Therapy ****
Take ten deep breaths twice per day connecting the inhale to the exhale while mentally repeating the affirmations for this problem.

Color Therapy
Radiate the following colors twice per day, one after the other: red for twenty minutes, orange for ten minutes, yellow for ten minutes.

Herbs

Western

Gotu kola/ kola vera **Damiana** **Lavender** **Rosemary**	1X 3 capsules 1:1 ratio daily or 15 drops of tincture 1:1 ratio 3 times daily in ½ glass of water.

Good formula for general lassitude.
Lime blossom *(Tilia europea):*   In infusion.v:1 ratio (teaspoon) three times daily or 15 drops of tincture three times daily in ½ glass of water.
Valeriana

Chinese ***

Ginseng, Longan and Bupleurum Combination *(Chia-wei-kuei-pi-tang):*   For depression and anxiety.

Astragalus Combination: General tonic formula.

Ignatia: 3 to 6 four times daily when due to worry or sudden changes in life.

Arsenicum album: 3 four times daily for anxiety and depression.

Spigelia: 3 four times daily when accompanied by chest distress.

Aurum: When there is a suicidal personality.

Sepia: When irritated by daily chores.

Hydrotherapy

Take an alternating hot-cold shower twice a day.

Reflexology **

Press the following points twice per day for three minutes each:

1—Sinus, 2—Pituitary, 3—Cerebrum, 13—Thyroid, 20—Adrenal Gland, 24—Liver, 51—Thymus, 52—Autonomic Nervous System, 54—Cranial Nerves

Schuessler Tissue Salts

Take the following remedy twice per day, one after the other, ten tablets each:

Natrum muriaticum 200X   **Ferrum phosphorica** 30X
Natrum sulphorica 30X

ANXIETY AND STRESS

SYMPTOMS

Feelings of panic, giving rise to palpitations and sweating, even vomiting and diarrhea. Often nighttime reactions in feelings of fear of death or insanity.

SUGGESTED TREATMENT

General: As in personality disorders, psychological treatment is recommended to solve the source of the stress.

Acupuncture and Acupressure **

1.   CV 14, CV 17, UB 15, GV 11, GV 19, HT 5, HT 6, HT 7, HT 8
2.   CV 14, UB 15, GB 19, GB 24, LiV 2, UB 58, LiV 5

For anxiety in children:
 K1 L, UB 64, ST 36, LiV 2
 Use mild pressure.
For anxiety and palpitations:
 PC 3, CV 14, CV 17, GV 24, LI 3, LI 4, LI 11, LiV 2, LiV 3, LiV 5,
HT 5, HT 6, HT 7, K 1, K 4, LU 9
 Ear—Subcortex, Neurogate, Shenen.

Applied Nutrition ***
The same diet therapy as in Personality Disorders.

Aromatherapy
Take the following extracts on a base of brown sugar tablets, five twice
per day: **basil** 4%, **bergamot** 4% **jasmine** 6%.

Autosuggestion ****
Repeat the same affirmations as in Personality Disorders and also the
following affirmations twice per day, ten times each:

 I joyously release the past and live joyously now.
 I release all stress of the past and live peacefully.

Breathing Therapy ****
The same exercise as in the case of depression. It is very helpful to
breathe deeply due to hard physical activity such as sport or physical
work.

Color Therapy **
Radiate the following colors one after the other twice per day until
condition improves: blue for thirty minutes, indigo for ten minutes,
green for ten minutes.

Herbs

Western

Valeriana and **skullcap:**   Excellent in pill form. The tea *doesn't* taste
good.
Lady's slipper *(Cypreipedium pubescens):*   Infusion is good for anxiety
associated with insomnia.

Homeopathy

Ignatia: 3 every two to three hours.
Magnesia Carbonica: 200X every four hours.
Pulsatilla: 3X to 30X for the anxious woman.

Hydrotherapy

Take twice per day alternating showers of cold/hot water. Alternate for a few seconds cold/hot water eight or ten times each shower.

Hypnotherapy

Can be very helpful to reduce anxiety and stress.

Reflexology

Press the following points twice per day until stress is relieved:

2—Pituitary for two minutes, 11—Parathyroid for two minutes, 13—Thyroid for two minutes, 20—Adrenal Gland for two minutes, 24—Liver for two minutes, 51—Thymus for two minutes, 52—Autonomic nervous system for five minutes.

Schuessler Tissue Salts

Take the following remedies one after the other twice a day, ten tablets each:

Calcarea phosphorica 30X   **Ferrum phosphorica** 30X
Kali phosphorica 200X

MANIC-DEPRESSION, SCHIZOPHRENIA, AND PSYCHOSIS

SYMPTOMS

Manic-depression: wild fluctuations in mood, with frenzied activity followed by depression and despondency.
Schizophrenia: behavior exhibiting poor logical associations, limited emotional responses, delusions, and ambivalence.

SUGGESTED TREATMENT

General: The treatment of schizophrenia should include psychological treatment by one of the systems of therapy in Personality Disorders.

Acupuncture **

For manic psychosis:
    CV 15, CV 13, GB 20, PC 8, LU 11, LI 4, LiV 3, N-HN-54 (Anmnian). Moxa GV 20.
For depressive psychosis:

GV 15, CV 11, PC 6, HT 5, SP 6, GV 20, K 5, GB 34, LiV 5, HT 7. Moxa LiV 1.

Ear acupuncture: Sympathetic, Shen-men, Neurogate, Liver, Subcortex, Endocrine, Occiput

Autosuggestion

Repeat the same affirmations as in Personality Disorders in the tape recorder cassette.

Color Therapy

The color therapy should be in the depressive cycle of the disease, one after the other twice per day: red for twenty minutes, orange for ten minutes, yellow for ten minutes. In the mania cycle of the disease, one after the other twice per day: blue for thirty minutes, indigo for ten minutes. After these colors use green for thirty minutes three times a day until condition improves.

Herbs

Chinese

Licorice and Jujube Combination

Homeopathy

Ambra grisea: 2X to 3X four to six times daily.
Belladonna: 30X three to four times daily.

Reflexology

Massage and press the same points as in Schizophrenia.

Schuessler Tissue Salts

Take twice per day the following remedies, ten tablets each:

Kali phosphorica 200X   **Natrum muriaticum** 30X
Calcarea phosphorica 30X   **Ferrum phosphorica** 30X

DRUG ADDICTION

SUGGESTED TREATMENT

General: A group support or group therapy is very important in the treatment of this problem.

Acupuncture and Acupressure ***

For alcoholism:

UB 18, UB 19, UB 21, ST 36, LiV 13, LiV 14, GB 8, CV 6, UB ₁ ⅄ UB 58, ST 40.

For sobering up:

K9, ST 25, ST 36, UB 38, UB 58, GV 25, ST 44 to minimize hangover.

Ear points for excessive alcohol consumption:

Brain, Forehead, Thirst, Kidney, Internal Secretion, Occiput, Shenmen, Mouth

For withdrawal of alcohol addiction:

PC 6, GB 30, LI 4, GB 24, UB 23, UB 24, UB 48, UB 58, HT 7, point zero (Nogier)

For drug addiction withdrawal:

UB 13 +

Ear points: Lung, Mouth, Shen-men

To stop smoking:

LU 7, LU 9, GB 15, GB 22, GB 37, CV 17, CV 22, HT 5, HT 7, SP 6, SP 9, K 10, LI 4, LI 20, LI 19

Ear points: Larynx, Pharynx, Mouth, Shen-men, Occiput, Lung

Applied Nutrition **

Commence the diet therapy with three days juice fasting; then continue with the same diet therapy as in Personality Disorders.

Also take every hour until the need for alcohol, drugs or smoking is over:

1,000 mg vitamin C, to a maximum of 12,000 mg per day
100 mg bioflavinoids, to a maximum of 1,200 mg per day
200 mg calcium, to a maximum of 3,000 mg per day
80 mg magnesium, to a maximum of 1,200 mg per day
100 mg pantothenic acid, to a maximum of 1,800 mg per day
50 mg niacinamid, to a maximum of 600 mg per day

Aromatherapy

Take twice per day the following extracts on brown sugar base: **fennel** 12%, **rose** 8%, **eucalyptus** 4%

Autosuggestion ****

Repeat the same tape cassette as in Personality Disorders, twice per day.

Bach Flowers ***

Crabapple: For cleansing for all types of addictions.
Cherry plum: For desperation.

Cerato: To gain confidence in breaking the habit.
Agrimony: To aid anxiety.

Herbs

Western

Coffee: The seeds of the pl ints are known as antinarcotic and will help dispel the feeling of drowsiness resulting from narcotic poisoning.

Chinese

Siler and Platycodon: For those with delicate constitution, alcoholics.

Homeopathy

Coffee, nicotine, and alcohol can be taken in homeopathic dilutions made to order in homeopathic pharmacies. A correct prescription by a qualified practitioner is recommended.

Sulph: A single dose is given for alcoholic habit.

Nux vomica: 3X four to six times daily. For those who try to get off alcohol and vomit in the early morning.

Quercus: 3X six times daily for chronic drunks.

Nux vomica: When getting off tobacco, take 3 every four to five hours.

Camphor: Chew a pilule when craving a cigarette.

Hypnotheray

Hypnotherapy is very efficient when done properly to solve addiction problems of any kind.

Reflexology **

Press the following points, three minutes each point in the hand and foot twice per day:

2—Pituitary, 20—Adrenal Gland, 21—Kidney, 24—Liver, 52—Autonomic nervous system

Also press the following points in both ears for five minutes each point:

73—Alcoholism, 74—Stop Smoking and Drug Addiction, 73—Alcoholism—is located in the cymba of conchae above midpoint of crus of Helix, 74—Stop Smoking—near center of Cavum of Concha.

Schuessler Tissue Salts

For any kind of addiction take the following remedies, five tablets each, three times per day. In the first two or three days take five tablets of each every hour until the need for a drug, smoking, or alcohol is over. Then continue three times per day with the same remedies:

Ferrum phosphorica 200X   **Calcarea sulphorica** 30X
Natrum muriaticum 30X   **Calcarea fluorica** 30X

INSOMNIA

SYMPTOMS

Prolonged sleeplessness or sense of tiredness upon awakening, whether justified or not by duration of sleep. Often, fear of death or functional problems (breathing, etc.) during sleep can cause sleep disorders.

SUGGESTED TREATMENT

General: Psychological treatment is important to find the mental reason for these problems.

Acupressure and Acupuncture **
With acupressure, touch back first. Start pressing or Moxa on these stiff points:
   UB 10, UB 17, UB 18, UB 23.
Then:
   CF 15, CV 14, ST 1i, LiV 14, LiV 13, K 16, ST 27, CV 4, K 1.
With acupuncture:
   HT 7, K 3, SP 6, PC 6.
If person is tired, anemic, add:
   UB 20, UB 15, UB 17 and Moxa SP 1.
For anxious, angry, and nervous person, add:
   UB 18, UB 19, GB 12.
For those with digestion disorders, add:
   ST 36, UB 21. Also tap cutaneous needle on extra points sishencong and huatu yiayi from above downward 203 times.

Applied Nutrition
Take the same diet therapy as in Personality Disorders. Avoid heavy meals before sleep.

Aromatherapy **
In case of insomnia take five tablets of brown sugar as a base for the following extracts: **basil** 4%, **camomile** 4%, **lavender** 4%, **rose** 6%.

In case of oversleeping take five tablets of brown sugar as a base for the following extracts: **marjoram** 4%, **pennyroyal** 8%, ·**peppermint** 4%.

Autosuggestion

Before going to sleep use the tape recorder cassette as in Personality Disorders.

Herbs

Western ***

Valeriana: Baths before bed are recommended. Pour one liter (two pints) of boiling water over two handfuls of the dried root of the herb and leave it for twenty-five minutes. Strain liquid and add to bath.

California poppy *(Eschsolizia california):*   In infusion or two to four ml of tincture or two capsules before bedtime.

Jamaican dogwood *(Piscidia erythrina):*   In decoction, can be combined with **hops** *(Humulus lupulus)* and **valeriana.**

Passion flower *(Passiflora):*   A relaxant.

Gelsemium *(Jasmine):*   Decoction or one to two grains of powdered root is an effective sedative for insomnia.

Chinese

Pinellia and Magnolia Combination: For insomnia accompanied by anxiety and emotional instability.

Gentiana Combination: For insomnia due to pain, herpes, hypertension, boils, and carbuncles of vertibular or external auditory canal.

Bamboo and Hoelen Combination *(Wen-tan-tang):*   For restlessness, timidity, palpitations, and dizziness.

Cinnabar Formula *(Zhu-shan-an-shen-wan):*   For insomnia accompanied by forgetfulness, palpitations, and shortness of breath.

Coptis and Gelatin: For insomnia accompanied by restlessness, dry throat, and dry mouth.

Homeopathy **

Coffee: Take 3X to 200X for insomnia following too much coffee drinking.

Camomile: For children, use three.

Nux vomica: For wakefulness in the middle of the night, use 6X to 12X.

Passiflora: For restless sleep, use 3 to 6.

Cocculus: For overtiredness and exhaustion, use 12X.

Hypnotherapy

Hypnotherapy is very useful in solving this problem.

Meditation

Meditation is also very useful to alleviate sleeping problems by relaxing before going to sleep.

Reflexology **

Massage the following points before going to sleep for five to six minutes each:

3, 4, 9, 17, 20, 52.

Schuessler Tissue Salts **

Take the following remedies for the various disorders, ten tablets each twice per day until condition improves.

For insomnia:

Natrum muriaticum 30X   **Kali phosphorica** 12X

For oversleeping:

Natrum sulphorica 12X

For nightmares:

Natrum sulphorica 12X

For awake screaming:

Kali phosphorica 12X

For crying out in sleep:

Calcarea phosphorica 12X

For tiredness in the morning:

Natrum muriaticum 12X   **Calcarea phosphorica** 12X

For those hard to wake in the morning:

Calcarea phosphorica 12X

For constant desire to sleep in the morning:

Natrum muriaticum 30X

For sleep that does not refresh:

Natrum muriaticum 12X

For great drowiness in old persons:

Silica 30X

For jerking of limbs during sleep:

Silica 30X   **Natrum muriaticum** 20X

For anxious dreams:

Natrum muriaticum 12X

For vivid dreams:

Kali sulphorica 12X

APPENDIX

CONTENTS

REJUVENATING DIET

This diet is for 30 days only. It should be prolonged only after being checked by an expert in nutrition.

General Instructions

1. The quantities of the food in the Diet Program depend, (as in any other diet), on your: weight, age, physical condition, daily physical activities, and your sex. For example, for a 35 year-old man, average weight of 170 pounds, average physical activities. He should eat between 1,800 to 2,400 calories per day.

2. Never overeat. When you finish your meal, you should feel that you could eat more (about 25–35%).
3. You can have between 2 to 5 meals per day, it's up to you, but we recommend the 3 meals per day schedule.
4. Drink in-between meals only. Do not eat and drink at the same time. Usually 15 to 30 minutes break would be a good waiting time.
5. Use organically grown products in your meals. That means natural foods without pesticides, preservatives, hormones, antibiotics, artificial colors added to the food, etc.
6. Do not add salt in your diet. If you want salt, then take the 60-40% mixture of sodium and potassium chloride, as a salt substitute.

The Diet

Morning: When you wake up, drink 1 to 2 glasses of mountain spring pure water.

20–30 Minutes Later: One of the following.

1. Any raw fruit—fresh—such as: Apples, oranges, grapefruit, pears, grapes, etc.
2. Or: Any fresh raw vegetables, whole or cut, as a salad, such as carrots, broccoli, cabbage, celery, cucumbers, tomatoes, cauliflower, lettuce, etc.—if it is a salad, you can add: 1 spoon of olive/sunflower oil and fresh lemon juice.
3. Or: Especially if you have any medical problem, it is a good idea to drink after the water one glass of juice from whole wheat-germ, mixed 50% with pure water, in place of the Number 1 and 2 items of the Diet.
4. If you choose Number 2 (salad), you can add to the breakfast, whole rice biscuits, crackers or whole wheat bread.
5. In place of Item Number 4, you can take low fat plain yogurt, together with the salad. But only if you are not allergic to dairy products and not suffering from any allergic disease problem or any rheumatic condition.

Lunch: The meal should be at least 30–50% vegetables.

1. A big, fresh raw salad made with a lot of green and red vegetables such as: Cucumbers, lettuce, cabbage, broccoli, celery, green onions, cauliflower, asparagus, carrot, green peppers, tomatoes, red peppers, squash, and a lot of sprouts.

A a dressing to the salad, take 1 to 2 spoons of vegetable oil, such as olive oil, sunflower oil, sesame seed oil, etc., unheated and natural. Add fresh lemon juice and salt substitute if you so desire.
Also, as a dressing, you can add ground sesame seeds, unsalted and unheated, mixed with water and lemon.
After the salad, you can eat one of the following:

2.   Raw nuts, almonds, or ground sesame seeds, sunflower seeds, etc. (All unsalted and unroasted). (Do not eat peanuts or peanut butter in place of the nuts/almonds).

Or: Whole rice, cooked or steamed, with or without cooked vegetables, together with one of the following: peas, beans, soybeans, lima beans, etc.

Or: Any other cereal boiled or steamed such as: grits, whole wheat, corn, barley, rye, or potatoes. Eat the cereals also with legumes, as in 2(a).

Dinner: The best time for dinner is about sunset, but not more than 2 to 3 hours before going to sleep. The dinner, as the lunch, should consist of at least 30–50% vegetables.

1.   A fresh raw salad, as in the lunch time. Use the same dressings as in the lunch or whole vegetables, eaten separately.
     Eat one of the following, together with the salad:
2.   Whole rice or wild rice as in the lunch, together with legumes.
2(a)   Any other cereal, boiled or steamed, together with the legumes, as in the lunch time.
3.   In place of Number 2, a cup of whole plain yogurt. (The same restrictions apply as in the morning).

Or: Raw unroasted and unsalted almonds or nuts.

4.   Or: In place of Numbers 1, 2 and 3, you can eat fresh raw fruits, as a sole substitute for the dinner.

In-Between Meals: Eat a fresh vegetable or a fresh fruit, or a fruit/vegetable juice mixed with 50% pure water; or drink herb tea with rice biscuits/crackers.

The food supplements (Vitamins and Minerals) should be taken with the meals, and as follows:

• 6 days per week-take the food supplements—one day stop.
• 3 weeks per month-take the food supplements—one week stop.
• Every 5 months-one month stop taking the food supplements. And then continue with any diet as recommended specifically.

Use *exactly the same way as the basic vitamins and minerals formula.*

Food Supplements to the Rejuvenating Diet

Follow the Basic Formula of Vitamins/Minerals (see p. 316) or use the following Vitamins/Minerals:

10,000 I.U.	Beta Carotene
1,000 I.U.	Vitamin E
1,000 mg.	Vitamin C
500 mg.	Bioflavonoids
25 mg.	Thiamine-Vitamin B_1
25 mg.	Riboflavin-Vitamin B_2
50 mg.	Niacin
50 mg.	Niacinamid
20 mg.	Pyridoxine-Vitamin B_6
50 mcg.	Cobalcamine-Vitamin B_{12}
400 Mcg.	Folic Acid
150 mcg.	Biotin
50 mg.	Pantothenic Acid
100 mg.	Choline
50 mg.	Inositol
50 mg.	Paba-Para Aminobenzoic Acid
1,000 mg.	Calcium-Amino Chelated
10 mg.	Iron
500 mg.	Magnesium
10 mg.	Zinc
50 mg.	Potassium
1,200 mg.	Lecithin

BASIC HEALTH DIET

General Instructions

The Basic Health Diet is a diet to keep after you are in balance and after healing of your health problems.

The same instructions as in the Rejuvenating Diet (p. 309) apply in this diet too, with the following additions, which should also be added to any other diet:

- Eat only when you are relaxed and happy. Do not eat while you are angry or under stress. Try to relax first and then eat.
- Chew your food well. Do not swallow large quantities of any food or drink.

- Drink as much as you feel your needs are, but at least a few cups of water per day.
- The best temperature of the drinks or foods should be room temperature (not too hot or too cold).
- As this diet is for a long time, many combinations are offered. But you still have to eat according to your basic needs. In this diet, your body and weight should be maintained, as this is not a weight gain or loss program.

Morning:
1.   One cup of pure water;
2.   Or one cup of water and one cup of vegetable/fruit juice mixed with 50% water. (Two glasses).

15–30 Minutes Later (Breakfast):
1.   Fresh salad with a lot of green vegetables. As a dressing to the salad: 1 to 2 spoons of vegetable oil, fresh lemon slice and salt substitute if so desired.
2.   Whole wheat bread, or whole rice biscuits or crackers.
3.   In place of Number 2—One boiled egg. (Maximum 3 to 4 eggs per week). Or: Low fat yogurt and low fat cottage cheese.
4.   Or: In place of Numbers 1, 2, 3 and 4—any fresh raw fruits.
5.   Or: 1–2 sandwiches of whole wheat bread, with vegetables and avocado, or vegetables and ground whole sesame seeds with lemon and salt substitute, or tofu cheese and vegetables.
N.B. Do not eat bread and dairy products or bread and meat/poultry products at the same time.

Lunch:
1.   Salad with a lot of fresh green vegetables with the same dressing as in the morning.
Or: In place of the salad, or in addition to the salad, a vegetable soup, made with fresh vegetables of all kinds.
Eat one of the following together with the above:
2.   Whole cereal, such as whole rice, whole wheat, corn, or potatoes, boiled/steamed with legumes such as: beans, soy beans, lima beans, peas, etc.
Or: In place of Number 2—Nuts or almonds or whole sesame seeds (ground), unsalted and unroasted.
Or: Sea-Fish of any kind, boiled, steamed, broiled or baked, but not fried.
Or: If you want meat, then eat naturally grown poultry with no hormones, antibiotics, etc., boiled, steamed, broiled or baked, but not fried.

FOOD SUPPLEMENTS

Use Master Vitamin and Mineral Formula (p. 316). Also, the following vitamins and minerals in addition to the master formula:

Vitamin A—as Beta Carotene	10,000 I.U.
Vitamin E	100 I.U.
Vitamin K	50 mg.
Vitamin D	200 I.U.
Vitamin C	500 mg.
Bioflavonoids	250 mg.
Folic Acid	400 mcg.
Vitamin B_1 (Thiamine)	50 mg.
Vitamin B_2 (Riboflavin)	50 mg.
Niacin	50 mg.
Niacinamid	50 mg.
Vitamin B_6 (Pyridoxine)	50 mg.
Vitamin B_{12} (Cobalcamine)	50 mcg.
Biotin	50 mcg.
Pantothenic Acid	50 mg.
Choline	50 mg.
Inositol	50 mg.
Paba-Para Aminobenzoic Acid	50 mg.

Minerals

Calcium	500 mg.
Iron	10 mg.
Magnesium	250 mg.
Zinc	5 mg.
Manganese	25 mg.
Potassium	20 mg.
Chromium	20 mg.

Digestive Aids

Ox Bile	50 mg.
Bromelain	25 mg.
Pancrelipase	30 mg.
Papain	30 mg.
Betaine (Hydrochloric Acid)	30 mg.
Lecithin	1,200 mg.

Or: In place of 2, 2(a), 2(b), and 2(c)—Dairy products such as plain yogurt and low fat cottage cheese, farmer cheese or ricotta cheese.

3.   A few slices of whole wheat bread with the salad in place of Number 2.

Dinner: The dinner can be with the same products as in the lunch. You can substitute also a dinner with the choices of the breakfast, or you can have fresh fruit, raw or cooked.

As a dessert to the lunch and dinner you can eat fresh raw/cooked fruits, or dried fruits: but at least 30 minutes or more after each meal. NOT IMMEDIATELY AFTER THE MAIN MEAL.

As a food supplement to this diet (Vitamins and Minerals) take the Master Formula (Basic Formula of Vitamins and Minerals).

GLUTEN-FREE DIET

General Instructions

In this diet, you should *exclude* all sources of gluten, such as, wheat, rye, oats, and barley, in any foods. Also avoid dried peas, cucumbers, cabbage, turnips, beans, prunes, plums and their juices. Also avoid ale, beer of any kind, instant coffee, malted milk, Postum products containing cereals.

Recommended Foods

Beverages: Pure spring water, fruit/vegetable raw juice mixed with 50% water, herb tea, milk, and yogurt (plain).
Breads: Breads made with: Corn meal, potato, rice, or special Gluten-Free wheat.
Cereals: Rice, grits, and corn.
Dairy Products: Milk, cottage cheese, and yogurt.
Eggs: 2 to 4 eggs per week.
Oils: Corn oil, cottonseed oil, olive oil, sesame, soybean and sunflower oil.
Fruits: All cooked and their juices. Avoid initially all seeds and skin of the fruits. Fresh fruits as tolerated.
Meat: Sea-Fish, poultry—baked, broiled or boiled.
Vegetables: As the fruits, cooked, or as a salad with a lot of green and red raw vegetables.
Sweets: Honey, molasses, brown sugar. Do not over-eat sweets.

MASTER VITAMIN AND MINERAL FORMULA

Vitamins		*Minerals (Amino Chelated Basis)*	
Beta Carotene	10,000 I.U.	Calcium	500 mg.
as Vitamin A		Iodine	150 mcg.
Vitamin D	400 I.U.	Iron	15 mg.
Vitamin E	200 I.U.	Magnesium	250 mg.
Vitamin K	50 mcg.	Copper	2 mg.
Vitamin C	200 mg.	Zinc	15 mg.
Bioflavonoids	100 mg.	Manganese	15 mg.
Rutin	25 mg.	Potassium	50 mg.
Hesperidin	25 mg.	Chromium	50 mcg.
Folic Acid	400 mcg.	Selenium	20 mcg.
Vitamin B$_1$		*Digestive*	
(Thiamine)	10 mg.	*Aids*	
Vitamin B$_2$		Iron Ox Bile	10 mg.
(Riboflavin)	10 mg.	Bromelain	10 mg.
Niacin	20 mg.	Pancrelipaze	15 mg.
Niacinamid	20 mg.	Papain	10 mg.
Vitamin B$_6$		Betain HCI	10 mg.
(Pyridoxine)	10 mg.		
Vitamin B$_{12}$		Lecithin	600 mg.
(Cobalamine)	30 mcg.		
Biotin	150 mcg.		
Pantothenic Acid	50 mg.		
Choline	50 mg.		
Inositol	50 mg.		
Para Aminobenzoic			
Acid (Paba)	30 mg.		

All vitamins and minerals should be taken as follows: 6 days per week-take continuously; one day-stop taking; then 3 weeks per month—take continuously; one week-stop taking; then 5 months take continuously; one month—stop taking—and then continue with the food supplements.

THE MACROBIOTIC DIET

The objective in this way of eating is to maintain a good balance of yin and yang in all levels of life, including your diet. According to George Ohsawa, there are ten basic diets in the macrobiotic diet. They are as follows:

Diet No.	Cereals	Fresh Vegetables	Soup	Animal Meat & Fish	Fruists	Sweet Desert	Beverage
7	100%						As little
6	90	10%					as you feel
5	80	20					you need.
4	70	20	10%				
3	60	30	10				
2	50	30	10	10%			
1	40	30	10	20			
−1	30	30	10	20	10%		
−2	20	30	10	25	10	5%	
−3	10	30	10	30	15	5	

Consult your nutritionist as to what diet number you should start at. As a general rule: the more severe the disease/problem the higher in number of diet you should start at.

The macrobiotic approach to organically grown foods is very similar to the vegetarian way of natural foods. As your health improves you can add foods to your diet according to the table of diets.

ORTHOMOLECULAR THERAPY (MEGA VITAMIN THERAPY)

The administration of large doses of vitamins and minerals was first introduced in 1968 by the American scientist, Professor Linus Pauling, 1945 Nobel prize winner in chemistry for the treatment of psychiatric disorders such as schizophrenia.

Shortly after 1968, many physicians found out that most of the diseases and maladies of the human body could be treated and cured by proper nutrition, which includes: natural foods and large doses of vitamins and minerals. In order to ensure the optimum nutrients in the body, the quantities of vitamins and minerals were much larger than the R.D.A. Some of the vitamins such as vitamin C, or the B vitamins group, were given a thousand times more than the R.D.A., with excellent results.

Today, there are two approaches to orthomolecular therapy:

1. The administration of maximum levels of vitamins and minerals, for a short time and under the supervision of a trained physician/ nutritionist in the field of orthomolecular therapy.

2. Lower quantities of vitamins and minerals (but still much higher than the R.D.A. recommendations) for a longer period of time. This should be done under the supervision of a trained physician/nutritionist.

In this manual we recommend the first approach for each disease mainly to illustrate the quantities of vitamins and minerals that can be taken for each problem. Both approaches have their advantages and disadvantages. Consult your physician/nutritionist for your optimum levels of vitamins and minerals recommended for your personal needs, as the optimum needs and level of nutrients may vary from person to person.

We also recommend, in any case of taking large doses of vitamins and minerals, to rest from taking the mega doses as follows: one day per week, one week per month, and one month per six months. This will ensure that you do not overdose with the added nutrients.

Juice Fasting

If your physical condition permits, it is very important to commence any diet in this manual with a juice fasting for a period of three to six days. Check with your physician/nutritionist for recommendations on how long you should use this fast.

The materials you will need daily in the juice fasting:
1. 1 to 2 pounds of fresh lemons (organically grown).
2. 2 to 4 pounds of fresh whole beets, including root and top.
3. ½ to 1 gallon of distilled water.
4. Dietary fiber tablets (14–18 tablets daily).
5. If your health permits, 1 to 2 teaspoons of pure honey daily.
6. One tablet of multi-vitamins and minerals.

First Day of Fasting

Start with a cup of pure distilled water. Then take a cup of fresh-squeezed lemon juice mixed with two parts of water and a cup of juice made of beets (tops and roots) with two parts of water (2 to 3 cups in the morning).

You can drink during the first day, as much as you want from these juices, but at least six cups daily minimum. Two cups of pure distilled water and the rest fresh juices mixed with water.

Take 7–9 tablets of dietary fiber and 1 tablet of multi-vitamins and minerals each morning with the juice. In the afternoon take only the dietary fiber (7–9 tablets) with the juices. It is recommended to help your first day of fasting with a colon enema. Once per day for the first three days. It is important to take breathing therapy and mental affirmations as part of the fasting.

Second Day

The same as the first day. But today increase the beet juice mixed with water. Two cups per day.

If you feel weak or too tired take one to two teaspoons of pure honey if your condition permits. Also take the dietary fiber tablets and multi-vitamins and minerals as you did on the first day.

Third Day

The third day is the same as the second day, only increase the quantity of beets to three cups per day mixed with two parts of water.

Fourth, Fifth and Sixth Day of Fasting

These next three days of fasting are usually much easier on the body. The water and juices should be the same as the first day of fasting. You can discontinue with the multi-vitamin and mineral tablet and the beet juice. In place of beet juice you can take carrot juice mixed with two parts of water and other vegetable juices such as cucumber, tomatoes, wheat sprouts or any other sprout juices mixed with two parts water. Also discontinue with the enema. Continue with the breathing exercises and the mental affirmations.

When juice fasting is over, start gradually with the rejuvenating diet or other diets recommended in this manual. The first day after the fast, eat one-third of the food quantitites only. The second day you may consume two-thirds of the food quantitites. On the third day eat 100% of the full diet.

HYPNOTHERAPY AND SELF HYPNOSIS

Hypnotherapy is the help of emotional, mental and physical problems when the patient is in a state of hypnosis.

According to Gil Boyne, certified hypnotherapist and founder, director and teacher of the largest training institute for hypnotherapists and hypnotism in U.S.A., H.T.I.:

The state of hypnosis is a natural state of mind with special identifying characteristics:

1. An extraordinary quality of relaxation.
2. An emotionalized desire to satisfy the suggested behavior. The person feels like doing what the hypnotherapist suggests provided that what is suggested does not generate conflict with his belief system.
3. The organization becomes self-regulating, it produced normalization of the nervous systems (voluntary and involuntary systems).
4. Heightened and selective sensitivity to stimuli being received by the five senses and four basic perceptions.
5. Immediate softening of psychic defenses.

Hypnosis can be induced either by a hypnotherapist or by yourself. For the treatment of the various problems in this manual it is recommended to start the hypnosis state with the instructions of a certified hypnotherapist* then continue with self-hypnosis. Actually, any disease/problem can be cured or helped with hypnosis as primary or secondary therapy.

YOGA AND OTHER BREATHING THERAPIES

The various breathing therapies are well known among the people who practice: Yoga, Hinduism, Confucianism, Taoism, Zen Buddhism, Shintoism. In recent years, a breathing therapy technique was developed by Mr. Leonard Orr, in Sierraville, California, called "Rebirthing."

The main purpose of most of the breathing exercises is: To regulate and harmonize various functions of the body, mind and *Ki. (*Ki is the life energy of our body). Also, each part of our body has a Ki (life energy) of its own.

This harmony can be achieved by breathing in a very specific way, according to the various exercises.

Breathing Exercise Precaution

Usually, it is a good idea to practice the breathing therapy exercises under the supervision of a trained Yoga teacher, Rebirther, or other breathing instructors. This is especially important to the beginner, who without being watched during the exercise may commence his or her practice by breathing too hard, too deep or too quick. And as a result,

---

*Hypnotherapist is an occupational title in the U.S.A. and a respected profession by itself (the same as psychologist, physician or electrician). The hypnotherapist helps the patient by means of hypnosis only. Other therapists may use hypnosis as a part of their professional services.

he or she may feel sick, feel bad, nauseated, dizzy, have pain, strong heart beat, fast pulse, stiffness of the limbs, abnormal feelings on the skin, etc.

Therefore, breathing therapy must be performed in a proper manner. It must be started easy, not too forceful or too tense. The amount of air you inhale while breathing, the speed of the breathing and the force of breathing should be a matter of your sound judgment. But in any case, if you feel any of the above-mentioned symptoms, stop the exercise and continue with a professional teacher.

Basic Postures For Breathing Therapy

When practicing the various breathing therapies, you should maintain a proper posture. The three basic postures are:

1. The erect position—standing position;
2. The sitting position—either on a chair or on the floor;
3. Lateral position—lying on the floor, or floating in a tank of water or swimming pool.

Exercise Number 1: Inhale and exhale through the nose for 10 times, normally. Then breathe in (inhale) deeply. Hold your breath for the count of 3 (approximately 3 seconds). Then exhale all the air from your lungs (through the nose) as much as you can. Count to 3 and then repeat it by inhaling. Do this breathing exercise 5 times continuously, every day for one week. But each day add one breathing exercise until you reach 10 exercises of breathing per day. Then continue with the 10 breathing exercises every day.

Exercise Number 2: While sitting in a comfortable chair: Inhale through your nose for the count of 4 (approximately 4 seconds). Hold your breath for the count of 2. Then exhale for the count of 4. Now, hold your breath for the count of 2. Then repeat this exercise by inhaling again for the count of 4. Holding the air in your lungs for the count of 2, exhale for the count of 4 and stop breathing to the count of 2. Repeat this exercise 5 times per day after the first one.

Exercise Number 3: While lying on the floor, breathe deeply in and out continuously. In this exercise, you connect the inhale to the exhale without stopping the breathing, in a continuous rhythm of breathing. You can start with 5 connected breathings per day for a week, then increase slowly the number of exercises for 15 to 20 minutes, and with experience, it can be prolonged to one hour every other day. (This is the Rebirthing Technique) It should be practiced with another person trained in Rebirthing supervising you, as you practice, because this practice brings out many reactions, both emotionally and physically.

CHINESE HERBAL PRESCRIPTIONS

Most of the basic formulas used in Chinese herbal medicine come from Chang Chung-ching's classics: *Treatise on Febrile Diseases* and *Summaries of Household Remedies*. Over the two thousand years of use, however, doctors and patients have altered and amended formulas and made up new ones.

Areca Seed Combination (Chiu-pin-wu-fu-tang)

Objectives: beriberi, fatigue, weak legs, gasping, edema, swollen feeling under the heart, tendon pain, cardiac neurosis—difficult breathing, palpitation, insomnia, heart pain, nervousness, cold arms and legs, cold sweat, headache, diarrhea, and general body pain
Composition:

3.0g cinnamon twigs
3.0g Mandarin orange peel
4.0g betel seeds (areca)

3.0g ginger rhizome
3.0g magnolia bark
3.0g China root (hoelen)

Atractylodes Combination (Yueh-pi-chia-chu-tang)

Objectives: dry throat, edema or severe bullae, and occasional excessive secretion
Indications: nephritis, nephrosis, beriberi, arthritis, rheumatism, dermatitis, eczema, dacryocystitis, colitis, ocular eczema, keratitis, glaucoma, and nocturia
Composition:

6.0g ma-huang
8.0g gypsum
3.0g ginger rhizome
3.0g jujube fruit

2.0g licorice root
4.0g *paichu* (white atractylodes rhizome)

Atractylodes and Hoelen Combination (Ling-kuei-chu-kan-tang)

Objectives: dizziness, severe palpitation, flushing, headache, facial redness, anemia, increased urinary frequency but decreased volume, and dry lips.
Indications: tuberculosis, irregular pulse, cardiac neurosis, valvular

disease, hypertension, hypotension, weakness, hysteria, conjunctivitis, ocular eczema or bleeding, corneal inflammation, dacryocystitis, cataract, rhinitis, suppuration, and Ménière's syndrome
Composition:

6.0g China root (hoelen)
4.0g cinnamon twigs
2.0g licorice root

3.0g *paichu* (white atractylodes rhizome)

Bupleurum and Cinnamon Combination (Chai-hu-kuei-chih-tang)

Objectives: sweating, slight fever, chills, distressed heart, headache, joint and occasional stomach pain, nausea, and severe abdominal pain with loss of appetite
Indications: cold pleurisy, gastric spasm or ulcer, cholelithiasis, cholecystitis, appendicitis, nephritis, nephrosis, pyelonephritis, petechiae, and intercostal neuralgia
Composition:

5.0g hare's ear root (bupleurum)
2.0g skullcap root (scute)
2.5g peony root
1.0g ginger rhizome
4.0g pinellia rhizome

2.0g ginseng root
2.5g cinnamon twigs
2.0g jujube fruit
1.5g licorice root

Bupleurum, Cinnamon, and Ginger Combination (Chai-hu-kuei-chih-kan-chiang-tang)

Objectives: delicate health, moderate fever, head and night sweats, distressed chest, malaise, loss of appetite, periumbilical spasms, a tendency towards weakness, insomnia, soft stools, decreased urine, dry mouth, and dry cough
Indications: cold, tuberculosis, pleurisy, pulse irregularities, cardiac disorders, endocarditis, valvular disease, cardiac asthma, hepatitis, cholecystitis, pancreatitis, peritonitis, weakness, nephritis, neophrosis, anemia, goiter, insomnia, hysteria, menopausal problems, and allergies
Composition:

6.0g hare's ear root (bupleurum)
3.0g cinnamon twigs
2.0g ginger rhizome
3.0g snake gourd root (trichosanthes)

3.0g skullcap root (scute)
3.0g oyster shell
2.0g licorice root

Bupleurum and Dragon Bone Combination (Chai-hu-chia-lung-ku-mu-li-tang)

Objectives: mental instability with a tendency to be frightened, cardiac hyperfunction, chest distress, vertigo, flushing, insomnia, occasional periumbilical palpitation, heart distress with constipation, and decreased urine

Indications: cardiac distress, valvular disease, cardiac asthma, angina pectoris, arteriosclerosis, hypertension, nephritis, nephrosis, kidney atrophy, impotence, sexual neurasthenia, goiter, insomnia, noctiphobia, menopausal disorders, and glaucoma

Composition:

5.0g hare's ear root (bupleurum)
4.0g pinellia rhizome
2.5g skullcap root (scute)
2.5g ginger rhizome
2.5g jujube fruit
2.5g ginseng root

3.0g cinnamon twigs
2.5g oyster shell
3.0g China root (hoelen)
1.0g rhubarb rhizome
2.5 dragon bone

Bupleurum and Schizonepeta Formula (Shih-wei-pai-tu-san)

Objectives: chronic symptoms with slight secretion

Indications: furuncles, anthrax, lymphadenitis, anal ulcers, eczema, hives, infected suppurative crusts, warts, facial boils, mastitis, styes, blepharitis, otitis externa or media, and rhinitis

Composition:

3.0g hare's ear root (bupleurum)
3.0g balloon flower root (platy-codon)
1.0g ginger rhizome
3.0g China root (hoelen)
2.0g siler root
2.0g angelica root *(tang-kuei)*

1.0g *chinchieh* herb (schizone-peta)
1.0g licorice root
3.0g Szechuan lovage rhizome (cnidium)
1.0g Pseudocerasi bark (cherry bark)

Bupleurum and Scute Combination (Chai-hsien-tang)

Objective: chest or back pain or chest fluid, distressed chest or stomach, and occasional cough

Indications: bronchial dilation, bronchitis, pleurisy, and intercostal neuralgia

Composition:

5.0g hare's ear root (bupleurum)
3.0g skullcap root (scute)
3.0g ginger rhizome
3.0g jujube fruit
2.0g ginseng root
1.5g licorice root

5.0g pinellia rhizome
3.0g snake gourd fruit and seeds (trichosanthes)
1.5g goldenthread rhizome (coptis)

Capillaris Combination (Yin-chen-hao-tang)

Objectives: dry throat, chest distress with constipation—suitable for patients with jaundice
Indications: hepatitis, nephritis, nephrosis, hives, and stomatitis
Composition:

1.0g capillary artemisia herb
2.0g gardenia fruit

1.0g rhubarb rhizome

Cardamon and Fennel Formula (An-chung-san)

Objectives: chills and psychoneurosis with stomach pain or heart distress
Indications: gastritis, prolapsed and weak stomach, and gastric and duodenal ulcers
Composition:

4.0g cinnamon twigs
3.0g corydalis rhizome
3.0g oyster shell
1.5g fennel fruit

0.5g lesser galangal rhizome
0.5g licorice root
1.0g cardamon seeds

Cimicifuga Combination (I-tzu-tang)

Objectives: constipation with minor bleeding, severe local pain
Indications: hemorrhoids, prolapsed rectum, and vaginal itching
Composition:

1.0g rhubarb rhizome
6.0g Chinese angelica root *(tang-kuei)*
3.0g skullcap root (scute)

2.0g licorice root
5.0g hare's ear root (bupleurum)
1.5g bugbane rhizome (cimicifuga)

Cinnamon Combination (Kuei-chih-tang)

Objectives: chills, fever, headache, weak pulse, and sweating. It is good for those of delicate health.

Indications: colds, neuralgia, headache, rheumatism, abdominal pain, neurasthenia, impotence, and emissions
Composition:

4.0g cinnamon twigs	4.0g ginger rhizome
4.0g jujube fruit	2.0g licorice root
4.0g peony root	

Cinnamon, Atractylodes, and Aconite Combination (Kuei-chih-chia-chu-fu-tang)

Objectives: chilled and numb feeling with pain or difficulty moving
Indications: neuralgia, rheumatism, stiff shoulders in persons over fifty, and paralysis on one side
Composition:

4.0g cinnamon twigs	2.0g licorice root
4.0g peony root	4.0g *paichu* (white atractylodes
4.0g ginger rhizome	rhizome)
4.0g jujube fruit	1.0g mugwort root (aconite)

Cinnamon, Hoelen, and Atractylodes Combination (Kuei-chih-chia-ling-chu-tang)

Objectives: same as for Cinnamon Combination along with palpitation and difficult urination
Indications: heart failure, ear and digestive disorders, beriberi, ocular neuralgia, lower back pain, rheumatism, and arthritis
Composition:

4.0g cinnamon twigs	5.0g *paichu* (white atractylodes
3.0g peony root	rhizome)
3.0g ginger rhizome	3.0g jujube fruit
5.0g China root (hoelen)	1.5g licorice root

Cinnamon and Dragon Bone Combination (Kuei-chih-chia-lung-ku-mu-li-tang)

Objectives: psychoneurosis with headache, flushing, tinnitus, tendency to fatigue, spasms at the umbilicus, and polyuria
Indications: sexual weakness, nocturia, night fears, falling hair, and penile atrophy
Composition:

4.0g cinnamon twigs	4.0g ginger rhizome
4.0g peony root	4.0g jujube fruit

2.0g licorice root
3.0g dragon bone

3.0g oyster shell

Cinnamon and Hoelen Formula (Kuei-chih-fu-ling-wan)

Objectives: flushing, headache, stiff shoulders, dizziness with chills, and pain in the lower abdomen
Indications: difficult menstruation, endometritis, swelling of uterine muscles, oophoritis, salpingitis, menopausal disorders, sterility, orchitis, appendicitis, hepatitis, arthritis, sciatic neuralgia, chilblains, hemorrhoids, eczema, hives, facial vesicles, maculae, styes, ocular eczema, and iritis
Composition:

4.0g cinnamon twigs
4.0g peony root
4.0g China root (hoelen)

4.0g tree peony bark
4.0g peach seeds (persica)

Cinnamon and Peony Combination (Kuei-chih-chia-shao-yao-tang)

Objectives: abdominal distress with frequent pain—usually periumbilical or in lower abdomen; diarrhea with muddy and mucous stools while suffering from a cold; abdominal pain; intestinal catarrh; peritonitis with nodules; acute or chronic appendicitis—unsuitable for peritonitis with fluid and exudate
Indications: delicate health, diarrhea from weakness, abdominal distention and pain
Composition:

4.0g cinnamon twigs
6.0g peony root
4.0g ginger rhizome

2.0g licorice root
4.0g jujube fruit

Cnidium and Rhubarb Formula (Chiung-huang-san)

Objectives: moderate purgative for habitual constipation in the elderly or persons with delicate health
Indications: constipation, headache, and heavy head
Composition:

1.1g Chinese lovage rhizome (cnidium)

1.0g rhubarb rhizome

Coix Combination (I-yi-jen-tang)

Objectives: general pain in the muscles and joints, numbness, pain in the feet and hands, and stiffness occasionally associated with swelling or fever. Also for stiff shoulders caused by extravasated blood or cold.
Indications: neuralgia, rheumatism, and arthritis
Composition:

8.0g Job's tears seeds (coix)
4.0g Chinese angelica root *(tang-kuei)*
3.0g cinnamon twigs
2.0g licorice

4.0g ma-huang herb
4.0g *paichu* (white atractylodes rhizome)
3.0g peony root

Coptis and Rhubarb Combination (San-huang-hsieh-hsin-tang)

Objectives: flushing, mental instability, stomach distress with severe constipation, and an occasional tendency towards hyperemia or hemorrhaging
Indications: hemoptysis, hemorrhoidal bleeding, chronic constipation, hypertension, arteriosclerosis, excessive or vicarious menstruation, conjunctivitis, cataract, and eye hemorrhage
Composition:

1.0 g goldenthread rhizome (coptis)

1.0g skullcap root (scute)
1.0g rhubarb rhizome

Coptis and Scute Combination (Huang-lien-chieh-tu-tang)

Objectives: flushing, distressed stomach or soft stools with constipation, and ocular hyperemia
Indications: tuberculosis, stomatitis, gastritis, hemoptysis, intestinal, uterine or hemorrhoidal bleeding, hepatitis, hypertension, weakness, insomnia, and bleeding eyelids
Composition:

3.0g goldenthread root (coptis)
2.0g skullcap root (scute)

2.0g phellodendron bark
1.0g gardenia fruit

Cyperus and Perilla Formula (Hsiang-su-san)

Objectives: psychoneurosis, headache, melancholia, and loss of appetite

Indications: cold, headache, migraine, hives, hysteria, menopausal disorders, and difficult menstruation
Composition:

4.0g nutgrass rhizome (cyperus)
1.0g perilla leaf
2.5g citrus peel

3.0g ginger rhizome
1.0g licorice root

Dragon Bone and Oyster Shell Combination (Lung-ku-mu-li-tang)

Objectives: a sedative for palpitation and an astringent for night sweats
Indications: hypersecretion of gastric acid, neuralgia, chronic gastritis, and difficult urination
Composition:

1.0 g dragon bone
0.1g gum arabic

1.0g oyster shell

Eriocheir and Viper Formulas (Po-chou-san)

Objectives: subacute or chronic dermatosis with suppuration
Indications: bone ulcers, nodules, crusts, anal ulcers, hemorrhoids, dermatosis with suppuration, mastitis, dacryocystitis, otitis media, and gum abscess
Composition:

1.0g eriocheir
1.0g viper

1.0g deer horn

Ginseng and Astragalus Combination (Pu-chung-i-chi-tang)

Objectives: decreased stomach and intestinal function, fatigue, severe loss of appetite; and occasional headache, chills, night sweats, and slow bleeding
Indications: tuberculosis; pleurisy; weak digestion; prolapsed stomach, rectum, or uterus; peritonitis; hypotension; involuntary emission; impotence; anemia; hysteria; insomnia; osseous ulcers; endometritis; and increased sweating
Composition:

4.0g ginseng root
3.0g Chinese angelica
1.5g licorice root

4.0g *paichu* (white atractylodes rhizome)
2.0g Mandarin orange peel

1.0g hare's ear root (bupleurum)
0.5g bugbane rhizome (cimicifuga)

4.0g Chinese milk vetch root (astragalus)
0.5g ginger rhizome

Ginseng and Ginger Combination (Jen-sheng-tang)

Objectives: weak digestion, pale face, wet tongue, polyuria with low specific gravity, cold arms and legs, oversecretion of saliva, tendency towards diarrhea, occasional vomiting, dizziness, headache, gastric pain, irregular pulse, and abdominal distention
Indications: acute or chronic gastritis, weak digestion, stomach dilation, nausea, pale face from renal atrophy, edema, polyuria, tendency towards diarrhea, intoxication in children
Composition:

3.0g ginseng root
3.0g *paichu* rhizome (white atractylodes)

2.0-3.0g ginger rhizome
3.0g licorice root

Ginseng and Gypsum Combination (Pai-hu-chia-jen-sheng-tang)

Objectives: severe thirst with a constant desire to drink or a strong feverish sensation
Indications: diabetes mellitus, pneumonia, measles, sunstroke, and cold
Composition:

5.0g anemarrhena rhizome
15.0g gypsum
10.0g rice

2.0g licorice root
3.0g ginseng root

Ginseng Nutritive Combination (Jen-sheng-yang-yung-tang)

Objectives: slender physique with chronic fever, chills, chronic cough, fatigue, loss of appetite, mental instability, night sweats, and tendency towards constipation
Indications: tuberculosis, pleurisy, penile atrophy after sickness, postpartum weakness and constipation
Composition:

3.0g ginseng root
2.5g Chinese milk vetch root (astragalus)
4.0g white *paichu* rhizome (atractylodes)

4.0g China root (hoelen)
4.0g Chinese angelica root *(tang-kuei)*
2.5g cinnamon twigs
4.0g Chinese foxglove root and

rhizome (rehmannia)
4.0g peony root
2.5g citrus peel
2.0g Chinese milkwort root (po-
lygala)

1.5g schizandra fruit
1.5g licorice root

Ginseng and Tang-kuei Formula (Jen-sheng-tang-shao-san)

Objectives: cold arms and legs, psychoneurosis, dry skin, tired eyes, headache, dizziness, tinnitus, menopausal complaints, weakness, stiff shoulders, and neuroasthenia
Indications: chronic nephritis, kidney disease during pregnancy, and lower back pain
Composition:

3.0g Chinese angelica root *(tang-kuei)*
2.5g Chinese lovage rhizome (cnidium)
3.0g peony root
3.0g water plantain rhizome (alisma)

1.5g cinnamon twigs
3.0g *paichu* rhizome (white atractylodes rhizome)
3.0g China root (hoelen)
3.0g ginseng root
1.0g licorice root

Hoelen Combination (Fu-ling-yin)

Objectives: distressed stomach with swollen feeling, hypersecretion of gastric fluid, nausea, loss of appetite, and decreased urine
Indications: prolapsed stomach, weak digestion, gastric disorders, and stomach dilation
Composition:

5.0g China root (hoelen)
4.0g *paichu* rhizome (white atractylodes rhizome)
3.0g ginseng root

3.0g ginger rhizome
1.5g immature citrus peel
3.0g Mandarin orange peel

Hoelen Five Herb Formula (Wu-ling-san)

Objectives: excessive dry throat, decreased urinary volume, heavy head, head sweats, nausea, vomiting—occasionally associated with swelling
Indications: watery dysentery, acute gastroenteric catarrh, vomiting, drunkenness, sunstroke, hepatitis, cirrhosis of the liver, jaundice, cholelithiasis, cholecystitis, peritonitis, valvular diseases, nephritis, ne-

phrosis, pyelonephritis, cystitis, urethritis, diabetes mellitus, trigeminal neuralgia, dacryocystitis, and night blindness
Composition:

3.0g cinnamon twigs
4.5g *paichu* (white atractylodes rhizome)
4.5g grifola (polyporus)

6.5g China root (hoelen)
6.0g water plantain rhizome (alisma)

Hoelen and Ginger Combination (Ling-chiang-chu-kan-tang)

Objectives: cold waist and feet, pain, fatigue, polyuria, and cold sweat or watery secretions
Indications: lower back pain, cold waist and feet, sciatic neuralgia, leukorrhea, urinary retention, nocturia in children, eczema, and ulcers
Composition:

6.0g China root (hoelen)
3.0g ginger rhizome
3.0g *paichu* (white atractylodes rhizome)

2.0g licorice root

Lithospermum Ointment (Tzu-yun-kao)

Objectives: to promote granulation of tissue and to prevent dermal erosion
Indications: burns, chilblain, anal ulcers, hemorrhoids, facial vesicles, infected crusts, and athlete's foot
Composition:

100.0g Chinese angelica root
(tang-kuei)
100.0g Asiatic groomwell root
(lithospermum)

1000.0g flax oil
25.0g lard
380.0g beeswax

Magnolia and Ginger Formula (Ping-wei-san)

Objectives: stomach pain with indigestion, abdominal discomfort, diarrhea, loss of appetite, and gas after meals; relief follows diarrhea
Indications: stomatitis, gastritis, weak digestion, gastric dilation, and diarrhea
Composition:

3.0g magnolia bark
4.0g *tsangchu* (atractylodes rhizome)
3.0g Mandarin orange peel

1.0g ginger rhizome
1.0g licorice root
2.0g jujube fruit

Ma-huang Combination (Ma-huang-tang)

Objectives: severe fever or chills with pain, rheumatoid discomfort, stuffy nose in infants, and acute dermal suppuration
Indications: influenza, bronchitis, bronchial asthma, pneumonia, rhinitis, acute arthritis, muscular rheumatism, stuffy nose, and acute dermatosis in infancy with suppuration
Composition:

5.0g ma-huang herb	1.5g licorice root
4.0g cinnamon twigs	5.0g apricot seeds

Ma-huang and Apricot Seed Combination (Ma-hsing-kan-shih-tang)

Objectives: severe cough with dry throat, head sweating, and stridor
Indications: bronchitis, whooping cough, bronchial and childhood asthma, and pneumonia
Composition:

4.0g ma-huang herb	10.0g gypsum
2.0g licorice root	4.0g apricot seeds

Ma-huang and Asarum Combination (Ma-huang-hsi-hsin-fu-tzu-tang)

Objectives: moderate fever, fatigue, headache, chills and body pain
Indications: delicate health, colds in the elderly, bronchitis, acute fever, asthma, suppuration, and cough from poor health
Composition:

4.0g ma-huang herb (ephedra)	1.0g wolfsbane root (aconite)
3.0g wild ginger herb (asarum)	

Ma-huang and Coix Combination (Ma-hsing-i-kan-tang)

Objectives: acute or chronic arthritis and muscular pain
Indications: joint and muscular rheumatism, warts, athlete's foot, chronic nephritis, and nephritis in pregnancy
Composition:

4.0g ma-huang herb	10.0g Job's tears seeds (coix)
3.0g apricot seeds	2.0g licorice root

Ma-huang and Magnolia Combination (Shen-mi-tang)

Objectives: chronic cough with small volume of sputum
Indications: bronchial asthma
Composition:

5.0g ma-huang herb
4.0g apricot seeds
2.0g licorice root
1.5g perilla leaves

2.5g citrus peel
3.0g magnolia bark
2.0g bupleurum root

Major Bupleurum Combination (Ta-chai-hu-tang)

Objectives: heart distress, pain and pressure in the chest or around the abdomen, severe constipation, occasional tinnitus aurium, stiff shoulders, and loss of appetite
Indications: bronchial asthma, gastritis, gastric or duodenal ulcer, chronic dysentery, habitual constipation, hepatitis, cholelithiasis, cholecystitis, hypertension, arteriosclerosis, insomnia, involuntary emission, impotence, sexual neurasthenia, obesity, diabetes mellitus, intercostal neuralgia, furunculosis, anthrax, bleeding hemorrhoids, rectocele, eczema, hives, facial vesicles, keratitis, iritis, tinnitus aurium, otitis media, suppuration, tonsillitis, and alveolar pyorrhea
Composition:

6.0g hare's ear root (bupleurum)
3.0g skullcap root (scute)
4.0g pinellia rhizome
3.0g peony root

2.0g immature citrus peel
1.0-2.0g rhubarb rhizome
3.0g jujube fruit
4.0g ginger rhizome

Minor Blue Dragon Combination (Hsiao-ching-lung-tang)

Objectives: decreased urinary volume after acute fever, chest distress, sensation of fluid in the stomach, coughing of watery sputum with stridor or rhinitis with copious nasal drainage, and opthalmological disorders with tearing
Indications: bronchitis, rhinitis, bronchial asthma, whooping cough, bronchial enlargement, pleurisy, nephritis, nephrosis, arthritis, conjunctivitis, ocular eczema, keratitis, and dacryocystitis
Composition:

3.0g ma-huang herb
3.0g peony root
3.0g ginger rhizome
3.0g licorice root

3.0g wild ginger root (asarum)
3.0g schizandra fruit
3.0g cinnamon twigs
6.0g pinellia rhizome

Minor Bupleurum Combination (Hsiao-chai-hu-tang)

Objectives: distressed chest or abdomen, slight fever with alternating chills, loss of appetite with bitter taste, occasional white tongue coating, nausea, vomiting, and cough.

Indications: cold, bronchitis, whooping cough, bronchial and childhood asthma, pneumonia, tuberculosis, pleurisy, gastritis, stomach and duodenal ulcers, hepatitis, cirrhosis of the liver, cholelithiasis, cholecystitis, pancreatitis, peritonitis, nephritis, nephrosis, pyelonephritis, kidney and gall stones, anemia, tonsillitis, otitis media, measles, childbirth fever, mastitis, ocular eczema, keratitis, iritis, rhinitis, and suppuration

Composition:

7.0g hare's ear root (bupleurum)　3.0g jujube fruit
3.0g skullcap root (scute)　2.0g licorice root
5.0g pinellia rhizome　3.0g ginseng root
4.0g ginger rhizome

Minor Cinnamon and Peony Combination (Hsiao-chien-chung-tang)

Objectives: poor health with a tendency toward fatigue, flushing, abdominal pain or palpitation, chills with warm arms and legs, frequent urination

Indications: gastroptosis, indigestion, reduction of acid, childhood dysentery, peritonitis, childhood constipation, rickets, noctiphobia, nocturia, bone ulcers, prolapsed rectum, ocular eczema, keratitis, iritis, and tonsillitis

Composition:

4.0g cinnamon twigs　4.0g ginger rhizome
6.0g peony root　4.0g jujube fruit
2.0g licorice root　20.0g maltose

Ophiopogon Combination (Mai-men-tung-tang)

Objectives: cough with flushing up and usually a small volume of sticky sputum, or flushing up with dryness and odd sensation in the throat

Indications: bronchitis, whooping cough, bronchial or childhood asthma, laryngitis, pneumonia, tuberculosis, and diabetes mellitus

Composition:

5.0g pinellia rhizome　10.0g ophiopogon root
2.0g ginseng root　2.0g licorice root
3.0g jujube fruit　5.0g rice

Peony and Licorice Combination (Shao-yao-kan-tsao-tang)

Objectives: muscular pain and tension, pain in the feet, and muscular rheumatism; bronchial asthma; pain in the abdomen; and cholelithiasis
Indications: rheumatoid pain, sciatic neuralgia, and lower back pain
Composition:

4.0-8.0g peony root   4.0-8.0g licorice

Persica and Rhubarb Combination (Tao-ho-cheng-chi-tang)

Objectives: violet or dark pink lips or gums, and tendency toward headaches or flushing
Indications: habitual constipation, hypertension, arteriosclerosis, nephritis, nephrosis, kidney atrophy, cystitis, enlarged prostate, hypertrophy, sciatic neuralgia, chilblains, hemorrhoids, menstrual disorders, endometritis, swelling of uterine muscles, oophoritis, salpingitis, menopausal disorders, eczema, hives, facial vesicles, tinea, ocular eczema, iritis, glaucoma, ocular bleeding, periodentitis, and alveodental suppuration
Composition:

5.0g peach seeds (persica)   1.5g licorice root
4.0g cinnamon twigs   2.0g nitrous sulfate
3.0g rhubarb rhizome

Pinellia Combination (Pan-hsia-hsieh-hsin-tang)

Objectives: distressed stomach, nausea, and vomiting
Indications: prolapsed stomach, stomatitis, gastritis, weak digestion, diarrhea, enteritis, nausea, gastric and duodenal ulcers
Composition:

1.0g goldenthread rhizome (coptis)   3.0g ginseng root
3.0g jujube fruit
3.0g skullcap root (scute)   3.0g licorice root
6.0g pinellia rhizome   3.0g ginger roots

Pinellia and Ginseng Six Combination (Pan-hsieh-liu-chun-tzu-tang)

Objectives: distended or tense stomach, pain, nausea, distressed heart, gas, diarrhea, anemia, loss of appetite, vomiting, fatigue, painful hunger, and gastric spasms or dilation

Indications: gastric or intestinal catarrh, hypersecretion of gastric acid, prolapsed stomach, stomach and duodenal ulcers, and gastric weakness

Composition:

4.0g pinellia rhizome
4.0g ginseng root
3.0g skullcap root (scute)
3.0g goldenthread rhizome (coptis)
1.0g ginger rhizome

3.0g licorice root
9.0g China root (hoelen)
3.0g *paichu* (white atractylodes rhizome)
3.0g Mandarin orange peel
4.0g oyster shell

Pinellia and Magnolia Combination (Pan-hsia-hou-pu-tang)

Objectives: mental instability, distressed throat and chest, stomach distention, weak digestion, occasional nausea, and vomiting

Indications: bronchitis, tonsillitis, pharyngitis, whooping cough, bronchial asthma, tuberculosis, esophageal stricture, gastric neurosis, poor digestion, prolapsed stomach, irregular pulse, cardiac nerve disorders, cardiac asthma, hypotension, neurasthenia, phobias, insomnia, nausea, menopausal disorders, uterine bleeding, and absence of menses

Composition:

6.0g pinellia rhizome
5.0g China root (hoelen)
3.0g magnolia bark

2.0g perilla leaves
4.0g ginger rhizome

Platycodon and Chih-shih Formula (Pai-nung-san)

Indications: tumors with suppuration and pain, muscle spasms, nodules, crusts, and lymphadenitis. Note: Unsuitable for chronic tumors and cold sores.

Composition:

5.0g immature citrus fruit *(chih-shih)*
5.0g peony root

2.0g balloon flower root (platycodon)

Platycodon and Gypsum Combination (Chieh-keng-shih-kao-tang)

Objectives: thirst and chronic expectoration
Indications: expectoration

Composition:

1.1g balloon flower root (platy- ,   1.0g gypsum
codon)

Polyporus Combination (Chu-ling-tang)

Objectives: dry throat, painful urination, dysuria, and hematuria
Indications: pyelonephritis, kidney or gall stones, cystitis, urethritis,
and gonorrhea
Composition:

3.0g water plantain rhizome   3.0g talc
(alisma)   3.0g grifola (polyporus)
3.0g China root (hoelen)   3.0g gelatin

Pueraria Combination (Ko-ken-tang)

objectives: headache; fever; chills without sweating; pain in the neck,
shoulders, and back; chronic dental pain; stuffy nose; suppuration; stiff
shoulders; and neuralgia
Indications: cold, otitis media, rhinitis, suppuration, trachoma, tonsillitis, styes, conjunctivitis, ocular eczema, iritis, dacryocystitis, cataract, eczema, hives, mastitis, alveodental suppuration, measles, trigeminal neuralgia, muscular rheumatism, enteritis, and hemicrania
Composition:

8.0g common kudzu root (puer-   4.0g jujube fruit
aria)   3.0g cinammon twigs
4.0g ma-huang herb   3.0g peony root
1.0g ginger rhizome   2.0g licorice root

Pueraria Nasal Combination (Ching-pi-tang)

Indications: stuffy nose, headache, chronic nasal suppuration, supraorbital neuralgia, melancholia, rhinitis, and postoperative nasal diseases
Composition:

Pueraria Combination   gypsum
Cnidium and Rhubarb Formula   Job's tears seeds (coix)
balloon flower root (platycodon)   magnolia flowers

Rehmannia Eight Formula (Pa-wei-ti-huang-wan)

Objectives: a tendency towards fatigue; cold, or sometimes hot, arms and legs; occasional lower back pain; dry throat; frequent urination with decreased volume and sensation of retention; and occasional polyuria at night

Indications: hypertension, arteriosclerosis, nephritis, kidney nephrosis, atrophy, pyelitis, kidney and gall stones, urethritis, enlargement of the prostate, involuntary emissions, impotence, genital neuralgia, beriberi after childbirth, menopausal disorders, eczema, hives, weak eyesight, cataract, glaucoma, and pyorrhea

Composition:

4.0g yam (dioscorea)
4.0g Asiatic cornelian cherry fruit (cornus)
3.0g water plantain rhizome (alisma)
3.0g China root (hoelen)

1.0g cinnamon twigs
8.0g Chinese foxglove roots and rhizome (rehmannia)
1.0g wolfsbane root (aconite)
3.0g tree peony bark

Rhubarb and Moutan Combination (Ta-huang-mu-tan-pi-tang)

Objectives: distressed pain or constipation of the upper colon, hard stools, purplish or dark red skin, hyperemia, or tendency to bleed

Indications: appendicitis, chronic constipation, arteriosclerosis, kidney or gall stones, cystitis, urethritis, enlarged prostate, tendonitis, menstrual irregularity, endometritis, oopharitis, salpingitis, orchitis, menopausal problems, eczema, facial vesicles, ringworm, infected crusts, and iritis

Composition:

2.0 rhubarb rhizome
4.0g nitrous sulfate
4.0 tree peony bark (moutan)

6.0g wax gourd seeds
4.0g peach seeds

Rhubarb Five Formula (Wu-huang-san)

Objectives: flushing, dark red face, distressed heart, mental instability, occasional insomnia, dizziness, stiff shoulders, and a rough feeling in the mouth

Indications: hypertension, arteriosclerosis, tinnitus, stiff shoulders, stomach ulcer, gastritis, menopausal disorders, insomnia, nosebleed,

uterine bleeding, headache from habitual constipation, hyperemia, dry lips, bitter tongue, and alcoholism
Composition:

4.5g goldenthread rhizome (coptis)
9.0g rhubarb rhizome

3.5g skullcap root (scute)
3.5g phellodendron bark
3.5g gardenia fruit

Siler and Platycodon Formula (Fang-feng-tung-sheng-san)

Objectives: obesity with constipation and decreased urine volume
Indications: stomach and duodenal ulcers, habitual constipation, irregular pulse, cardiac neurosis, angina pectoris, valvular disease, cardiac asthma, fatty heart, arteriosclerosis, hypertension, nephrosis, kidney and bladder stones, involuntary emission, impotence, sexual weakness, obesity, stiff shoulders in persons over fifty, arthritis, neuralgia, nodules, crusty skin, eczema, hives, rosacea, athlete's foot, loss of hair, corneal inflammation, iritis, cataract, otitis media, suppuration and gingival abscess
Composition:

1.2g Chinese angelica root *(tang-kuei)*
1.2g Chinese lovage rhizome (cnidium)
1.2g peony root
1.2g gardenia fruit
1.2g ginger rhizome
1.2g forsythia fruit
3.0g siler root
2.0g licorice root
1.2g *chinchieh* herb (schizonepeta)

1.5g nitrous sulfate
1.2g ma-huang herb (ephedra)
2.0g *paichu* (white atractylodes rhizome)
1.5g rhubarb rhizome
1.2g field mint herb
2.0g balloon flower root (platycodon)
2.0g skullcap root (scute)
2.0g gypsum
3.0g talc

Sophora and Schizonepeta Formula (Ku-chin-san)

Indications: ecxema
Composition:

1.0g sophora root
1.0g *chinchieh* herb (schizonepeta)

Stephania and Astragalus (Fang-chi-huang-chi-tang)

Objectives: edema; clear, pale skin; and a tendency toward swelling and sweating

Indications: obesity, arthritis, joint rheumatism, and sweating
Composition:

5.0g stephania root
5.0g Chinese milk vetch root (astragalus)
3.0g ginger rhizome

3.0g *paichu* (white atractylodes rhizome)
3.0g jujube fruit
1.5g licorice root

Stephania and Ginseng Combination (Mu-fang-chi-tang)

Objectives: distressed heart, difficult breathing with asthmatic breath sounds, occasional edematous swelling with decreased urine, and thirst
Indications: endocarditis, valvular diseases, cardiac asthma, chronic nephritis, and nephrosis
Composition:

4.0g stephania root
3.0g ginseng

10.0g gypsum
3.0g cinnamon twigs

Tang-kuei and Arctium Formula (Hsiao-feng-san)

Objectives: chronic dry or secreting dermatosis which aggravates during summer or warm weather
Indications: hives and eczema
Composition:

3.0g Chinese angelica root *(tang-kuei)*
3.0g Chinese foxglove root and rhizome (rehmannia)
3.0g gypsum
2.0g siler root
2.0g *tsangchu* rhizome (atractylodes)

1.0g *chinchieh* herb (schizonepeta)
2.0g birthwort
2.0g burdock (arctium)
1.5g anemarrhena rhizome
1.5g flax seeds
1.0g cicada
1.0g sophora root

Tang-kuei and Bupleurum Formula (Hsiao-yao-san)

Objectives: tendency toward fatigue, headache, stiff shoulders, dizziness, chest distress, red face with hot sensation, turbid urine, urinary retention, bad temper, and mental instability
Indications: women with delicate health; psychoneurosis, neurasthenia, hysteria, insomnia, menstrual irregularity, tuberculosis, dermatosis, leukorrhea, chronic endometritis, and hypertensive palpitation
Composition:

3.0g Chinese angelica root *(tang-kuei)*
3.0g peony root
3.0g hare's ear root (bupleurum)
3.0g China root (hoelen)

3.0g *paichu* (white atractylodes rhizome)
2.0g ginger rhizome
1.5g licorice root
1.0g field mint

Tang-Kuei, Evodia, and Ginger Combination (Tang-kuei-szu-ni-chia-wu-chu-yu-sheng-chiang-tang)

Objectives: severely cold arms and legs, tendency towards anemia, and occasional chills with lower back pain or lower abdominal pain
Indications: sciatic neuralgia, chilblains, and lower abdominal pain in women
Composition:

3.0g Chinese angelica root *(tang-kuei)*
3.0g cinnamon twigs
3.0g peony root
2.0g licorice root

4.0g ginger rhizome
2.0g asarum
3.0g akebia
5.0g jujube fruit
2.0g evodia fruit

Tang-kuei Four Combination (Szu-wu-tang)

Objectives: one of the choicest drugs for gynecological problems; used for anemia and as a tranquilizer for psychosomatic complaints
Indications: menstrual irregularity, menopausal disorders, leukorrhea, pre- or post-partum illnesses
Composition:

4.0g Chinese angelica root *(tang-kuei)*
4.0g Chinese lovage rhizome (cnidium)

4.0g peony root
4.0g Chinese foxglove roots and rhizome (rehmannia)

Tang-kuei and Gelatin Combination (Chiung-kuei-chiao-ai-tang)

Objectives: chills and anemia from excessive bleeding
Indications: hemoptysis, metrorrhagia, intestinal or hemorrhoidal bleeding, hemorrhage during pregnancy, chronic bleeding after childbirth, excessive menstruation, and petechiae
Composition:

4.5g Chinese angelica root *(tang-kuei)*
3.0g Chinese lovage rhizome (cnidium)
4.5g peony root

3.0g gelatin
6.0g rehmannia roots and rhizome
3.0g licorice root
3.0g mugwort leaves (artemisia)

Tang-kuei and Paeonia Formula *(Tang-kuei-shao-yao-san)*

Objectives: anemia with chills, pallor, dark color around the eyes, headache, dizziness, stiff shoulders, palpitation, urinary frequency but small volume, thirst, and pain or chills in the lower abdomen

Indications: irregular pulse, cardiac neurosis, valvular disease, hypotension, hypertension, nephritis, nephrosis, anemia, goiter, chilblains, hemorrhoids, prolapsed rectum or uterus, habitual abortion, nephritis in pregnancy, periodic menstrual irregularity, retroverted uterus, endometritis, congenital abnormalities, sterility, menopausal problems, hysteria, facial vesicles, athlete's feet, ringworm, ocular eczema, iritis, dacrycystitis, and cataract

Composition:

3.0g Chinese angelica root *(tang-kuei)*
3.0g Chinese lovage rhizome (cnidium)
4.0g peony root (paeonia)

4.0g water plantain rhizome (alisma)
4.0g *paichu* (white atractylodes rhizome)
4.0g China root (hoelen)

Vitality Combination *(Chen-wu-tang)*

Objectives: severely cold arms and legs, decreased urine, a tendency towards diarrhea, palpitation, and dizziness

Indications: chronic diarrhea, prolapsed stomach, peritonitis, appendicitis, hypertension, arteriosclerosis, and hypotension

Composition:

3.0g peony root
3.0g ginger rhizome
5.0g China root (hoelen)

3.0g *paichu* (white atractylodes rhizome)
1.0g wolfsbane root (aconite)

LISTS OF SUPPLIERS OF FOODS AND VITAMINS

Benowicz, Robert J., *Vitamins and You* (New York: Filmways Company Publishers, 1979). A selected list of multivitamin and single vitamin supplements, pp. 135—180.

Hulke, Malcolm, *The Encyclopedia of Alternative Medicine and Self-Help* (New York: Schocken Books, 1979). Contributors of the various healings and therapy systems, pp. 209–212. Associations, pp. 215–217. Products, nutrient manufacturers and distributors, pp. 218–225. Training and treatment centers, pp. 226–228. Health spas and resorts.

Pearson, Durk & Sandy Shaw, *Life Extension.* (New York: Warner Books, 1982). Nutrient supplies, pp. 618–621. Nutrient manufacturers, pp. 622–623. Devices (medical devices), pp. 624–625.

BIBLIOGRAPHY

GENERAL INFORMATION ON ALTERNATIVE MEDICINE

Ardell, Donald B., *High Level Wellness*. Emmaus, Pennsylvania: Rodale Press, 1977.

Berkeley Holistic Health Center, *The Holistic Health Hand Book*. Berkeley, California: Self Publishing, 1976.

Bricklin, Mark, *The Practical Encyclopedia of Natural Healing*. Emmaus, Pennsylvania: Rodale Press, 1976.

Eagle, Robert, *Alternative Medicine: A Guide to Medical Underground*. London: Futora, 1973.

Flatto, Edwin, *Revitalize Your Body with Nature's Secrets*. New York: Arco Publishers, 1972.

Fraser, J. Lloyd, *The Medicine Men: A Guide to Natural Medicine*. London: Thames TV/Methuen, 1981.

Fulder, Stephen, *The Handbook of Complementary Medicine*. London: Coronet Books, 1984.

Guirdham, Arthur, *A Theory of Disease*. London: Neville Spearman, 1980.

Hasting, A. C., *Health for the Whole Person*. Boulder, Colorado: Westview Press, 1981.

Hill, Ann, *A Visual Encyclopedia of Unconventional Medicine*. London: New England Library, 1979.

Hulke, Malcolm, *The Encyclopedia of Alternative Medicine and Self-Help*. New York: Schocken Books, 1979.

Inglis, Brian, *Fringe Medicine*. London: Faber & Faber, 1964.

———, *Natural Medicine*. London: Collins, 1979.

Jervis, D. C., *Folk Medicine*. New York: Ballantine Books, 1982.

Kaslou, Brian, *Wholistic Dimensions in Healing*. Garden City, N.Y.: Doubleday, 1978.

Law, Donald, *A Guide to Alternative Medicine*. Wellingborough, Great Britain: Turnstone, 1974.

Leshan, Lawrence, *Holistic Health: How to Understand and Use the Revolution in Medicine*. Wellingborough, Great Britain: Turnstone, 1984.

Pelletier, K. R., *Holistic Medicine: From Stress to Optimum Health*. New York: Delta, 1979.

Rodale, J. I., *Encyclopedia for Healthful Living*. Emmaus, Pennsylvania: Rodale Press, 1979.

Sobel, David, *Ways to Health: Holistic Approach in Ancient and Contemporary Medicine*. New York: Viking, 1976.

Space, Dossey L., *Time and Medicine*. London: Routledge & Kegan Paul, 1982.

Stanway, Andrew, *Alternative Medicine—A Guide to Natural Therapies*. New York: Penguin Books, 1982.

Tubesing, D. A., *Wholistic Health*. New York: Human Sciences Press, 1979.

Walker, B., *Encyclopedia of Metaphysical Medicine*. London: Routledge & Kegan Paul, 1978.

Wallis, R. and P. Morely, *Marginal Medicine*. London: Peter Owe, 1976.

Weil, A., *Health and Healing: Understanding Conventional and Alternative Medicine*. Boston: Houghton Mifflin, 1983.

HEALTH MAGAZINES

Accent on Living. Box 726, Bloomington, IL. Quarterly.

Allies of Animals. Suite 3H, 40 Waterside Plaza, New York, NY 10010.

American Dietetic Association Journal. 430 N. Michigan, Chicago, IL 60611. Monthly.

American Vegetarian Hygienist. Box 63, Duncannon, PA 17020. Bi-monthly.

Better Nutrition. 25 W. 45th St., New York, NY 10036. Monthly.

Cancer Control Journal. 2043 N. Berendo, Los Angeles, CA 90027. Monthly.

Fitness for Living. 33 Minor St., Emmaus, PA 18049. Bimonthly (Rodale Press).

The Health Letter. PO Box 326, San Antonio, TX 78292. Biweekly.

Healthways—American Chiropractic Association. 2200 Grand Avenue, Des Moines, IA 50312.

Health—PAC Bulletin. Policy Advisory Center, 17 Murray St., New York, NY 10007. Bimonthly.

The Herbalist. PO Box 62, Provo, UT 84601. Monthly (Biworld Publishing).

Holistic Health Review. PO Box 166, Berkeley, CA 94701. Quarterly.

Jewish Vegetarian. 855 Finchley Road, London NW11, England.

Let's Live. 444 N. Larchmont Blvd., Los Angeles, CA 90004. Monthly.

Mothering. PO Box 2046, Albuquerque, NM 87103. Quarterly.

Nutrition Today. 101 Ridgely Avenue, PO Box 465, Annapolis, MD. Bimonthly.

Prevention. 33 Minor St., Emmaus, PA 18049. Monthly.

Public Scrutiny. PO Box 1307, Monrovia, CA 91016. Monthly.

Sweet'n Low. 363 7th Avenue, New York, NY 10001. Monthly.

Today's Health. 535 N. Dearborn, Chicago, IL 60610. Monthly.

Vegetarian Courier. 227 Broadway, Room 1301, New York, NY 10007. Monthly.

Vegetarian Times. Suite 1838, 101 Park Ave., New York, NY 10017. Bimonthly.

Vegetarian Voice. 501 Old Harding Highway, Malaga, NJ 08328. Bimonthly.

ACUPUNCTURE/ACUPRESSURE

Academy of Traditional Chinese Medicine, *Essentials of Chinese Acupuncture*, rev. ed. Shanghai: Pergamon, 1985.

Bailey, Nathan, D.C., *Bailey's Atlas and Book on Acupuncture and Acupressure.* Cebu City, Philippines: n.d.

Chan, Dr. P., *Finger Acupressure.* Los Angeles: Price/Stern/Sloan, 1982.

de Schepper, Luc, M.D., C.A., *Acupuncture for the Practitioner.* Santa Monica, California: 1985.

Helm, Bill and Share Lew, Tui-Na, *Chinese Healing and Acupressure.* San Diego, California: Fellowship of the Tao, 1984.

Kapchuck, Ted, O.M.D., *The Web That Has No Weaver.* New York: Congdon a Weed, 1983.

Lawson-Wood, D., *Acupuncture and Chinese Massage*. Rostington: Health Science, 1965.

Lidell, Lucinda, *The Book of Massage* (A Fireside Book). New York: Simon & Schuster, 1986.

Low, Royston, *The Secondary Vessels of Acupuncture*. New York: Thorsons, 1983.

Lu, Henry, Ph.D., *Clinical Manual of Chinese Acupuncture: Diagnosis and Treatment*. Vancouver, British Columbia: Academy of Oriental Heritage, n.d.

————, *A Complete Textbook of Auricular Acupuncture*. Vancouver, British Columbia: no publisher, 1975.

Matsumoto, Kiko and Stephen Birch, *Five Elements and Ten Stems*. Brookline, Massachusetts: Paradigm, 1983.

Mori, Hiderato, *Introductory Acupuncture*. Ido-no-nippon-sha, Japan: no publisher, n.d.

Nickel, David, O.M.D., *Acupressure for Athletes*. Santa Monica, California: Health Acu-Press, 1985.

Ohashi, Wataru, *Do-it-Yourself Shiatsu*. New York: Dutton, 1976.

Stux, Stiller, Pothman, Yayasuriya, Drs., *Akupunktur-Lehrbuch und Atlas*. Berlin: Springer-Verlag, 1986.

Wiseman, Nigel, Andrew Ellis and Paul Zmiewski, *Fundamentals of Chinese Medicine*. Brookline, Massachusetts: Paradigm, 1985.

AROMATHERAPY

Genders, Roy, *Growing Herbs as Aromatics*. New Canaan, Connecticut: Keats Publishing, 1977.

Lautie, Raymond and Sandre Passeberg, *Aromatherapy—The Use of Plant Essences in Healing*. Wellingborough, Great Britain: Thorsons, 1984.

Maury, Marguerite, *The Secret of Life and Youth*. New York: MacDonald Publishing, 1964.

Price, Shirley, *Practical Aromatherapy*. Wellingborough, Great Britain: Thorsons, 1984.

Tisserand, Robert T., *The Art of Aromatherapy*. New York: C. W. Daniel Publishers, 1977.

AUTOSUGGESTION & HYPNOTHERAPY

Arons, Harry, *Handbook of Self Hypnosis*. Alhambra, California: Borden Publishing, 1964.

————, *Hypnosis in Criminal Investigation*. Alhambra, California: Borden Publishing, 1979.

————, *New Master Course in Hypnotism*. Alhambra, California: Borden Publishing, 1986.

————, *Techniques of Speed Hypnosis*. Alhambra, California: Borden Publishing, 1963.

Barnett, Edgar A., *Unlock Your Mind and Be Free—A Practical Approach to Hypnotherapy*. Riverdale, California: Westwood Publishers, 1979.

Boyne, Gil, *Hypnosis—New Tool in Nursing Practice*. Glendale, California: Westwood, 1982.

Brokes, S. H., *The Autosuggestion—According to Emil-Qua Theory*. Tel Aviv: Alef Publications, 1978.

Cooke, C. E. and A. E. Van Vogt, *Hypnotism Handbook*. Alhambra, California: Borden Publishing, 1965.

Elman, Dave, *Hypnotherapy*. Riverdale, California: Westwood Publishing Co., 1970.

Foundation for Inner Peace, *A Course in Miracles*. Tiburon, California: Foundation for Inner Peace, 1985.

Furst, Arnold, *Hypnosis for Salesmen*. Alhambra, California: Borden Publishing, 1978.

————, *Rapid Induction Hypnosis and Self Hypnosis*. Alhambra, California: Borden Publishing, 1981.

Gindes, Bernard C., *New Concepts of Hypnosis*. Alhambra, California: Borden Publishing, 1978.

Hay, Louise L., *Heal Your Body—The Mental Causes for Physical Illness and the Metaphysical Way to Overcome Them*. Los Angeles: Louise L. Hay Publication, 1981.

Hollander, Bernard, *Hypnosis and Self Hypnosis*. Alhambra, California: Borden Publishing, 1981.

Jampolsky, Garard G., *Love is Letting Go of Fear*. Berkeley, California: Celestial Arts Publishing, 1979.

Kuhn, Lesley and Salvatore Russo, *Modern Hypnosis*. Los Angeles: Wilshire Publishing, 1972.

Lecron, Lesle and Jean Bordeaux, *Hypnotism Today*. Los Angeles: Wilshire Publishing, 1953.

McGill, Ormand, *Art of Stage Hypnotism*. Los Angeles: Wilshire Publishing, 1974.

Orton, Louis, *Hypnotism Made Practical*. Los Angeles: Wilshire Publishing, 1968.

Powers, Melvin, *Advance Techniques of Hypnosis*. Los Angeles: Wilshire Publishing, 1965.

————, *Mental Power through Sleep Suggestion*. Los Angeles: Wilshire Publishing, 1962.

————, *Practical Guide to Self Hypnosis*. Los Angeles: Wilshire Publishing, 1960.

————, *Self-Hypnosis*. Los Angeles: Wilshire Publishing, 1961.

Rhodes, Raphael H., *Therapy Through Hypnosis*. Los Angeles: Wilshire Publishing, 1974.

Sextus, Carl, *Hypnotism*. Los Angeles: Wilshire Publishing, 1972.

Sparks, Laurence, *Self Hypnosis: A Conditioned Response Technique*. Los Angeles: Wilshire Publishing, 1974.

Van Pelt, S. J., *Secrets of Hypnotism*. Los Angeles: Wilshire Publishing, 1970.

BREATHING THERAPY

Bragg, Paul C. and Patricia, *Super Brain Breathing*. New York: Health Science Publications, 1974.

Josephson, Emmanual M., *Breathe Deeply and Avoid Colds*. New York: Chenny Press, 1973.

Journal of the Exploration Institute, "Personal Growth," *Journal of the Exploration Institute*, 1978.

Kofler, Leo, *Art of Breathing*. New York: Wehman Bros., 1982.

Nakamura, Takashi, *Oriental Breathing Therapy*. Tokyo: Japan Publications, 1981.

Orr, Leonard and Sondra Ray, *Rebirthing in the New Age*. Millbrae, California: Celestial Arts, 1977.

Ramacharaka Yogi, *Science of Breath*. Honesdale, Pennsylvania: Himalayan International Institute, 1981.

Rank, Otto and John Man, *Way of Growth*. New York: Viking Press, 1967.

Rush, Anne Kent, *Getting Clear*. New York: Random House, 1973.

Swami Rama, Rudolph Ballentine et al., *Science of Breathing—A Practical Guide*. New York: Himalayan Institute, 1981.

COLOR THERAPY

Anderson, Mary, *Color Healing*. New York: Samuel Weiser, 1975.

Clark, Zinda, *Colour Therapy*. Tel Aviv: OrAmi, 1975.

Copen, Bruce, *Character Analysis with Color*. West Sussex, Great Britain: Academic Publications, 1959.

————, *Chromo-Therapy Course*. West Sussex, Great Britain: Academic Publications, 1949.

————, *The Coloring Handbook*. West Sussex, Great Britain: Academic Publications, 1955.

————, *A Rainbow of Health*. West Sussex, Great Britain: Academic Publications, 1975.

Dane, Victor, *Colours and Their Effects on Health*. West Sussex, Great Britain: Academic Publishers, 1956.

Eaves, Osborne A., *The Colour Cure*. London: Phillip Welby, 1980.

Heline, Corine, *Healing and Regeneration Through Colour*. West Sussex, Great Britain: Academic Publishers, 1956.

Hessey, J. Dodson, *Colour Treatment of Disease*. West Sussex, Great Britain: Academic Publishers, 1956.

Hunt, Roland, *The Seven Keys to Colour Healing*. West Sussex, Great Britain: Academic Publishers, 1952.

Irwin, Beatrice, *The New Science of Colour*. West Sussex, Great Britain: Academic Publishers, 1923.

Mayer, Gladys, *Colour and Healing*. New Delhi: Krishna Press, 1973.

Sturzaker, James, *The Twelve Rays*. Wellingborough, Great Britain: The Aquarian Press, 1977.

Wright, W. D., *The Measurement of Colour*. London: Adam Hilger Ltd, 1944.

CHINESE HERBS

American College of Traditional Chinese Medicine, journals published at San Francisco, California.

Bensky-Gamble, with T. Kapchuck, *Chinese Herbal Medicine*. Seattle: Eastland Press, 1986.

Cheung, C. S., M.D., Yat Ki Lai, C.A., and U. Aik Kaw, B.A., *Mental Dysfunctions as Treated by T.C.M.* San Francisco: American College of Traditional Chinese Medicine, 1985.

Cheung, C. S., M.D., U. A. Kaw, H. Harrison, C.A., and Y. K. Lai, C.A., *Treatment of Toxic Side Effect Resulting from Radiation and Chemotherapy by T.C.M.* San Francisco: American College of Traditional Chinese Medicine, M.D.

Dharmananda, Subhuti, Ph.D., *Chinese Herbal Therapies for Immune Disorders.* Portland, Oregon: Institute for Traditional Medicine and Preventive Health Care, 1988.

Hsu, H. Yen, Ph.D., *The Way to Good Health with Chinese Herbs.* Long Beach, California: Ohai, 1982.

Hsu, H. Yen, Ph.D. (ed. & comp.), *Natural Healing with Chinese Herbs.* Long Beach, California: Ohai, 1981.

Hsu, H. Yen, Ph.D., and D. H. Easer, *A Practical Introduction to Major Chinese Herbal Formulas.* Long Beach, California: Ohai, 1980.

Hsu, H. Yen, Ph.D., and William G. Peacher, Ph.D., *Chinese Herb Medicine and Therapy.* Long Beach, California: Ohai, 1976.

Hsu, H. Yen, Ph.D., and M. M. Van Benschuten, C.A., *Index of Differentiation for Commonly Used Herb Formulas,* comp. by J. A. Rau, D.D.S. Long Beach, California: Ohai, 1984.

Lu, H. C., Ph.D., *Chinese Herbal Therapy: 30 Lessons.* Vancouver, British Columbia: Academy of Oriental Heritage, n.d.

Lucas, Richard, *Secrets of the Chinese Herbalists.* Englewood Cliffs, N.J.: Prentice-Hall, 1977.

Oriental Healing Arts Institute, bulletins published at Long Beach, California.

Roberts, Miles, C.A., *Lecture Series on Kampo.* Sacramento: n.d.

Teeguarden, Ron, *Chinese Tonic Herbs.* N.p.: Japan Publications, 1985.

Terashi, Bokuso, M.D., *Chinese Herbal Medicine and the Problems of Aging*. Long Beach, California: Ohai, 1984.

Yeung, Him-Che, C.A., O.M.D., *Handbook of Chinese Herbs and Formulas*, vols. 1, 2. Los Angeles: Institute of Chinese Medicine, n.d.

WESTERN HERBS

Coon, Nelson, *Using Plants for Healing*. Emmaus, Pennsylvania: Rodale Press, 1979.

Dextreit, Raymond, *Our Earth, Our Cure*. N.p.: Swan House, 1979.

Heinerman, John, *The Treatment of Cancer with Herbs*. Orem, Utah: Biworld Publishers, 1984.

Hulke, Malcolm (ed.), *The Encyclopedia of Alternative Medicine and Self Help*. New York: Schocken, 1979.

Law, Donald, *The Concise Herbal Encyclopedia*. New York: St. Martin's, 1976.

Lewis, Walter H. and Memory P. F. Elvin Lewis, *Medical Botany-Plants Affecting Man's Health*. New York: John Wiley, 1977.

Lust, John, *The Herb Book*. New York: Bantam, n.d.

Powell, Eric, Ph.D., *The Natural Home Physician*. N.p.: Health Science Press, 1975.

Thomson, Robert, *The Grosset Encyclopedia of Natural Medicine*. New York: Grosset and Dunlap, n.d.

Tierra, Michael, *The Way of Herbs*. Santa Cruz, California: Orenda/Unity Press, 1980.

Wren, R.C., *Potter's New Cyclopedia of Botanical Drugs and Preparations*. N.p.: Health Science Press, n.d.

HOMEOPATHY

Boericke, William, M.D., *Materia Medica with Repertory*. Philadelphia: Boericke & Runyon, 1927.

Clark, John H., M.D., *The Prescriber*. No location: Health Science Press, 1972.

Coats, Peter, *The Homeopathic Aide-Memoire*. London: C. W. Daniel, 1984.

Cowperthwaite, A., *A Text-Book of Materia Medica and Therapeutics*. New Delhi: Jain Publishing, 1976.

Cummings, Stephen and Dana Ullman, *Everybody's Guide to Homeo-pathic Medicines*. Los Angeles: Jeremy P. Tarcher, 1984.

Gibson, D., M.D., *First Aid Homeopathy in Accidents and Ailments*. St. Louis, Missouri: Formur International, 1975.

Kent, J. T., *Repertory of Homeopathic Materia Medica*. St. Louis, Missouri: Formur International, 1975.

Pratt, Noel, M.D., *Homeopathic Prescribing*. New Canaan, Connecticut: Keats Publishing, 1980.

Singh, Yuduir, Dr., *Homeopathic Cure for Common Diseases*. Delhi, India: Vision Books, 1983.

Stephenson, James H., *A Doctor's Guide to Helping Yourself with Homeo-pathic Remedies*. St. Louis, Missouri: Formur International, 1976.

Wheeler, C. E. and J. D. Kenyon, *An Introduction to the Principles and Practice of Homeopathy*. New York: British Book Center, 1975.

HYDROTHERAPY

Kovacs, R., *Electro Therapy and Light Therapy with Essentials of Hydro-therapy and Mechano Therapy*. Philadelphia: Kovac's R. Publishing, 1946.

Leibold, Gerhard, *Practical Hydrotherapy*. Wellingborough, Great Britain: Thorsons, 1980.

Lindlahr, Victor H., *The Natural Way to Health*. North Hollywood, California: New Castle, 1980.

MACROBIOTICS DIET THERAPY

Aihara, Cornelia, *Chico San Cookbook*. Chico, California: Chico San, 1979.

————, *The Do of Cooking*. Oroville, California: Oshawa Foundation, 1982.

Aihara, Herman, "Acids & Alkaline." Oroville, California: Oshawa Foundation, 1982.

Airola, Paavo O., *How to Keep Slim, Healthy and Young with Juice Fasting*. Chicago: Contemporary Books, 1971.

Buchinger, Otto H.F., *About Fasting*. Wellingborough, Great Britain: Thorson Publishers, 1966.

Carrington, Hereward, *Fasting for Health and Long Life*. Mokelumne Hill, California: Health Research, 1963.

De Vries, Arnold, *Therapeutic Fasting*. Los Angeles: Chandler Book Co., 1963.

Esko, Edward and Wendy, *Macrobiotic Cooking for Everybody*. Tokyo: Japan Publishers, 1980.

Holt, Calvin and Patch Caradine, *A Zen Macrobiotic Cookbook*. New York: Pyramid Publishers, 1971.

Kohler, Jean and Mary Alice, *Healing Miracles from Macrobiotics*. West Nyack, N.Y.: Parker Publishing, 1974.

Kushi, Michio, *The Book of Do In*. Tokyo: Japan Publishers, 1978.

————, *The Book of Macrobiotics*. Tokyo: Japan Publishers, 1986.

————, *The Cancer Prevention Diet*. New York: St. Martin's Press, 1984.

————, *How to See Your Health: The Book of Oriental Diagnosis*. Tokyo, Japan Publishers, 1980.

————, *The Macrobiotic Approach to Cancer*. Wayne, N.J.: Avery Publishing, 1982.

————, *Natural Healing through Macrobiotics*. Tokyo: Japan Publishing, 1979.

————, *Visions of a New World: The Era of Humanity*. Brookline, Massachusetts: East West Journal, 1979.

Oshawa, George, *The Book of Judgment*. Oroville, California: Oshawa Foundation, 1980.

———, *Cancer and the Philosophy of the Far East*. Binghamton, NY: Swan house, 1981.

———, *Guide Book for Living*. Oroville, California: Oshawa Foundation, 1985.

———, *Zen Macrobiotics*. Tokyo: Japan Publishing, 1965.

Shelton, Herbert M., *Fasting Can Save Your Life*. Bridgeport, Connecticut: Natural Hygiene Press, 1981.

———, *Fasting for Renewal of Life*. Bridgeport, Connecticut: Natural Hygiene Press, 1978.

MEGAVITAMINS AND ORTHOMOLECULAR THERAPY

Adams, R. and F. Murray, *Megavitamin Therapy*. New York: Larchmont Books, 1973.

———, *Megavitamin Therapy*. New York: Pinnacle Books, 1975.

Airola, Paavo, *How to Get Well*. Phoenix: Health Plus Publishers, 1974.

Bendwicz, Robert J., *Vitamins and You*. New York: Grosset & Dunlap Publishers, 1979.

Brin, M., *Newer Methods of Nutritional Biochemistry*. New York: Academic Press, 1967.

Brody, Jane, *Jane Brody's Nutrition Book*. New York: Bantam Books, 1982.

Burros, Marian, *Pure and Simple*. New York: Berkley, 1978.

Cherasken, E.S. and W. H. Ringsdorf, *New Hope for Incurable Disease*. New York: Exposition Press, 1971.

Clark, Linda, *Get Well Nutritionally*. New York: Arco Publishing, 1982.

———, *Know Your Nutrition*. New Canaan, Connecticut: Keats Publishing, 1981.

Davis, Adelle, *Let's Eat Right to Keep Fit*. New York: Signet Publishers, 1972.

————, *Let's Get Well*. New York: Signet Publishers, 1972.

Fredricks, C., *Eating Right for You*. New York: Grosset & Dunlap Publishers, 1974.

————, *Psycho Nutrition*. New York: Publishing Group, 1982.

Gerras, Charles and Joseph Galant, *The Complete Book of Vitamins*. Emmaus, Pennsylvania: Rodale Press, 1977.

Hawkins, D. and L. Pauling, *Orthomolecular Psychiatry: Treatment of Schizophrenia*. San Francisco: W. H. Freeman, 1973.

Hewitt, Jean, *The New York Times Natural Foods Cookbook*. New York: Avon, 1972.

Himwich, H. E., *Metabolism and Cerebral Disorders*. Baltimore: Williams and Williams, 1951.

Jacobson, Michael F., *Eater's Digest: The Consumer's Factbook of Food Additives*. Garden City, N.Y.: Doubleday, 1976.

Kirban, Salem, *The Getting Back to Nature Diet*. New Canaan, Connecticut: Keats Publishing, 1979.

Kirschmann, John, *Nutrition Almanac*. New York: McGraw Hill, 1975

Kloss, B. Jethro, *Back to Eden*. New York: Woodbridge Press, 1975.

Kugler, Hans J., *Seven Keys to a Longer Life*. New York: Stein & Day Publishers, 1978.

Kunin, Richard A., *Mega Nutrition*. New York: New American Library, 1983.

————, *Mega Nutrition for Women*. New York: New American Library, 1984.

Lappe, Frances Moore, *Diet for a Small Planet*. New York: Ballantine Books, 1982.

Lelord, Kordel, *Health the Easy Way*. New York: Charter Books, 1982.

Leonard, Jon N., J. L. Hofer and N. Pritkin, *Live Longer Now*. New York: Charter Books, 1974.

Lindauer, Lois Lyons, *It's in to Be Thin*. New York: Charter Books, 1984.

Ludeman, K. and L. Henderson, *The Do It Yourself Allergy Analysis Handbook*. New Canaan, Connecticut: Keats Publishing, 1979.

Mackarness, Richard, *Eating Dangerously*. New York: Harcourt Brace Jovanovich, 1976.

Marks, John. *A Guide to Vitamins—Their Role in Health and Disease*. Lancaster, England: Medical & Technical Publishing, 1973.

Mayer, J., *Overweight*. Englewood Cliffs, N.J.: Prentice Hall, 1968.

McGee, Charles T., *How to Survive Modern Technology*. New Canaan, Connecticut: Keats Publishing, 1979.

Passwater, Richard, *Super Nutrition for Healthy Hearts*. Wellingborough, Great Britain: Thorsons, 1981.

Pearson, D. and S. Shaw, *Life Extension*. New York: Warner Books, 1983.

Philpott, William and Dwight K. Kalita, *Brain Allergies*. New Canaan, Connecticut: Keats Publishing, 1980.

Price, Weston A., *Nutrition and Physical Degeneration*. La Mesa, California: The Price Pottenier Nutrition Foundation, Inc., 1979.

Randolph, Theron G. and Ralph W. Mos, *Allergy—Your Hidden Enemy*. Wellingborough, Great Britain: Turnstone Press, 1982.

Robinson, C., *Fundamentals of Normal Nutrition*. New York: Macmillan, 1972.

Roger, William T., *Nutrition against Disease—Health Is Wealth*. Huntington Beach, California: International Institute of Natural Health Sciences, 1985.

Rosenberg, Harold and A. N. Feldzahen, *The Book of Vitamin Therapy*. New York: Berkley Publishers, 1975.

Schroeder, H. A., *The Poisons around Us*. New Canaan, Connecticut: Keats Publishing, 1979.

————, *The Trace Elements and Man*. Old Greenwich, Connecticut: Devin Adair, 1973.

Schutte, Karl H. and John A. Myers, *Metabolic Aspects of Health*. Kentfield, California: Discovery Press, 1979.

Selye, Hans, *The Stress of Life*. New York: McGraw Hill, 1956.

Smith, Lendon H., *The Encyclopedia of Baby and Child Care*. New York: Warner Books, 1980.

————, *Feed Your Kids Right*. New York: Dell, 1979.

Stone, I., *The Healing Factor: Vitamin C against Disease*. New York: Grosset and Dunlap, 1972.

Thurston, Emory W., *The Parents Guide to Better Nutrition for Tots to Teens*. New Canaan, Connecticut: Keats Publishing, 1979.

Tracer, J., *The Belly Book*. New York: Grossman, 1972.

Walker, Morton, *Chelation Therapy: How to Prevent or Reverse Hardening of the Arteries*. Seal Beach, California: AG Press. 1980.

————, *How Not to Have a Heart Attack*. New York: Franklin Watts Inc., 1980.

————, *Total Health*. New York: Everest House, 1979.

Waston, G., *Nutrition and Your Mind: The Psychochemical Response*. New York: Harper & Row, 1972.

Williams, Roger J., *Nutrition Against Disease*. New York: Pitman, 1971.

Winter, Ruth, *Beware of the Food You Eat*. New York: American Library, 1972.

Yudkin, John, *Sweet and Dangerous*. New York: Bantam Press, 1972.

Underwood, E.J., *Trace Elements in Human and Animal Nutrition*. New York: Academic Press, 1971.

NUTRITION AND DIET THEORY

Bender, A. E., *Dietetic Foods*. London: Leonard Hill Books, 1973.

Briggs, George M., *Nutrition and Physical Fitness*. Philadelphia: Saunders College Publishers, 1979.

Burgstrom, G., *Principles of Food Science*. New York: The Macmillan Company, 1968.

Calloway, D. H., "Human Responses to Diets Very High in Protein," *Abstract of Federal Protocol*, 27(1968), 725.

Davidson, S., R. Passmore, J. F. Brock and A. S. Truswell, *Human Nutrition and Dietetics*. London: 1979.

FAO/WHO, "Handbook on Human Nutritional Requirements," *Nutritional Review*, 33(1975), 147.

FAO/WHO, "Recommendation on Protein and Energy Requirements," *Food & Nutrition*, 1:2(1975), 11.

Food & Nutrition Board, *Recommended Dietary Allowances*, 8th ed. Washington D.C.: National Research Council, National Academy of Science, 1974.

Goodhart, Robert S., *Modern Nutrition in Health and Disease*. Philadelphia: Lea & Febiger Publishers, 1980.

Guggenheim, Y. K., *Human Nutrition*. Jerusalem: Magnes Press, 1981.

Harper, H. A. & W. V. Rodwell, *Review of Physiological Chemistry*. Los Altos, California: Lange Medical Publications, 1979.

McCollum, E. V., *History of Nutrition*. Boston: Houghton Mifflin Company, 1957.

Perkins, E. G., *Modification of Lipid Metabolism*. New York: Academic Press, 1975.

Robin, Corine, H., *Basic Nutrition and Diet Therapy*. New York: Macmillan Publishers, 1980.

Sipple, H. L., *Sugars in Nutrition*. New York: Academic Press, 1974.

Spiller, G. A., *Fiber in Human Nutrition*. New York: Plenum Press, 1976.

Vergossen, A. J., *The Role of Fat in Human Nutrition*. New York: Academic Press, 1975.

Watt, B. K. & A. L. Marill, "Composition of Foods—Raw, Processed, Prepared," U.S. Department of Agriculture Handbook No. 8. Washington, D.C.: Government Printing Office, 1963.

West, E. S. et al., *Textbook of Biochemistry*. New York: Macmillan, 1966.

White, Abraham et al., *Principles of Biochemistry*. New York: McGraw Hill, 1978.

Williams, Sue Rodwell, *Nutrition and Diet Therapy*, St. Louis: The C. V. Mosby Company, 1981.

Yaakog, (Pingboin) Ilani, *All You Need to Know About Nutrition, Food and Diet*. Jerusalem: Shikmona Publishing, 1975.

PSYCHOTHERAPY

Alberti, Robert F., *Assertiveness, Innovations, Applications Issues*. San Luis Obispo, California: Impact, 1977.

Alvin, Juliette, *Music Therapy*. New York: Basic Books, 1975.

Ansbacher, H. L. and R. R. Ansbacher, *The Individual Psychology of Alfred Adler*. New York: Harper & Row, 1967.

Bernstein, Penny, *Theory and Methods in Dance Movement Therapy*. Dubuque, Iowa: Kendall/Hunt Publishers, 1975.

Bugental, J. F. T., *Psychotherapy and Process: The Fundamentals of an Existential Humanistic Perspective*. Reading, Massachusetts: Addison Wesley, 1979.

————, *The Search for Authenticity*. New York: Holt, Rinehart & Winston, 1965.

Craighiad, W. E., *Behavior Modification Principles: Issues and Applications*. Boston: Houghton Mifflin, 1976.

Gaston, E. T., *Music in Therapy*. New York: Macmillan, 1965.

Herink, Richie, *The Psycho Therapy Handbook—The A to Z Guide to More Than 250 Different Therapies in Use Today*. New York: New American Library, 1980.

Holder, E. M., "Physiological Changes in Primal Therapy," *Journal of the Association for Psychosomatic Research*, November 1976.

Janou, A. and E. M. Holden, *Primal Man*. New York: T. Y. Crowell, 1976.

Janou, A., *The Primal Scream*. New York: Putnam, 1978.

Johnson, D., *Diagnostic Implications of Dream Therapy*. Drama Book Specialists, 1978.

Mash, E. S. et al., *Behavior Modifications and Families*. New York: Brunner/Mazel, 1976.

Mosak, H. H. and Driekus, *Adlerian Psychotherapy*. Itasca, Illinois: Peacock Publishers, 1973.

Naumberg, Margaret M., *Dynamically Oriented Art Therapy: Its Principles and Practice*. New York: Grune & Stratton, 1966.

Perls, Frederick et al., *Gestalt Is*. Moab, Utah: Real People Press, 1975.

———, *Gestalt Therapy Verbatim*. Moab, Utah: Real People Press, 1969.

Schattner, G., *Drama in Therapy*. New York: Drama Book Specialists, 1973.

Schoop, Trudi, *Won't You Join the Dance: A Dancer's Essay into the Treatment of Psychosis*. Palo Alto, California: National Press, 1974.

Spotnitz, H., *Modern Psychoanalysis of the Schizophrenic Patient*. New York: Grune & Stratton, 1969.

Ulmen, E. and P. Dachinger, *Art Therapy in Theory and Practice*. New York: Schocken Books, 1975.

Whitmont, E. C., "Analysis in a Group Setting," *Journal of Analytic Psychology, Quadrant,* 16(Spring 1974).

Wolpe, Joseph, *The Practice of Behavior Therapy.* New York: Pergamon Press, 1973.

REFLEXOLOGY

Bean, Roy E., *Helping Your Health with Pointed Pressure Therapy.* New York: Parker Publishing, 1982.

Bendix, Gerard J., *Press Point Therapy.* Wellingborough, Great Britain: Thorsons, 1978.

Bergson, Anika and V. Tuchack, *Zone Therapy.* Tel Aviv: Or-Teva Publications, 1984.

Berkson, Devaki, *The Foot Book—Healing the Body Through Zone Therapy to Help Nature Help Yourself.* New York: Barnes and Noble Books, 1979.

Carter, M., *Hand Reflexology.* New York: Prentice Hall, 1975.

———, *Helping Yourself with Foot Reflexology.* New York: Prentice Hall, 1969.

Ingham, Eunice D., *Stories the Feet Can Tell Through Reflexology.* Miami: Ingham Publications, 1964.

———, *Stories the Feet Have Told Through Reflexology.* Miami: Ingham Publishing, 1963.

Kaye, Anna and Don Matchan, *Mirror of the Body.* Wellingborough, Great Britain: Thorsons, 1978.

Oliver, William H., *The Oliver Method of New Body Reflexology.* New York: Biworld Publications, 1978.

———, *New Body Reflexology.* New York: Biworld Publications, 1972.

Zwang, Moses, *Atlas of Reflexology.* Tel Aviv: Self Publication 1984.

———, *Atlas of Acupuncture and Shiatsu.* Tel Aviv: Self Publication, 1985.

SCHUESSLER TISSUE SALTS

Boerick, William, *The Twelve Tissue Remedies of Schuessler*. Philadelphia: Boerick & Takel Publishers, 1934.

Chapman, Esther, *How to Use the Twelve Tissue Salts*. Wellingborough, Great Britain: Thorsons, 1982.

Biochemic Pocket Guide—Physicians Quick Reference of Dr. Schuessler. New Delhi: Jain Publishing, 1981.

Goodwin, J. S., *The Biochemic Handbook*. Wellingborough, Great Britain: Thorsons 1982.

New Era Laboratories, *Biochemic Tissue Book*. London: New Era Laboratories, n.d.

ABOUT THE AUTHORS

Moshe Olshevsky, C.A, O.M.D., Ph.D., is chief acupuncturist and herbologist at the Holistic Medical Center in Tel Aviv. Shlomo Noy, M.D., is a graduate of the Hadassah Medical School, Jerusalem, and has published extensively in international medical journals. Moses Zwang, O.M.D., Ph.D., holds degrees in naturopathy, acupuncture and the natural sciences, and practices holistic medicine. Rogert Burger is the author of fifteen books and specializes in the areas of fitness and health.

INDEX